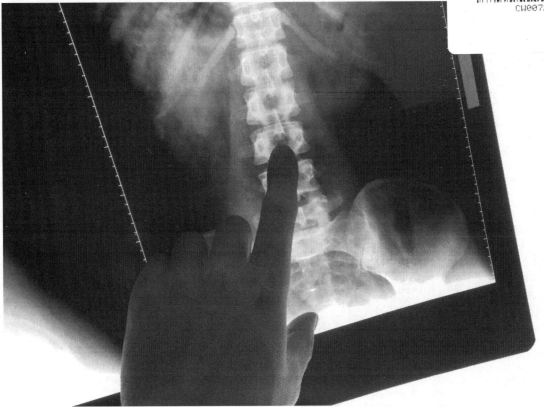

Succeeding in the FRCR Part 1 Anatomy Exam

An illustrated guide including 20 mock examinations comprising 400 images

Lorna Woodbridge, Dushyant Shetty, Sharif Abdullah & Grant Mitchell

Edited by
Harbir Sidhu, Gauraang Bhatnagar & Pervinder Bhogal

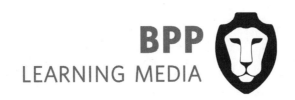

BPP
LEARNING MEDIA

First edition April 2012

ISBN 9781 4453 8167 1
e-ISBN 9781 4453 8581 5

British Library Cataloguing-in-Publication Data
A catalogue record for this book is available from the British Library

Published by
BPP Learning Media Ltd
BPP House, Aldine Place
London W12 8AA

www.bpp.com/health

Typeset by Replika Press Pvt Ltd, India
Printed in the United Kingdom

Your learning materials, published by BPP Learning Media Ltd, are printed on paper sourced from sustainable, managed forests.

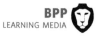

Contents

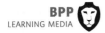

Contents

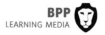

About the Publisher

BPP Learning Media is dedicated to supporting aspiring professionals with top quality learning material. BPP Learning Media's commitment to success is shown by our record of quality, innovation and market leadership in paper-based and e-learning materials. BPP Learning Media's study materials are written by professionally-qualified specialists who know from personal experience the importance of top quality materials for success.

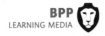

About the Authors

Lorna Woodbridge MBBS, MA (Cantab)

Lorna Woodbridge completed her pre-clinical studies at the University of Cambridge, having taken her part II in Pathology. She graduated from Barts and The London School of Medicine and Dentistry in 2008 with a MBBS before completing her foundation training in various hospitals around London. Lorna is currently a Radiology trainee on the Royal Free training programme.

Dushyant Shetty

Dr Dushyant Shetty graduated from Southampton Medical School in 2005. Before entering Radiology in the Peninsula Radiology Academy, he completed a two-year medical rotation during which time he completed his MRCP. He has a keen interest in medical education and was part of the very first cohort to successfully undertake the FRCR Part 1 Anatomy exam. Since then he has led the Peninsula structured FRCR anatomy teaching and achieved excellent results.

Sharif Abdullah

Sharif Abdullah is a Specialty Registrar in Radiology on the Royal Free training programme. He studied Medicine at University College London where he gained an intercalated BSc in Physiology. He entered Radiology in 2009 and passed the First FRCR Anatomy exam on his first attempt. During his training he has written and presented image-based educational posters at national and international levels, achieving a prize for his work.

Dr Grant Mitchell MBChB, MRCP, FRCR

Grant Mitchell trained at Leicester University. He worked in Peterborough, Leicester and Birmingham before joining the Peninsula Radiology Academy training scheme in 2005. He was subsequently appointed as a Consultant Radiologist at Derriford Hospital, Plymouth. His subspecialty Radiology interests are Cardiac CT, Cardiac MRI and Respiratory Imaging.

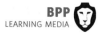

About the Editors

Harbir Sidhu

Harbir graduated from University College London Medical School in 2004. After undertaking basic surgical training in the Yorkshire deanery, he moved to the Southwest. He is currently working in the Peninsula training scheme as a radiology registrar.

Gauraang Bhatnagar

Gauraang qualified from Guy's King's and St Thomas' Medical School with MB BS and BSc in Anatomy and Biomedical Sciences in 2004. After completing basic surgical training in London he moved to the innovative Peninsula radiology academy where he is a post-FRCR registrar. He has a keen interest in medical education and is a Fellow of the Higher Education Authority.

Dr Pervinder Bhogal

Pervinder trained at Royal Free and University College London Medical School and graduated in 2004. After university he passed his MRCS Exam and is currently studying for a Masters Degree in Medical Education. He entered radiology training in 2007 and passed his FRCR Part 1 on the first attempt.

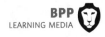

Acknowledgements

We gratefully acknowledge the following organisations that have allowed us to use images as follows:

Royal Free Hospital

Paper	Question
1	2, 6, 8, 11–15, 17, 19, 20
2	2, 4, 6, 8, 11–15, 17, 19
3	2, 4, 6, 8, 11–15, 17, 19, 20
4	2, 4, 6, 8, 11–15, 17, 19, 20
5	2, 4, 6, 8, 11–15, 17, 19, 20
6	2, 4, 6, 8, 11–15, 17, 19
7	2, 4, 6, 8, 11–15, 17, 19, 20
8	2, 4, 6, 8, 11–15, 17, 19, 20
9	2, 4, 6, 8, 11–15, 17, 19
10	2, 4, 6, 8, 11–15, 17, 19, 20
11	2, 4, 6, 8, 11–15, 17, 19, 20
12	2, 4, 6, 8, 11–15, 17, 19, 20
13	2, 4, 6, 8, 11–15, 17, 19
14	2, 4, 6, 8, 11–15, 17, 19, 20
15	2, 4, 6, 8, 11–15, 17, 19
16	2, 4, 6, 8, 11–15, 17, 19
17	2, 4, 6, 8, 11–15, 17, 19, 20
18	2, 4, 6, 8, 11–15, 17, 19, 20
19	2, 4, 6, 8, 11–15, 17, 19, 20
20	1, 2, 5, 7, 8, 11, 14–19

Derriford Hospital

Paper	Question
1	1, 3, 4, 5, 7, 9, 10, 16, 18
2	1, 3, 5, 7, 9, 10, 16, 18, 20
3	1, 3, 5, 7, 9, 10, 16, 18
4	1, 3, 5, 7, 10, 9, 16, 18
5	1, 3, 5, 7, 10, 9, 16, 18
6	1, 3, 5, 7, 9, 10, 16, 18, 20
7	1, 3, 5, 7, 9, 10, 16, 18
8	1, 3, 5, 7, 10, 9, 16, 18
9	1, 3, 5, 7, 9, 10, 16, 18, 20
10	1, 3, 5, 7, 9, 10, 16, 18
11	1, 3, 5, 7, 9, 10, 16, 18
12	1, 3, 5, 7, 9, 10, 16, 18
13	1, 3, 5, 7, 9, 10, 16, 18, 20
14	1, 3, 5, 7, 9, 10, 16, 18
15	1, 3, 5, 7, 9, 10, 16, 18, 20
16	1, 3, 5, 7, 9, 10, 16, 18, 20
17	1, 3, 5, 7, 9, 10, 16, 18
18	1, 3, 5, 7, 9, 10, 16, 18
19	1, 3, 5, 7, 9, 10, 16, 18
20	3, 4, 6, 9, 10, 12, 13, 20

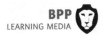

Dedication

To all the people that pick us up when we fall, pat us on the back when we have done well and stand by us in the face of adversity; without you we would be nothing.

About the exam and tips on passing it

The First FRCR Examination expects candidates to understand and demonstrate knowledge of the physical principles that underpin diagnostic medical imaging and of the anatomy needed to perform and interpret radiological studies. The examination is held three times a year and comprises a physics and a radiological anatomy module. All candidates will need to pass both modules in order to pass the examination overall but the modules can be sat separately. There is no limit on the number of times a candidate may sit the exam and no time limit to passing it.

Format of the test

The anatomy component of the examination lasts for 75 minutes and comprises 20 cases / images, with five questions about each. The cases are labelled 01 to 20 and the five questions are labelled (a) to (e). The cases / images will be presented digitally using computer workstations. Each workstation will comprise an Apple Mac Mini with a 19″ standard aspect ratio monitor and a mouse (right click disabled) but not a keyboard. You will also be provided with a question booklet into which you should write your answers. The images will be viewed using Osirix software.

Revision tips

Anatomy is not everyone's favourite subject and for those entering radiology with a principally medical background many may not have refreshed their knowledge of anatomy since medical school. This aside, regular study followed by self-assessment is the best way to prepare for this examination. In addition testing yourself on your anatomy knowledge while reporting at work is another excellent use of time. In order to give yourself the best chance of passing the examination at the first attempt start preparing approximately two to three months in advance.

This book should be used to test anatomy knowledge that will be principally gained from standard anatomy and texts and radiological anatomy atlases. This book will also be useful in determining areas of weakness, whether they be individual modalities such as CT or MRI or anatomical regions.

It is advisable that prior to the examination you become familiar with the Osirix software. This can be downloaded free for Apple Mac computers but will not run on a PC. If you own a PC it is advisable to practise on a Mac prior to the examination simply to aid your familiarity with the software and what to expect.

Tips for the exam
- Manage your time carefully
- Look at the labels carefully and try to be as accurate as possible
- If you are unsure skip the question and you can go back to it afterwards
- Guess any questions at the end because there is no negative marking and so it is worth putting an answer down
- Check for silly mistakes if you still have time – always get left and right correct!
- Keep watching the clock (100 labels in 75 minutes)

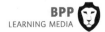

Paper 1

Question Bank

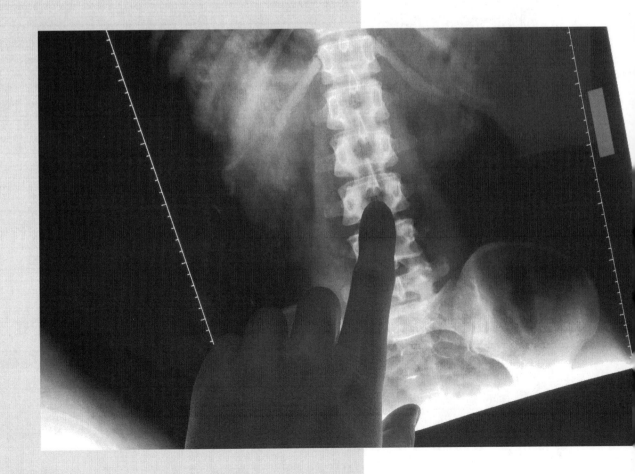

Question 1

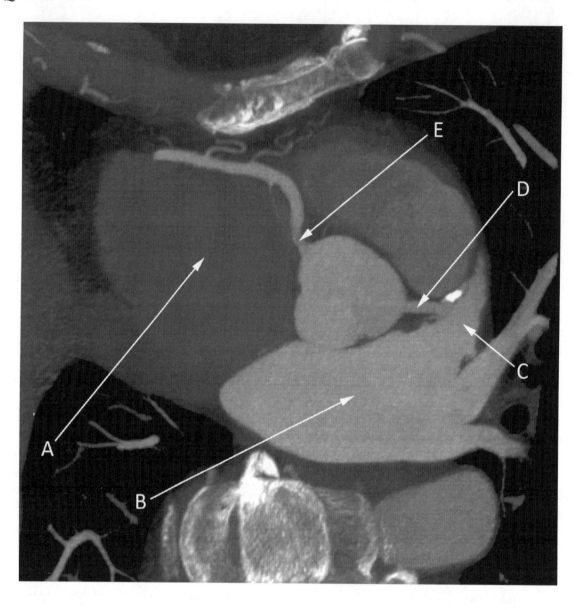

	QUESTION 1	WRITE YOUR ANSWER HERE
A	Name the structure labelled A	
B	Name the structure labelled B	
C	Name the structure labelled C	
D	Name the structure labelled D	
E	Name the structure labelled E	

Question 2

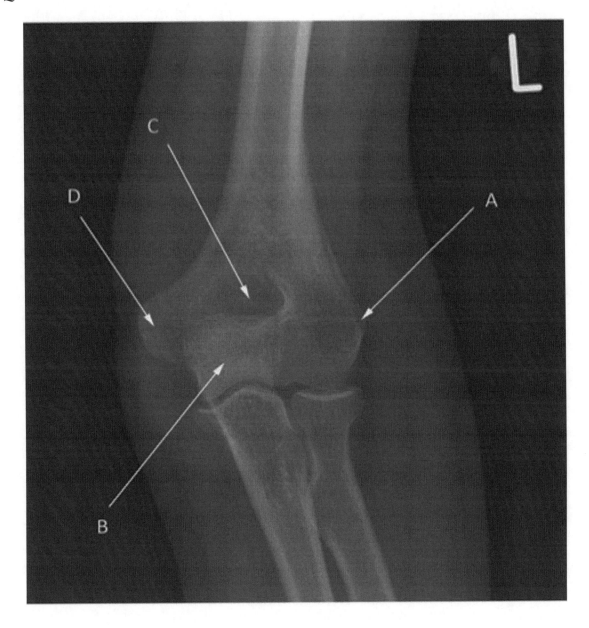

	QUESTION 2	WRITE YOUR ANSWER HERE
A	Name the structure labelled A	
B	Name the structure labelled B	
C	Name the structure labelled C	
D	Name the structure labelled D	
E	What attaches to D?	

Question 3

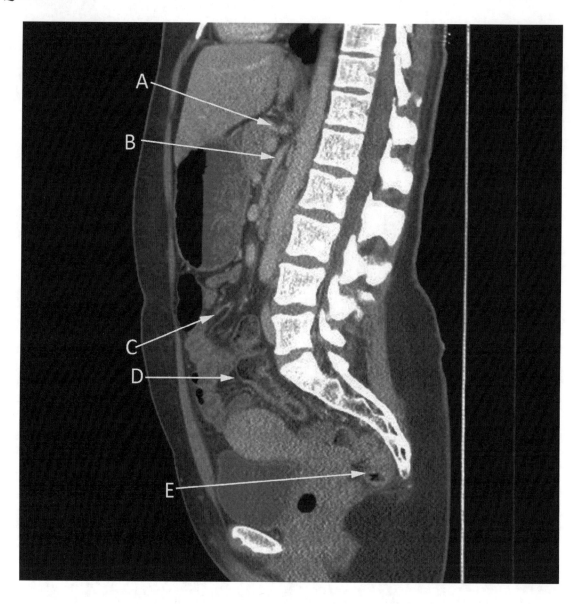

	QUESTION 3	WRITE YOUR ANSWER HERE
A	Name the structure labelled A	
B	Name the structure labelled B	
C	Name the structure labelled C	
D	Name the structure labelled D	
E	Name the structure labelled E	

Question 4

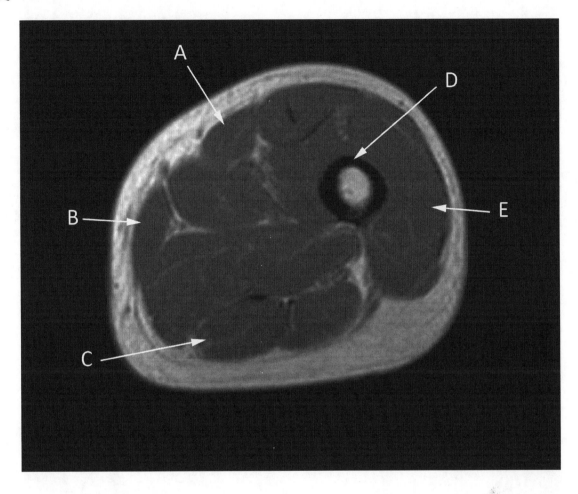

	QUESTION 4	WRITE YOUR ANSWER HERE
A	Name the structure labelled A	
B	Name the structure labelled B	
C	Name the structure labelled C	
D	Name the structure labelled D	
E	Name the structure labelled E	

BPP
LEARNING MEDIA

Question 5

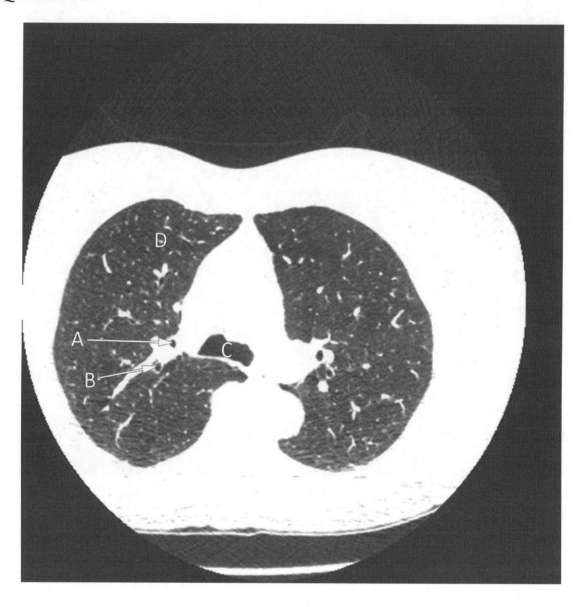

	QUESTION 5	WRITE YOUR ANSWER HERE
A	Name the segmental bronchus A	
B	Name the segmental bronchus B	
C	Name the bifurcation C	
D	Name the lobe and segment D	
E	Which lobe lies inferior to D?	

Question 6

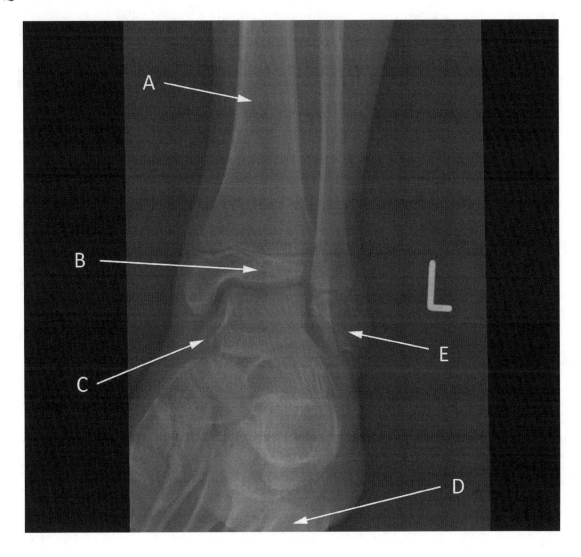

	QUESTION 6	WRITE YOUR ANSWER HERE
A	Name the structure labelled A	
B	Name the structure labelled B	
C	Name the structure labelled C	
D	Name the structure labelled D	
E	Name the structure labelled E	

Question 7

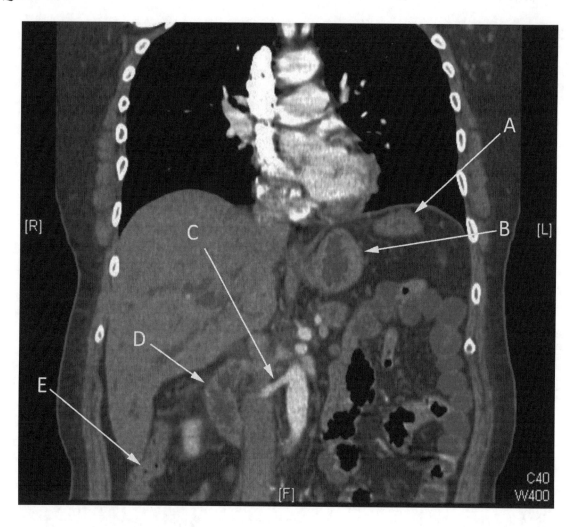

	QUESTION 7	WRITE YOUR ANSWER HERE
A	Name the structure labelled A	
B	Name the structure labelled B	
C	Name the structure labelled C	
D	Name the structure labelled D	
E	Name the structure labelled E	

Question 8

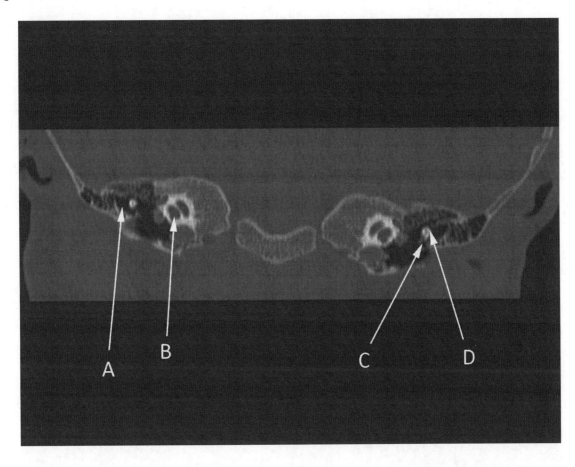

	QUESTION 8	WRITE YOUR ANSWER HERE
A	Name the structure labelled A	
B	Name the structure labelled B	
C	Name the structure labelled C	
D	Name the structure labelled D	
E	What ossicle connects to B?	

Question 9

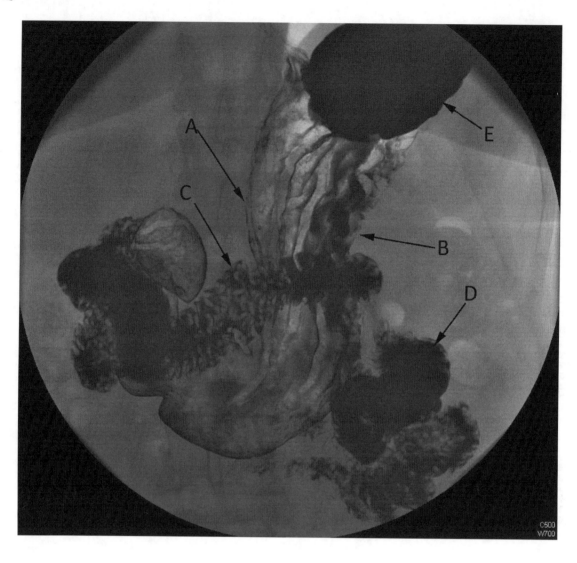

	QUESTION 9	WRITE YOUR ANSWER HERE
A	Name the structure labelled A	
B	Name the structure labelled B	
C	Name the structure labelled C	
D	Name the structure labelled D	
E	Name the structure labelled E	

Question 10

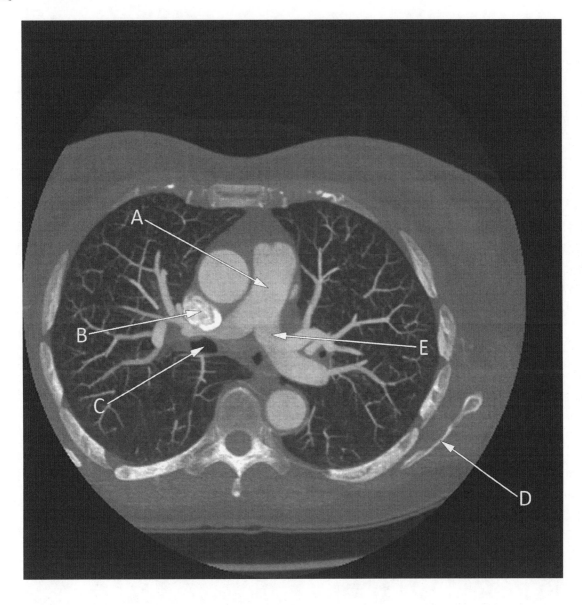

	QUESTION 10	WRITE YOUR ANSWER HERE
A	Name the structure labelled A	
B	Name the structure labelled B	
C	Name the structure labelled C	
D	Name the structure labelled D	
E	Name the structure labelled E	

Question 11

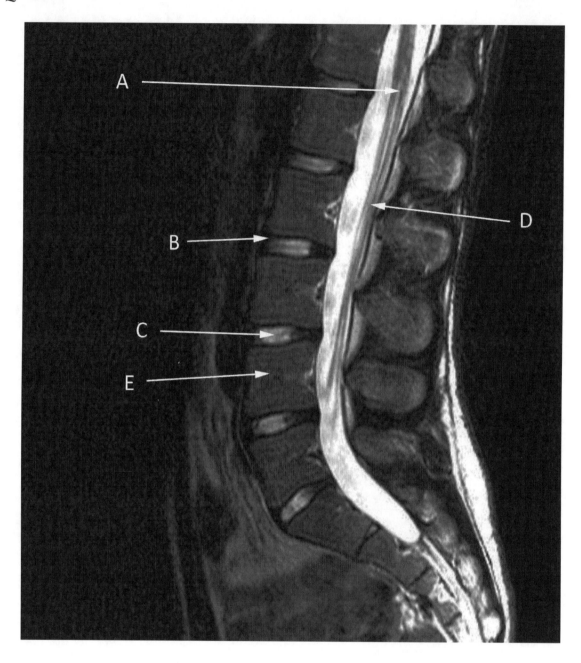

	QUESTION 11	WRITE YOUR ANSWER HERE
A	Name the structure labelled A	
B	Name the structure labelled B	
C	Name the structure labelled C	
D	Name the structure labelled D	
E	Name the structure labelled E	

Question 12

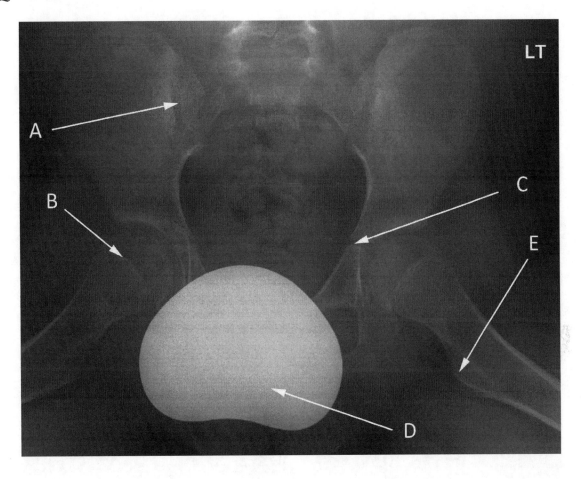

	QUESTION 12	WRITE YOUR ANSWER HERE
A	Name the structure labelled A	
B	Name the structure labelled B	
C	Name the structure labelled C	
D	Name the structure labelled D	
E	Name the structure labelled E	

Question 13

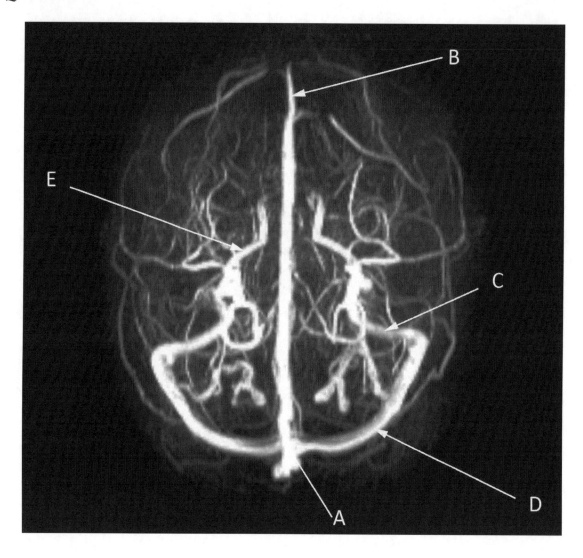

	QUESTION 13	WRITE YOUR ANSWER HERE
A	Name the structure labelled A	
B	Name the structure labelled B	
C	Name the structure labelled C	
D	Name the structure labelled D	
E	Through what does E exit the cranium?	

Question 14

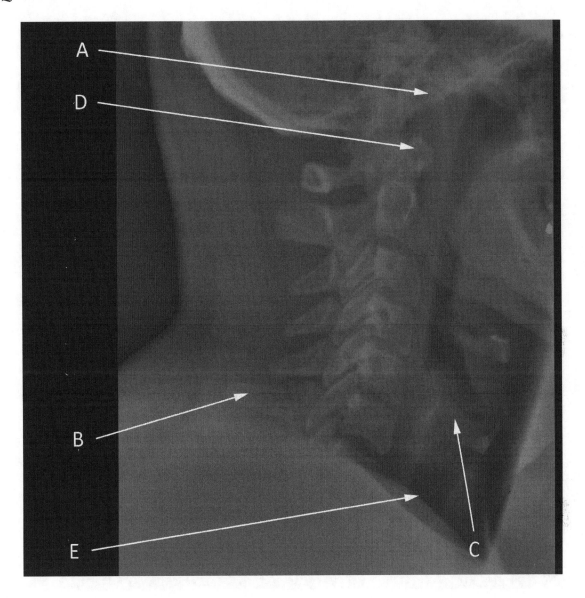

	QUESTION 14	WRITE YOUR ANSWER HERE
A	Name the structure labelled A	
B	Name the structure labelled B	
C	Name the structure labelled C	
D	Name the structure labelled D	
E	Name the structure labelled E	

BPP
LEARNING MEDIA

Question 15

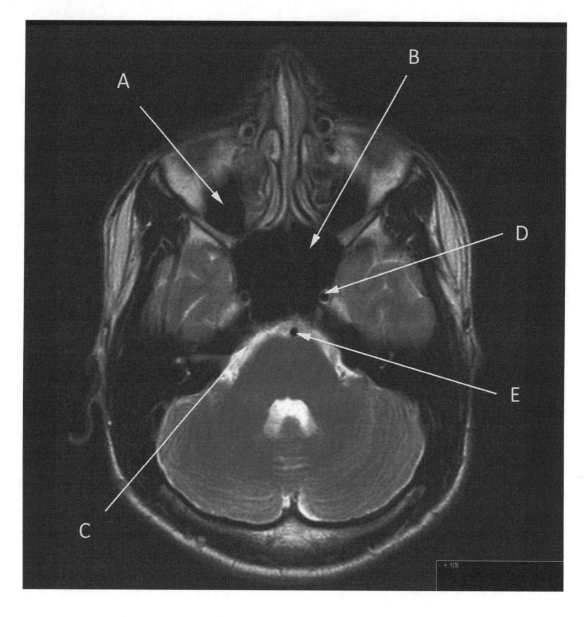

	QUESTION 15	WRITE YOUR ANSWER HERE
A	Name the structure labelled A	
B	Name the structure labelled B	
C	Name the structure labelled C	
D	Name the structure labelled D	
E	Name the structure labelled E	

Question 16

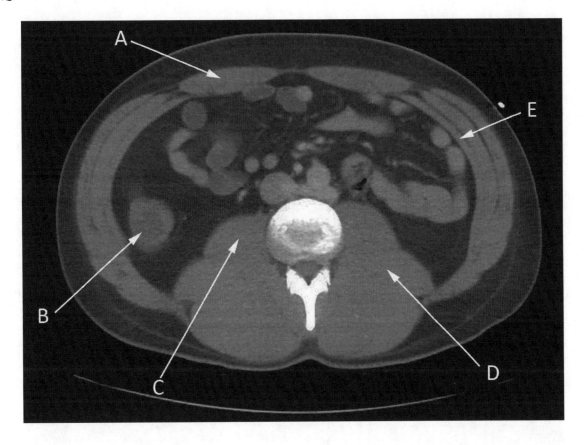

	QUESTION 16	WRITE YOUR ANSWER HERE
A	Name the structure labelled A	
B	Name the structure labelled B	
C	Name the structure labelled C	
D	Name the structure labelled D	
E	Name the structure labelled E	

Question 17

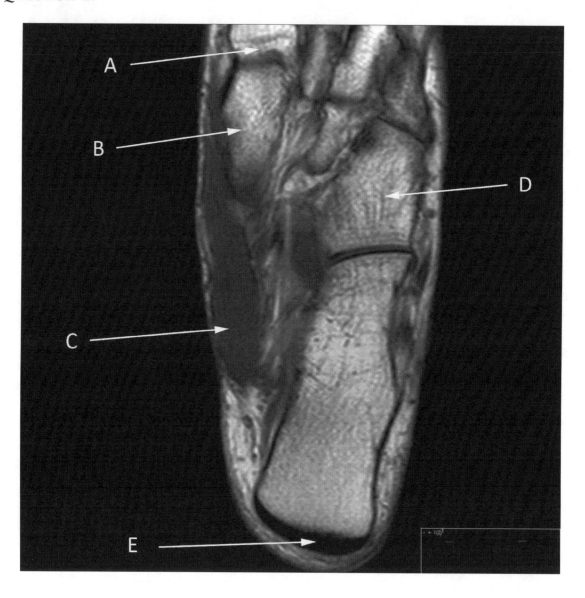

	QUESTION 17	WRITE YOUR ANSWER HERE
A	Name the structure labelled A	
B	Name the structure labelled B	
C	Name the structure labelled C	
D	Name the structure labelled D	
E	Name the structure labelled E	

Question 18

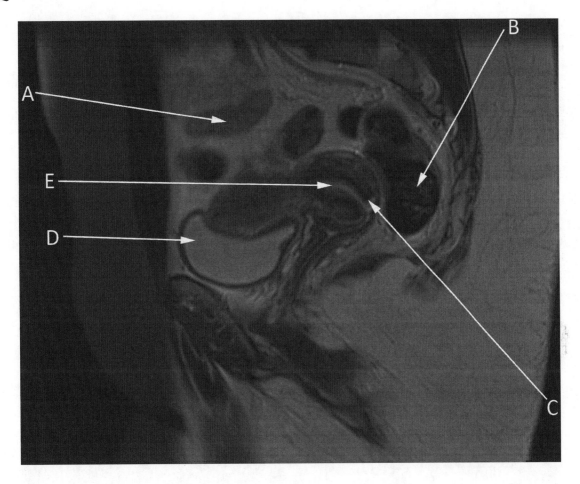

	QUESTION 18	WRITE YOUR ANSWER HERE
A	Name the structure labelled A	
B	Name the structure labelled B	
C	Name the structure labelled C	
D	Name the structure labelled D	
E	Name the structure labelled E	

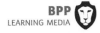

Question 19

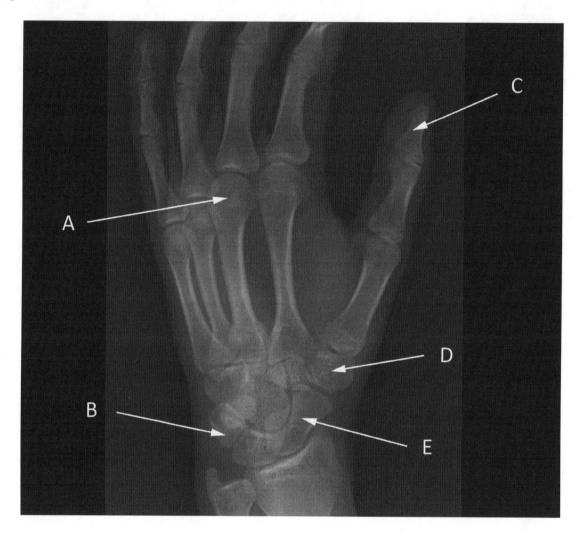

	QUESTION 19	WRITE YOUR ANSWER HERE
A	Name the structure labelled A	
B	Name the structure labelled B	
C	Name the structure labelled C	
D	Name the structure labelled D	
E	Name the structure labelled E	

Question 20

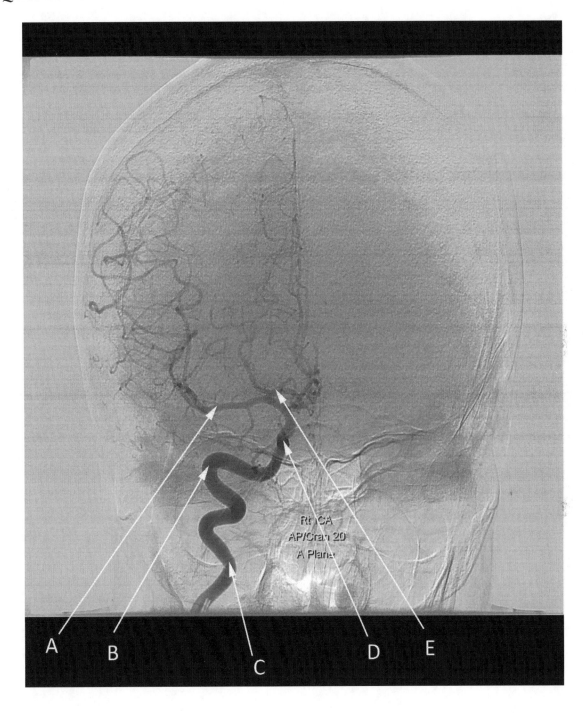

	QUESTION 20	WRITE YOUR ANSWER HERE
A	Name the structure labelled A	
B	Name the structure labelled B	
C	Name the structure labelled C	
D	Name the structure labelled D	
E	Name the structure labelled E	

Paper 1

Answers

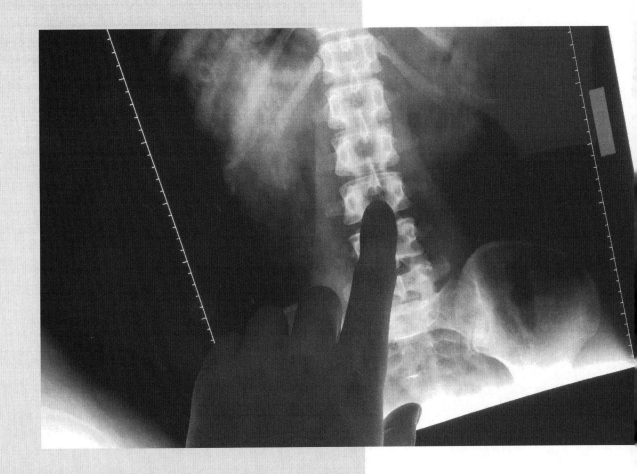

Question 1

A. Right atrium
B. Left atrium
C. Left atrial appendage
D. Left coronary artery / left main stem
E. Right coronary artery

Question 2

A. Left lateral epicondyle of humerus
B. Left trochlear
C. Left olecranon fossa
D. Left medial epicondyle of humerus
E. Common flexor origin

Question 3

A. Coeliac axis
B. Superior mesenteric artery
C. Mesenteric vessels
D. Descending colon
E. Sigmoid colon

Question 4

A. Sartorius muscle
B. Gracilis muscle
C. Semimembranosus muscle
D. Cortical bone of femur
E. Vastus lateralis muscle

Question 5

A. Right upper lobe apical segmental bronchus
B. Right upper lobe posterior segmental bronchus
C. The carina
D. Right upper lobe anterior segment
E. The (right) middle lobe

Question 6

A. Diaphysis of left tibia
B. Distal epiphysis of left tibia
C. Medial tubercle of left talus
D. Base of left fifth metatarsal
E. Left lateral malleolus

 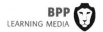

Question 7

A. Spleen
B. Stomach
C. Right renal artery
D. Duodenum
E. Ascending colon

Question 8

A. Right epitympanum
B. Right cochlea
C. Left incus
D. Head of left malleus
E. Stapes

Question 9

A. Lesser curvature
B. Greater curvature
C. Fourth part of duodenum
D. Jejunum
E. Gastric fundus

Question 10

A. Main pulmonary artery
B. Superior vena cava
C. Right main bronchus
D. Left scapula
E. Left pulmonary artery

Question 11

A. Conus medullaris
B. Annulus fibrosus of L2/3
C. Nucleus pulposus of L3/4
D. Cauda equina
E. L4 vertebral body

Question 12

A. Right sacroiliac joint
B. Right epiphyseal line
C. Left triradiate cartilage
D. Gonadal shield
E. Left lesser trochanter

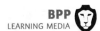

Question 13

A. Torcular Herophili (sinus confluence)
B. Superior sagittal sinus
C. Left sigmoid sinus
D. Left transverse sinus
E. Right jugular foramen

Question 14

A. Temperomandibular joint
B. Spinous process of C6
C. Thyroid cartilage
D. Anterior arch of C1 vertebra
E. Trachea

Question 15

A. Right maxillary antrum
B. Left sphenoid sinus
C. Pre-pontine cistern
D. Left internal carotid artery
E. Basilar artery

Question 16

A. Right rectus abdominis muscle
B. Ascending colon
C. Right psoas muscle
D. Left quadratus lumborum muscle
E. Left transversus abdominis muscle

Question 17

A. First metatarsal
B. Medial cuneiform
C. Abductor hallucis muscle
D. Cuboid
E. Achilles' tendon / tendo calcaneus

Question 18

A. Small bowel
B. Rectum
C. Posterior fornix
D. Urinary bladder
E. Cervical canal

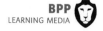

Question 19

A. Head of third metacarpal
B. Triquetral bone
C. Distal phalanx of the first finger
D. Trapezium bone
E. Scaphoid bone

Question 20

A. Right middle cerebral artery
B. Petrous part of the right internal carotid artery
C. Cervical part of the right internal carotid artery
D. Cavernous part of the right internal carotid artery
E. Right anterior cerebral artery

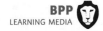

Paper 2

Question Bank

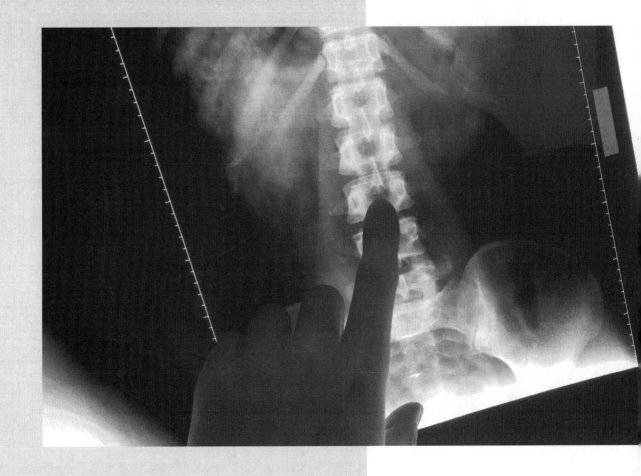

Question 1

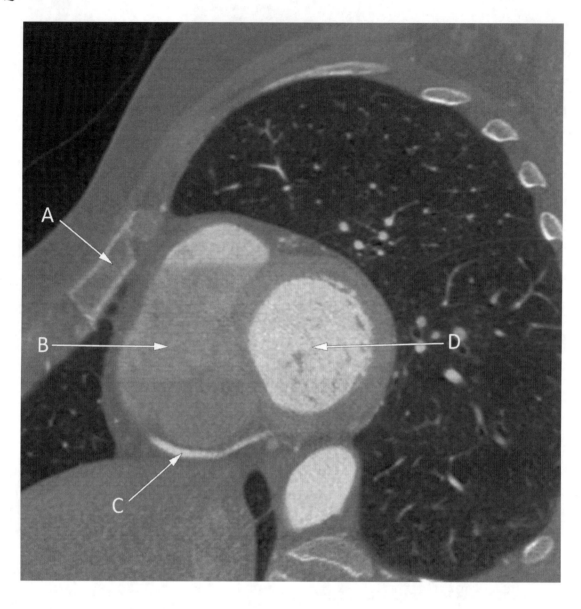

	QUESTION 1	WRITE YOUR ANSWER HERE
A	Name the structure labelled A	
B	Name the structure labelled B	
C	Name the structure labelled C	
D	Name the structure labelled D	
E	What 2 vessels arise from C?	

Question 2

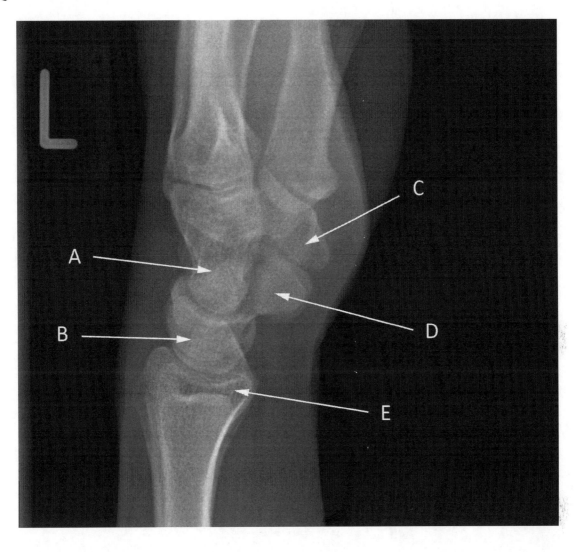

	QUESTION 2	WRITE YOUR ANSWER HERE
A	Name the structure labelled A	
B	Name the structure labelled B	
C	Name the structure labelled C	
D	Name the structure labelled D	
E	Name the structure labelled E	

Question 3

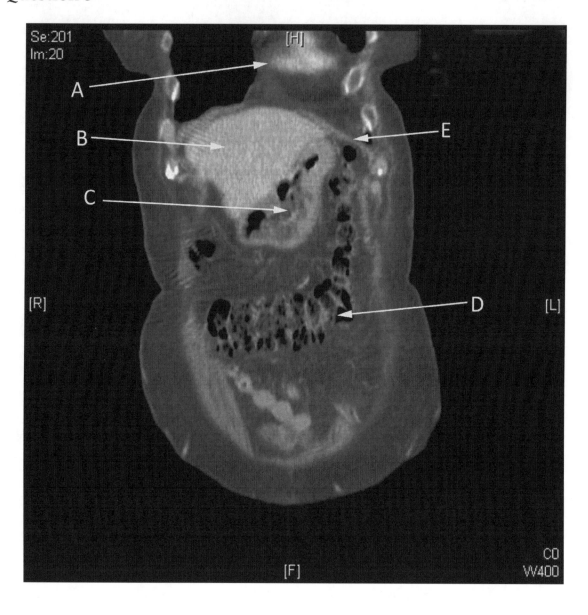

	QUESTION 3	WRITE YOUR ANSWER HERE
A	Name the structure labelled A	
B	Name the structure labelled B	
C	Name the structure labelled C	
D	Name the structure labelled D	
E	Name the structure labelled E	

Question 4

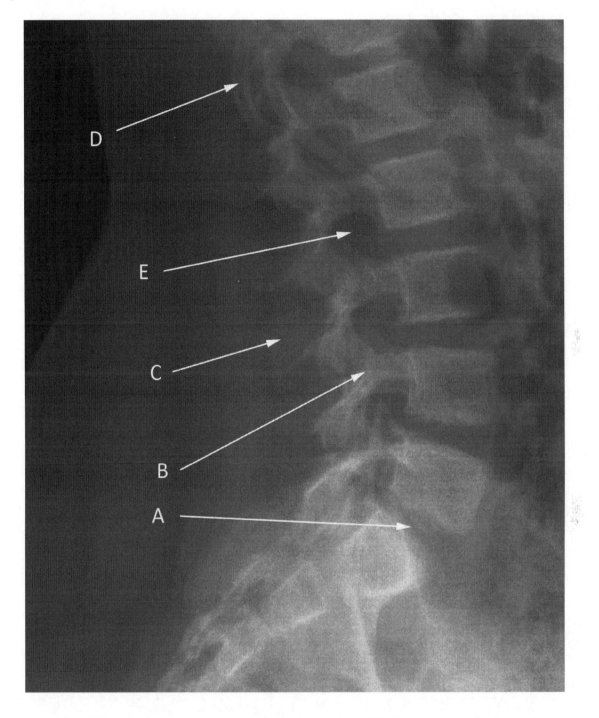

	QUESTION 4	WRITE YOUR ANSWER HERE
A	Name the structure labelled A	
B	Name the structure labelled B	
C	Name the structure labelled C	
D	Name the structure labelled D	
E	What exits through E?	

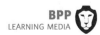

Question 5

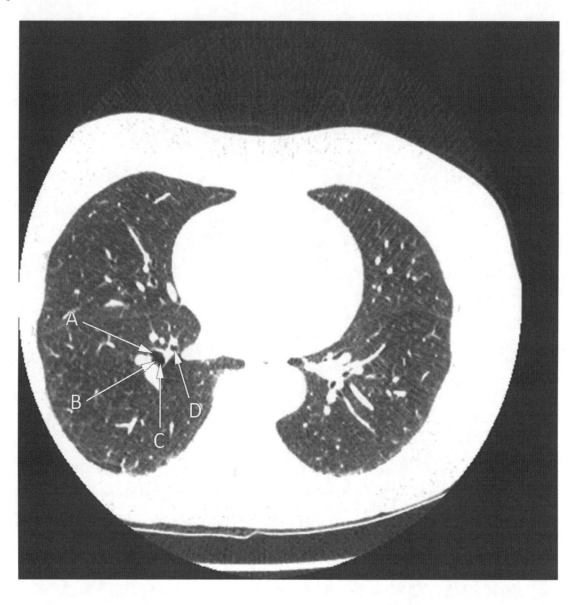

	QUESTION 5	WRITE YOUR ANSWER HERE
A	Name the segmental bronchus A	
B	Name the segmental bronchus B	
C	Name the segmental bronchus C	
D	Name the segmental bronchus D	
E	What is the 5th segmental bronchus (not visualised on the current slice) in the same lobe?	

Question 6

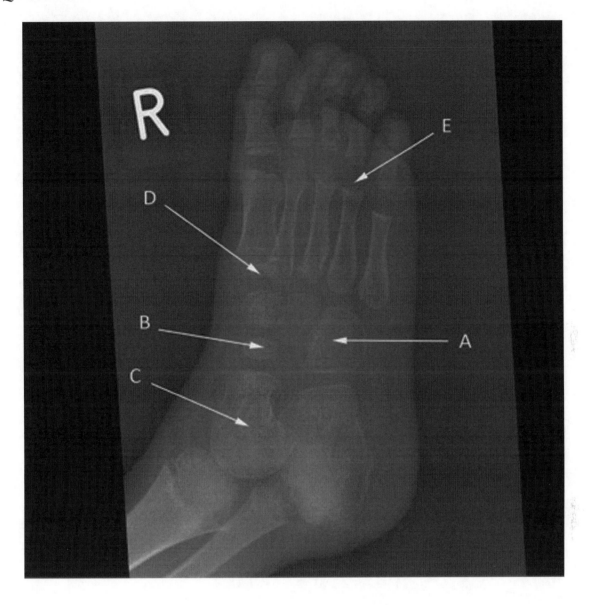

	QUESTION 6	WRITE YOUR ANSWER HERE
A	Name the structure labelled A	
B	Name the structure labelled B	
C	Name the structure labelled C	
D	Name the structure labelled D	
E	Name the structure labelled E	

Question 7

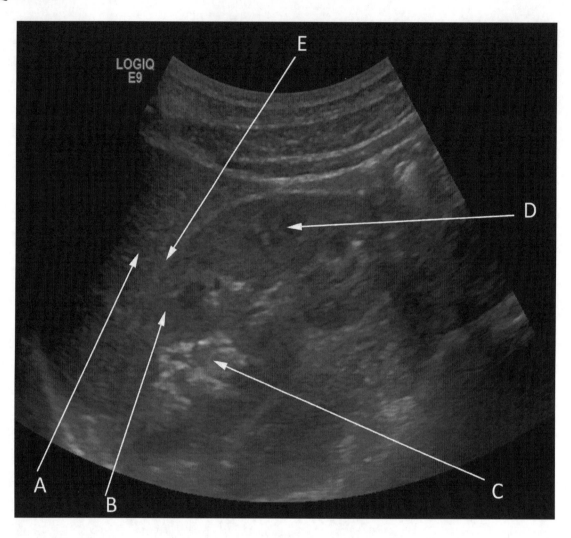

	QUESTION 7	WRITE YOUR ANSWER HERE
A	Name the structure labelled A	
B	Name the structure labelled B	
C	Name the structure labelled C	
D	Name the structure labelled D	
E	Name the anatomical space labelled E	

Question 8

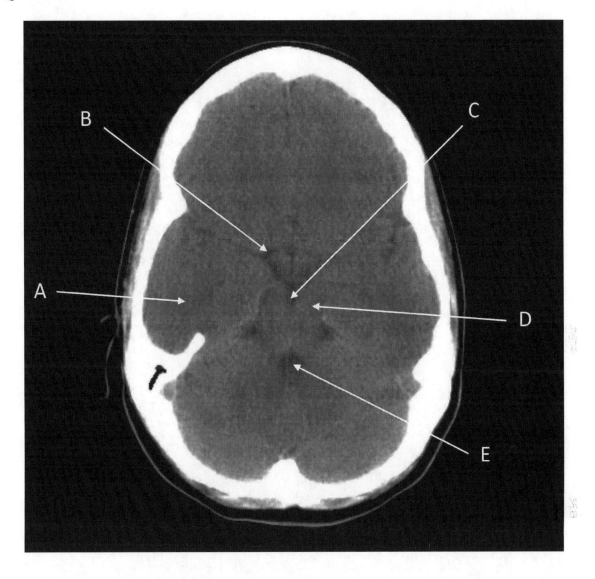

	QUESTION 8	WRITE YOUR ANSWER HERE
A	Name the structure labelled A	
B	Name the structure labelled B	
C	Name the structure labelled C	
D	Name the structure labelled D	
E	Name the structure labelled E	

Question 9

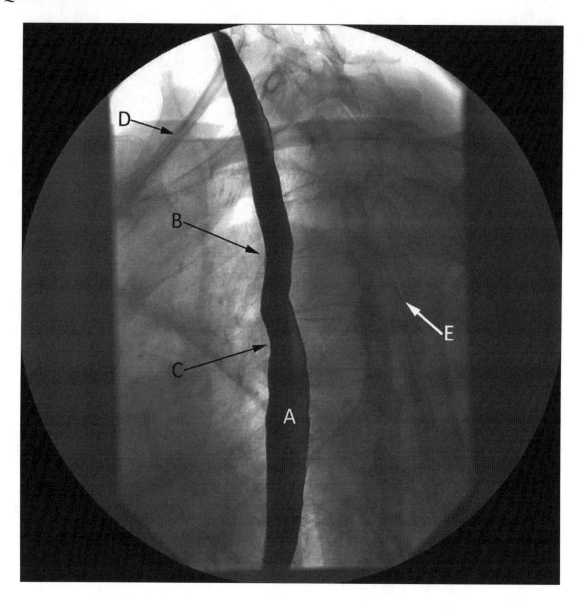

	QUESTION 9	WRITE YOUR ANSWER HERE
A	Name the structure labelled A	
B	Name the structure causing the impression labelled B	
C	Name the structure causing the impression labelled C	
D	Name the structure labelled D	
E	Name the structure labelled E	

Question 10

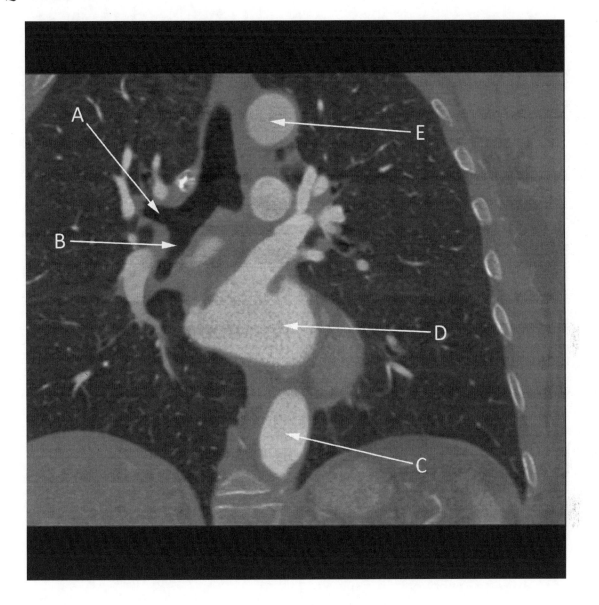

	QUESTION 10	WRITE YOUR ANSWER HERE
A	Name the structure labelled A	
B	Name the structure labelled B	
C	Name the structure labelled C	
D	Name the structure labelled D	
E	Name the structure labelled E	

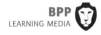

Question 11

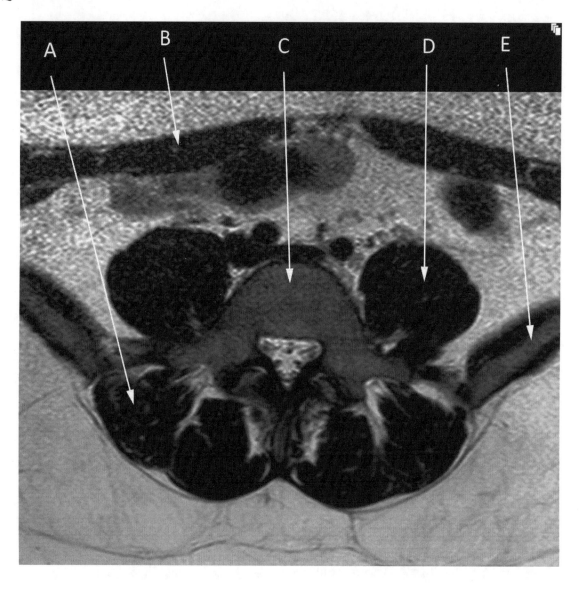

	QUESTION 11	WRITE YOUR ANSWER HERE
A	Name the structure labelled A	
B	Name the structure labelled B	
C	Name the structure labelled C	
D	Name the structure labelled D	
E	Name the structure labelled E	

Question 12

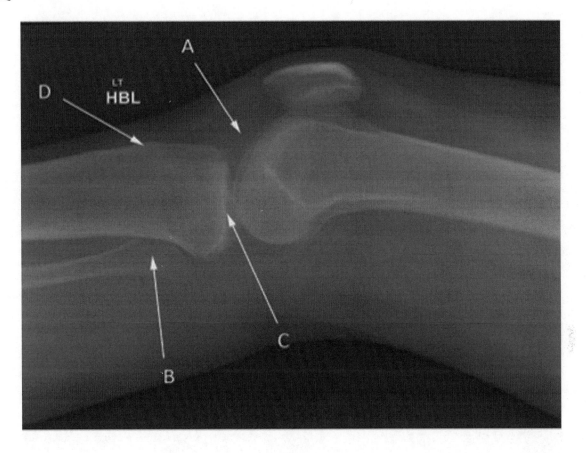

	QUESTION 12	WRITE YOUR ANSWER HERE
A	Name the structure labelled A	
B	Name the structure labelled B	
C	Name the structure labelled C	
D	Name the structure labelled D	
E	What attaches to D?	

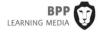

Question 13

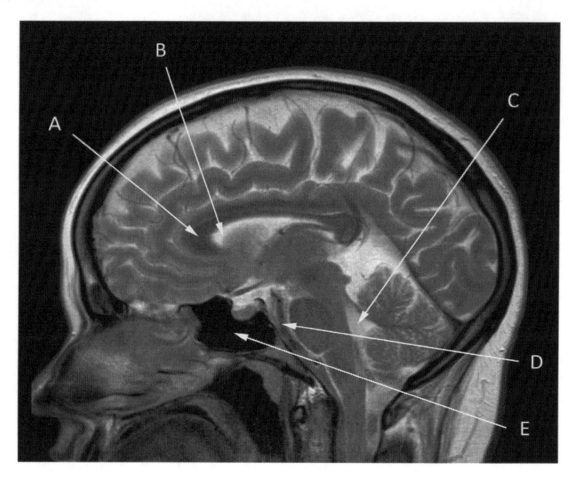

	QUESTION 13	WRITE YOUR ANSWER HERE
A	Name the structure labelled A	
B	Name the structure labelled B	
C	Name the structure labelled C	
D	Name the structure labelled D	
E	Name the structure labelled E	

Question 14

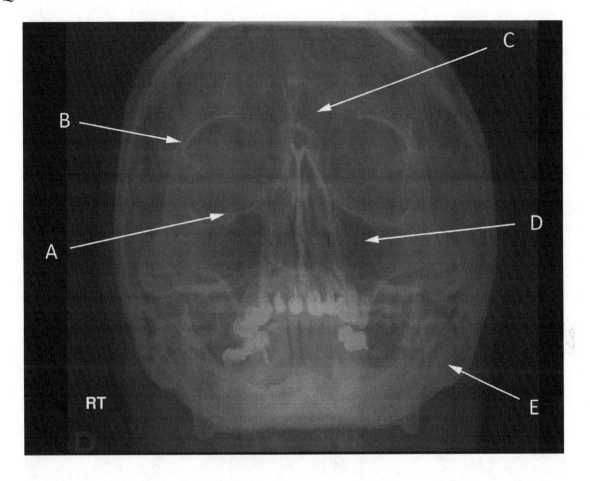

	QUESTION 14	WRITE YOUR ANSWER HERE
A	Name the structure labelled A	
B	Name the structure labelled B	
C	Name the structure labelled C	
D	Name the structure labelled D	
E	Name the structure labelled E	

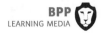

Question 15

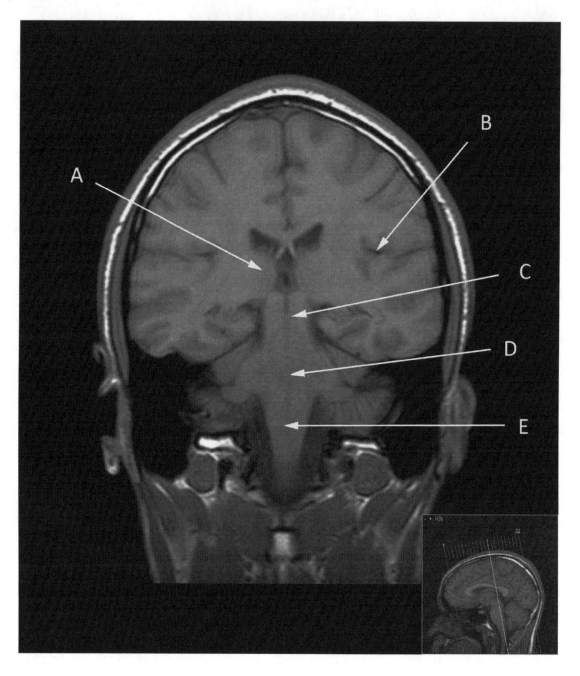

	QUESTION 15	WRITE YOUR ANSWER HERE
A	Name the structure labelled A	
B	Name the structure labelled B	
C	Name the structure labelled C	
D	Name the structure labelled D	
E	Name the structure labelled E	

Question 16

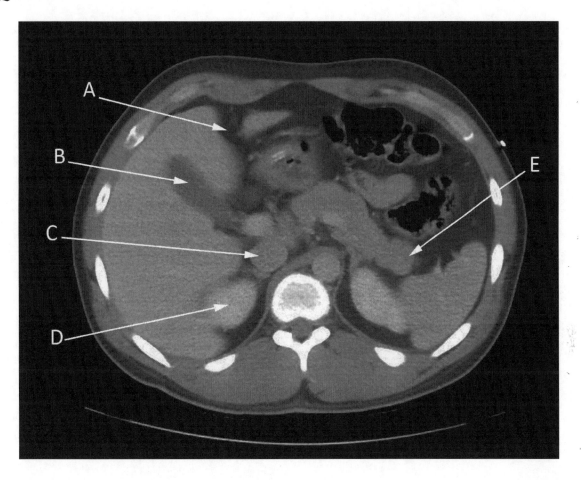

	QUESTION 16	WRITE YOUR ANSWER HERE
A	Name the structure labelled A	
B	Name the structure labelled B	
C	Name the structure labelled C	
D	Name the structure labelled D	
E	Name the structure labelled E	

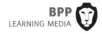

Question 17

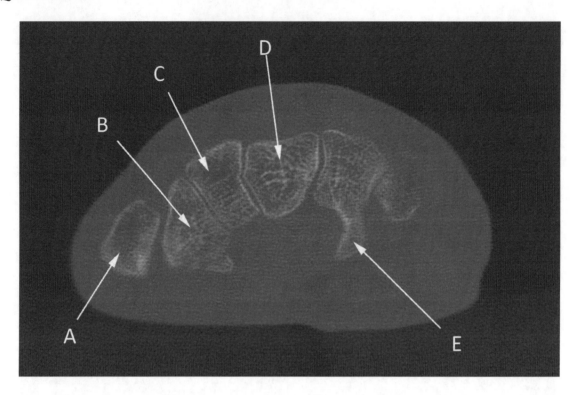

	QUESTION 17	WRITE YOUR ANSWER HERE
A	Name the structure labelled A	
B	Name the structure labelled B	
C	Name the structure labelled C	
D	Name the structure labelled D	
E	Name the structure labelled E	

Question 18

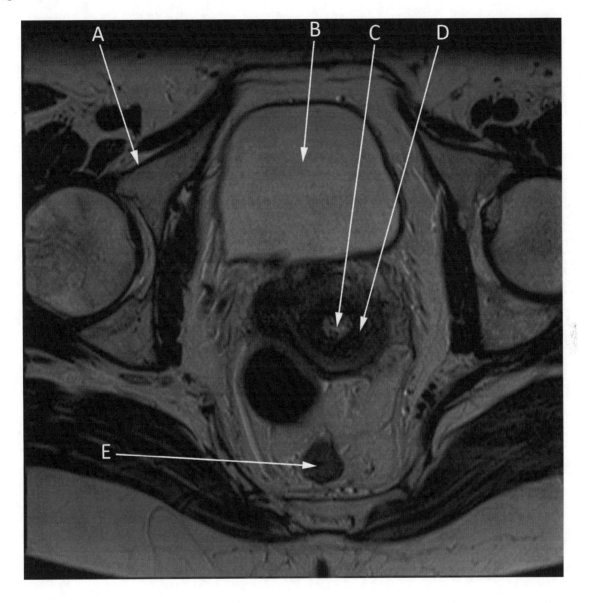

	QUESTION 18	WRITE YOUR ANSWER HERE
A	Name the structure labelled A	
B	Name the structure labelled B	
C	Name the structure labelled C	
D	Name the structure labelled D	
E	Name the structure labelled E	

Question 19

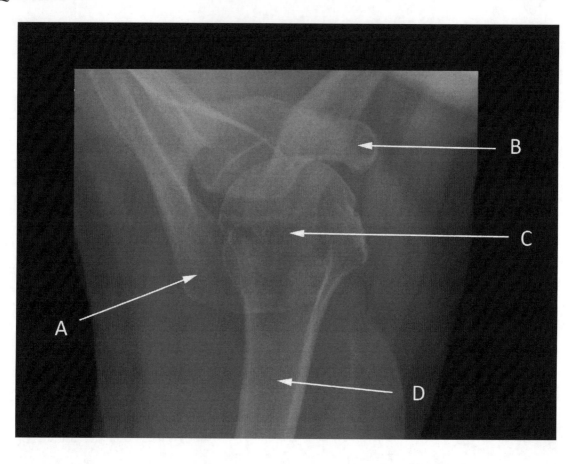

	QUESTION 19	WRITE YOUR ANSWER HERE
A	Name the structure labelled A	
B	Name the structure labelled B	
C	Name the structure labelled C	
D	Name the structure labelled D	
E	What attaches to A?	

Question 20

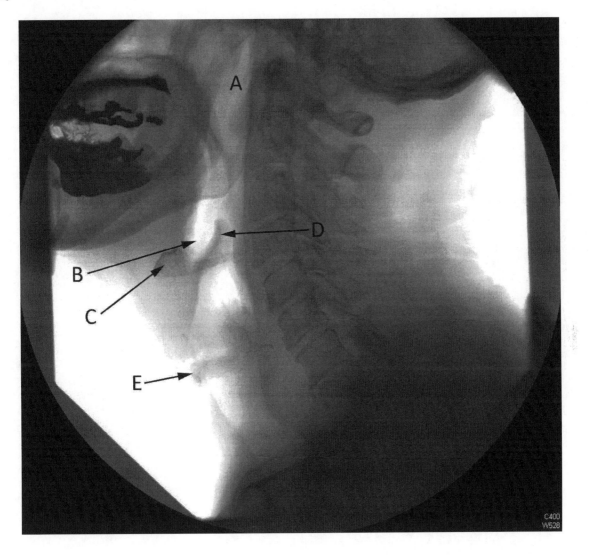

	QUESTION 20	WRITE YOUR ANSWER HERE
A	Name the structure labelled A	
B	Name the structure labelled B	
C	Name the structure labelled C	
D	Name the structure labelled D	
E	Name the structure labelled E	

Paper 2

Answers

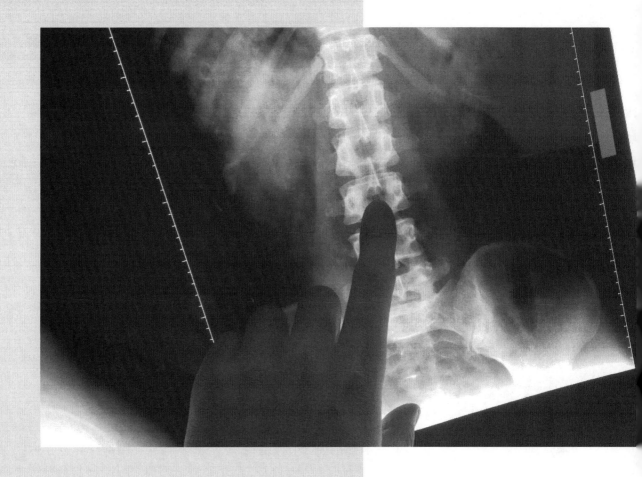

Question 1

A. Sternum
B. Right ventricle
C. Right coronary artery
D. Left ventricle
E. Posterolateral artery, posterior descending artery

Question 2

A. Left capitate bone
B. Left lunate bone
C. Left trapezium bone
D. Left scaphoid bone
E. Left distal radius

Question 3

A. Heart
B. Liver
C. Stomach
D. Transverse colon
E. Left diaphragm

Question 4

A. L5/S1 intervertebral disc space
B. Pars interarticularis
C. Spinous process of L3
D. 12th rib
E. L2 nerve root

Question 5

A. RLL anterior basal
B. RLL lateral basal
C. RLL posterior basal
D. RLL medial basal
E. RLL apical

Question 6

A. Right cuboid
B. Right navicular
C. Right talus
D. Growth centre for right first metatarsal
E. Growth centre for right fourth metatarsal

Question 7

A. Right lobe of liver
B. Renal cortex
C. Renal sinus fat
D. Medullary pyramid
E. Morrison's pouch

Question 8

A. Right temporal lobe
B. Suprasellar cistern
C. Interpeduncular cistern
D. Left cerebral peduncle
E. Fourth ventricle

Question 9

A.   Oesophagus
B. Aortic arch
C. Left main bronchus
D. Clavicle
E. Facet joint

Question 10

A. Right upper lobe bronchus
B. Bronchus intermedius
C. Descending aorta
D. Left atrium
E. Aortic arch

Question 11

A. Right erector spinae muscle
B. Right rectus abdominis muscle
C. L5 vertebral body
D. Left psoas major muscle
E. Left ilium

Question 12

A. Left Hoffa's fat pad
B. Head of left fibula
C. Left tibial plateau
D. Tuberosity of left tibia
E. Left patellar ligament

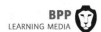

Question 13

A. Genu of corpus callosum
B. Third ventricle
C. Fourth ventricle
D. Basilar artery
E. Sphenoidal sinus

Question 14

A. Right inferior orbital wall
B. Right innominate line
C. Left frontal sinus
D. Left maxillary antrum
E. Left mastoid air cells

Question 15

A. Right thalamus
B. Left sylvian fissure
C. Midbrain
D. Pons
E. Medulla oblongata

Question 16

A. Fissure for ligamentum venosum
B. Gallbladder
C. Inferior vena cava
D. Right kidney
E. Tail of pancreas

Question 17

A. Base of fifth metacarpal
B. Trapezium
C. Trapezoid
D. Capitate
E. Hook of hamate

Question 18

A. Transversus abdominis muscle
B. Urinary bladder
C. Uterine endometrium
D. Uterine myometrium
E. Rectum

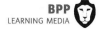

Question 19

A. Acromion of scapula
B. Coracoid process of scapula
C. Humeral head
D. Humeral shaft
E. Deltoid muscle

Question 20

A. Nasopharynx
B. Valleculae
C. Hyoid bone
D. Epiglottis
E. Cricoid cartilage

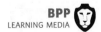

Paper 3

Question Bank

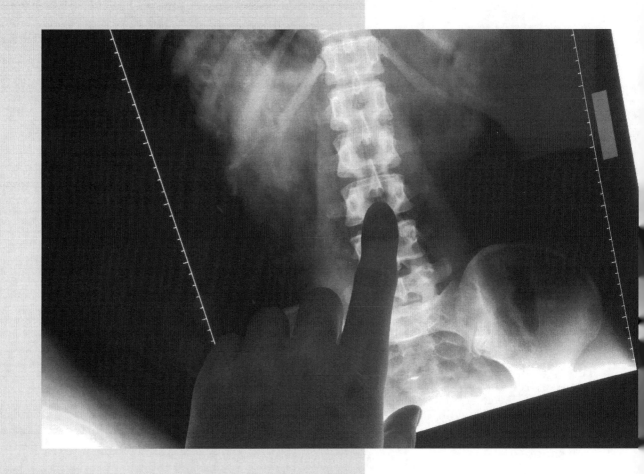

Question 1

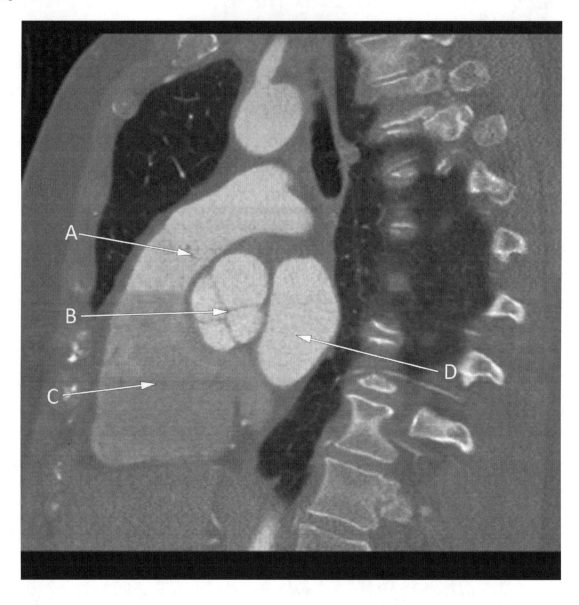

	QUESTION 1	WRITE YOUR ANSWER HERE
A	Name the structure labelled A	
B	Name the structure labelled B	
C	Name the structure labelled C	
D	Name the structure labelled D	
E	What structure lies between A and C?	

Question 2

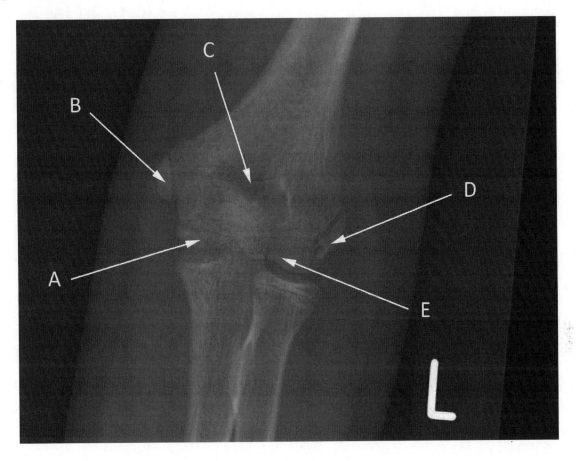

	QUESTION 2	WRITE YOUR ANSWER HERE
A	Name the structure labelled A	
B	Name the structure labelled B	
C	Name the structure labelled C	
D	Name the structure labelled D	
E	Name the structure labelled E	

Question 3

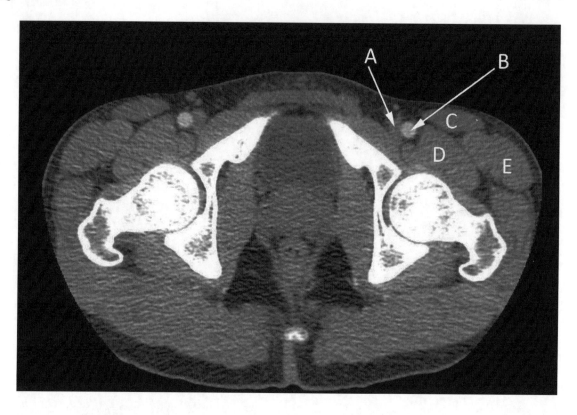

	QUESTION 3	WRITE YOUR ANSWER HERE
A	Name the structure labelled A	
B	Name the structure labelled B	
C	Name the structure labelled C	
D	Name the structure labelled D	
E	Name the structure labelled E	

Question 4

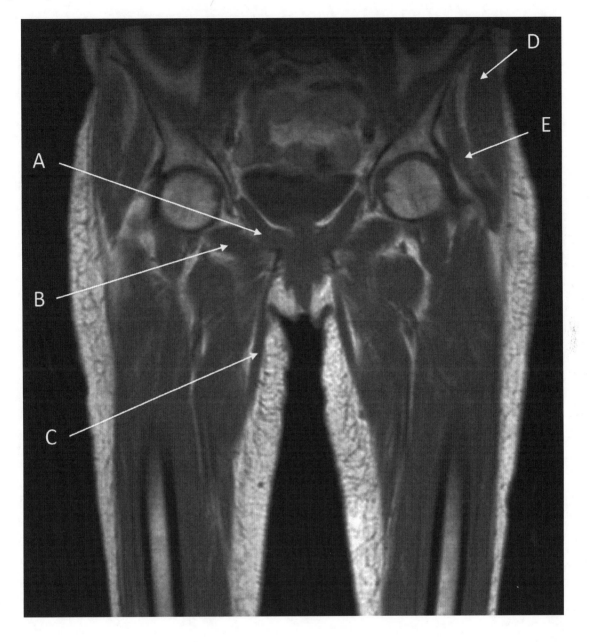

	QUESTION 4	WRITE YOUR ANSWER HERE
A	Name the structure labelled A	
B	Name the structure labelled B	
C	Name the structure labelled C	
D	Name the structure labelled D	
E	Name the structure labelled E	

Question 5

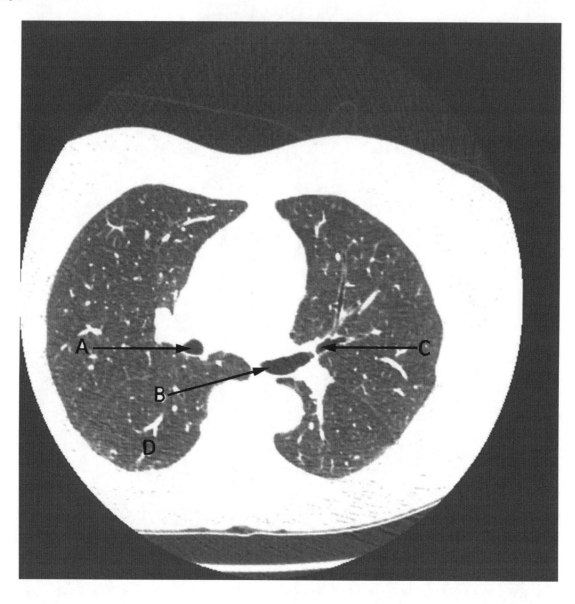

	QUESTION 5	WRITE YOUR ANSWER HERE
A	Name the bronchus labelled A	
B	Name the bronchus labelled B	
C	Name the segmental bronchus C	
D	Name the lobar segment D	
E	Which segment lies superior to that aerated by C?	

Question 6

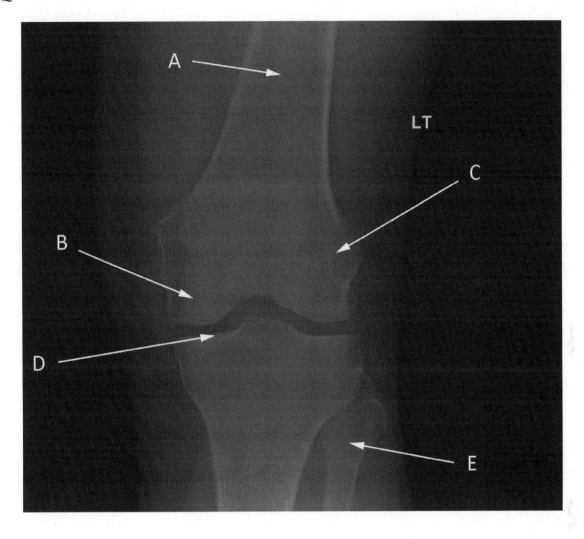

	QUESTION 6	WRITE YOUR ANSWER HERE
A	Name the structure labelled A	
B	Name the structure labelled B	
C	Name the structure labelled C	
D	Name the structure labelled D	
E	Name the structure labelled E	

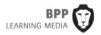

Question 7

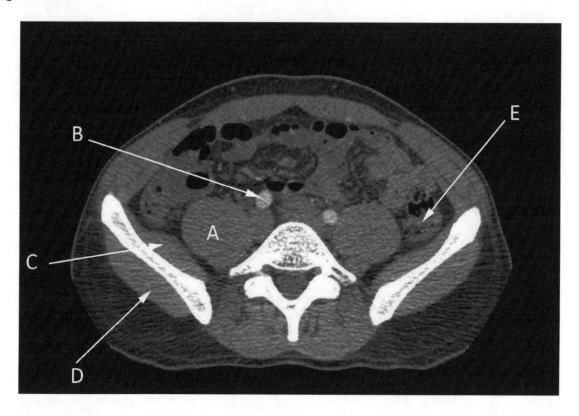

	QUESTION 7	WRITE YOUR ANSWER HERE
A	Name the structure labelled A	
B	Name the structure labelled B	
C	Name the structure labelled C	
D	Name the structure labelled D	
E	Name the structure labelled E	

Question 8

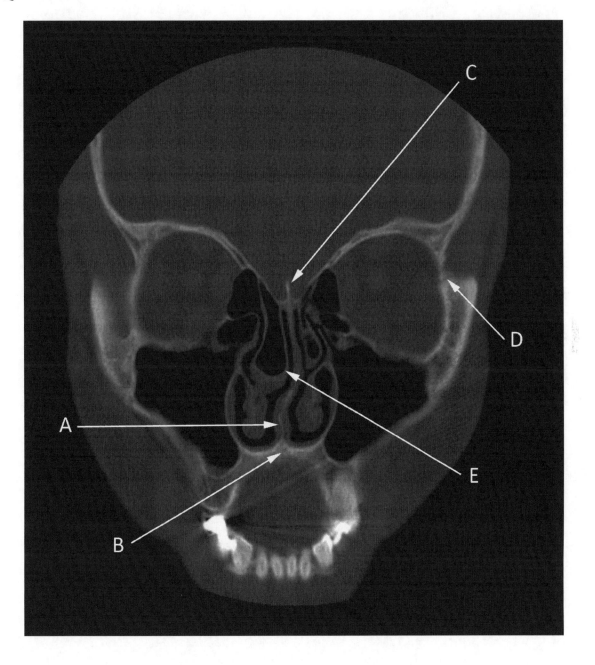

	QUESTION 8	WRITE YOUR ANSWER HERE
A	Name the structure labelled A	
B	Name the structure labelled B	
C	Name the structure labelled C	
D	Name the structure labelled D	
E	Name the normal variant labelled E	

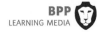

Question 9

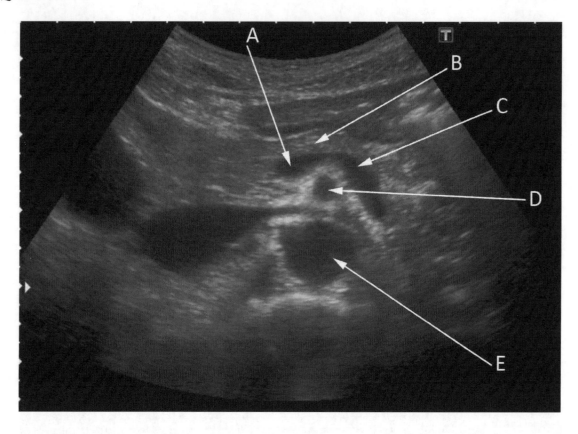

	QUESTION 9	WRITE YOUR ANSWER HERE
A	What two structures join to form A?	
B	Name the structure labelled B	
C	Name the structure labelled C	
D	Name the structure labelled D	
E	Name the structure labelled E	

Question 10

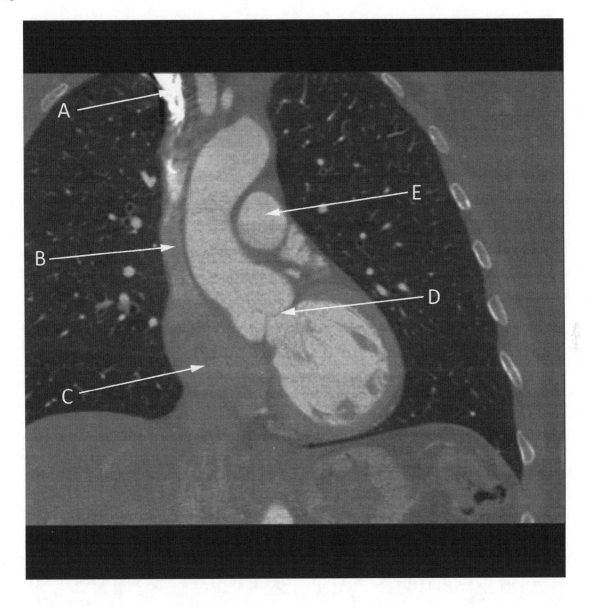

	QUESTION 10	WRITE YOUR ANSWER HERE
A	Name the structure labelled A	
B	Name the structure labelled B	
C	Name the structure labelled C	
D	Name the structure labelled D	
E	Name the structure labelled E	

Question 11

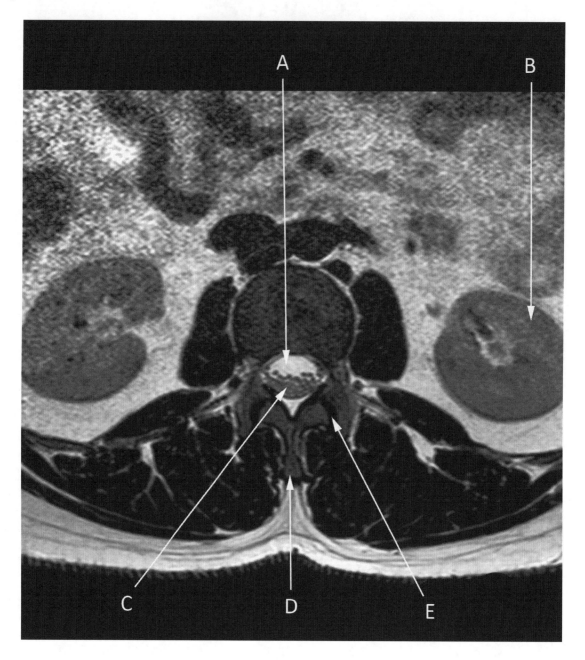

	QUESTION 11	WRITE YOUR ANSWER HERE
A	Name the structure labelled A	
B	Name the structure labelled B	
C	Name the structure labelled C	
D	Name the structure labelled D	
E	Name the structure labelled E	

Question 12

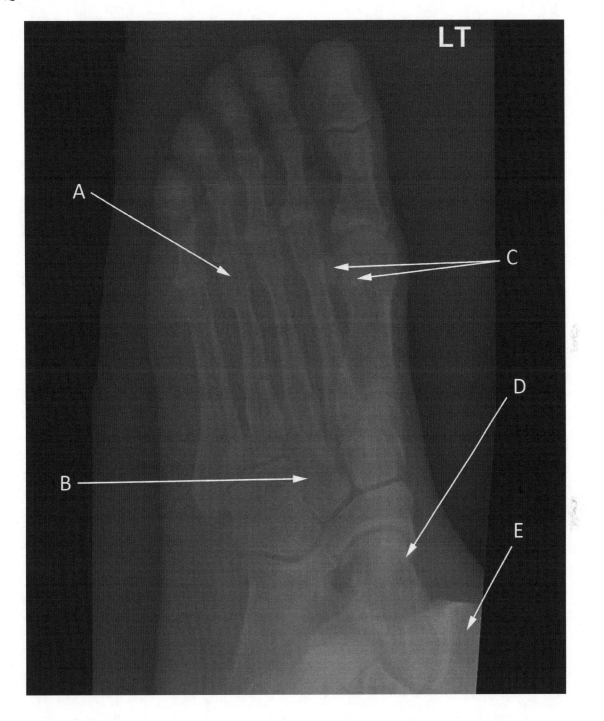

	QUESTION 12	WRITE YOUR ANSWER HERE
A	Name the structure labelled A	
B	Name the structure labelled B	
C	Name the structures labelled C	
D	Name the structure labelled D	
E	Name the structure labelled E	

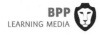

Question 13

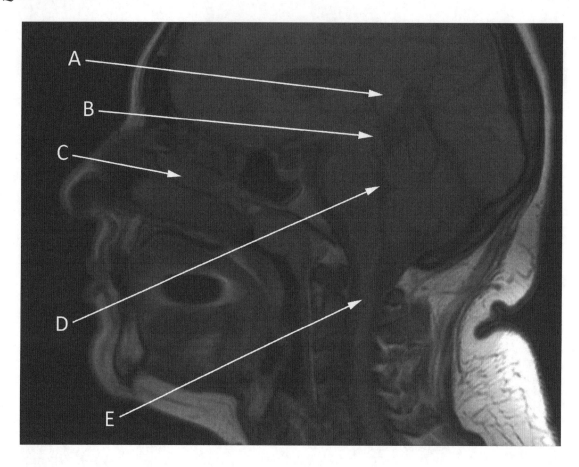

	QUESTION 13	WRITE YOUR ANSWER HERE
A	Name the structure labelled A	
B	Name the structure labelled B	
C	Name the structure labelled C	
D	Name the structure labelled D	
E	Name the structure labelled E	

Question 14

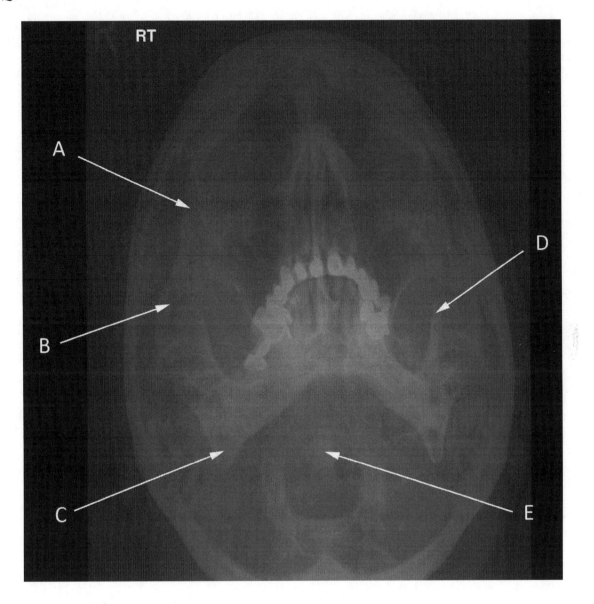

	QUESTION 14	WRITE YOUR ANSWER HERE
A	Name the structure labelled A	
B	Name the structure labelled B	
C	Name the structure labelled C	
D	Name the structure labelled D	
E	Name the structure labelled E	

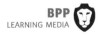

Question 15

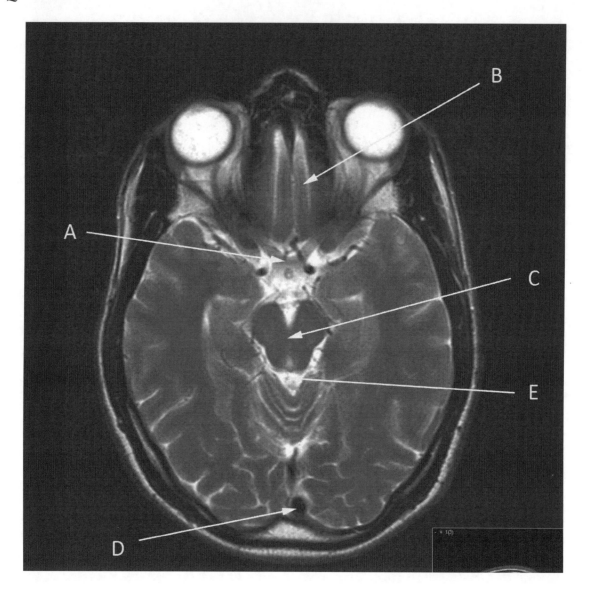

	QUESTION 15	WRITE YOUR ANSWER HERE
A	Name the structure labelled A	
B	Name the structure labelled B	
C	Name the structure labelled C	
D	Name the structure labelled D	
E	Name the structure labelled E	

Question 16

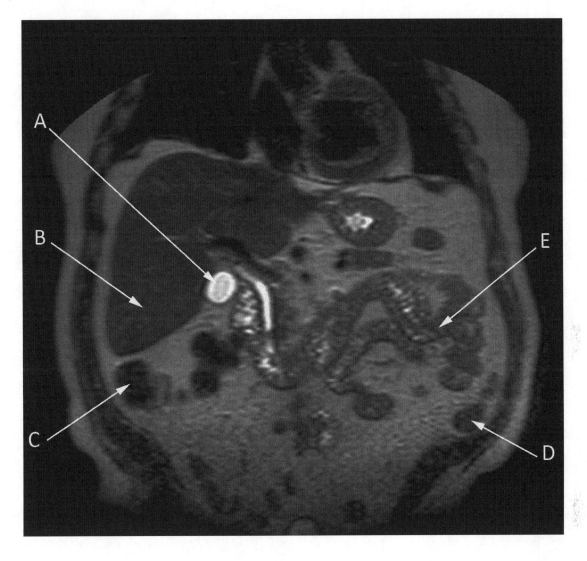

	QUESTION 16	WRITE YOUR ANSWER HERE
A	Name the structure labelled A	
B	Name the structure labelled B	
C	Name the structure labelled C	
D	Name the structure labelled D	
E	Name the structure labelled E	

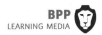

Question 17

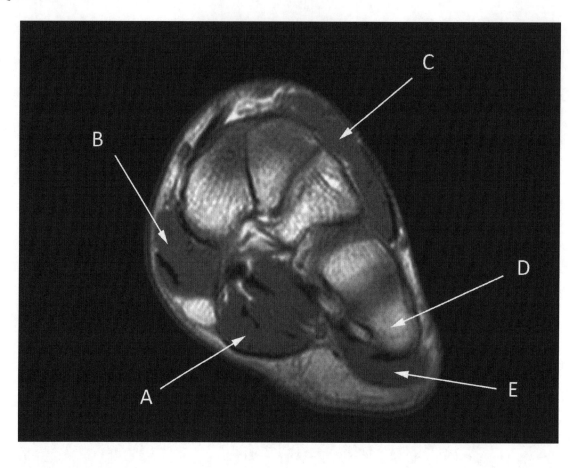

	QUESTION 17	WRITE YOUR ANSWER HERE
A	Name the structure labelled A	
B	Name the structure labelled B	
C	Name the structure labelled C	
D	Name the structure labelled D	
E	Name the structure labelled E	

Question 18

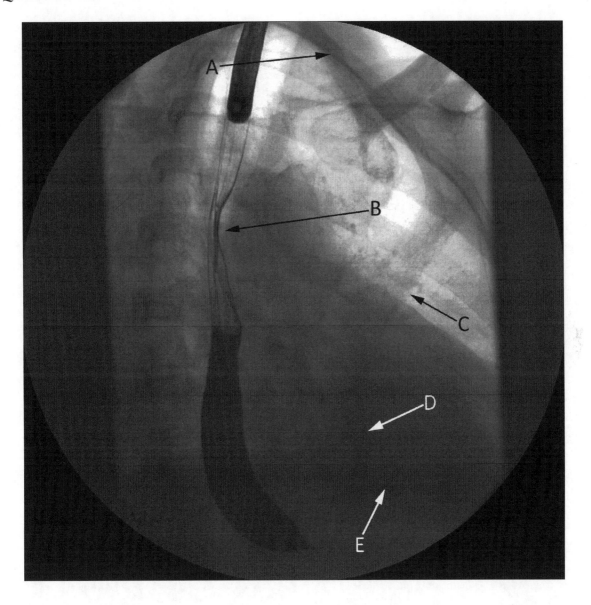

	QUESTION 18	WRITE YOUR ANSWER HERE
A	Name the structure labelled A	
B	Name the structure causing the impression labelled B	
C	Name the structure labelled C	
D	Name the structure labelled D	
E	Name the structure labelled E	

Question 19

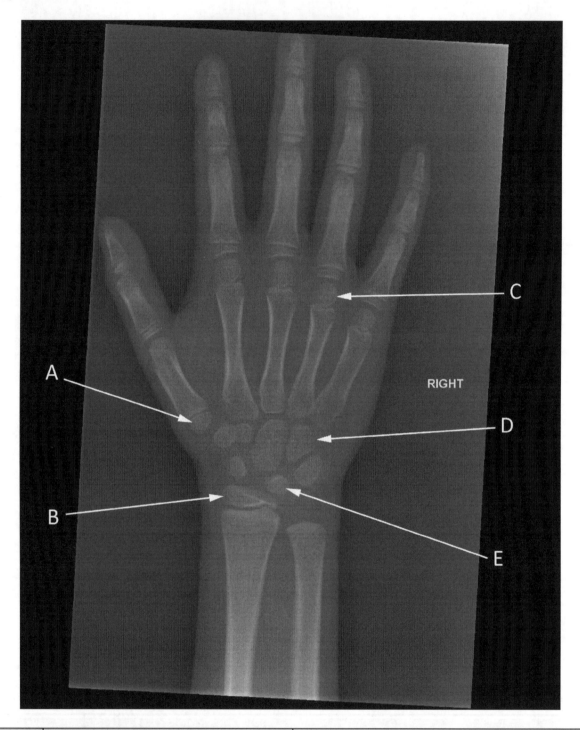

	QUESTION 19	WRITE YOUR ANSWER HERE
A	Name the structure labelled A	
B	Name the structure labelled B	
C	Name the structure labelled C	
D	Name the structure labelled D	
E	Name the structure labelled E	

Question 20

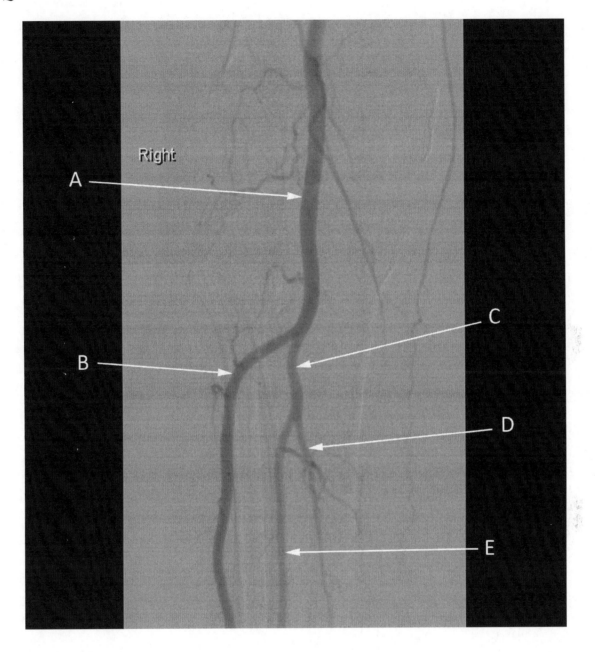

	QUESTION 20	WRITE YOUR ANSWER HERE
A	Name the structure labelled A	
B	Name the structure labelled B	
C	Name the structure labelled C	
D	Name the structure labelled D	
E	Name the structure labelled E	

Paper 3

Answers

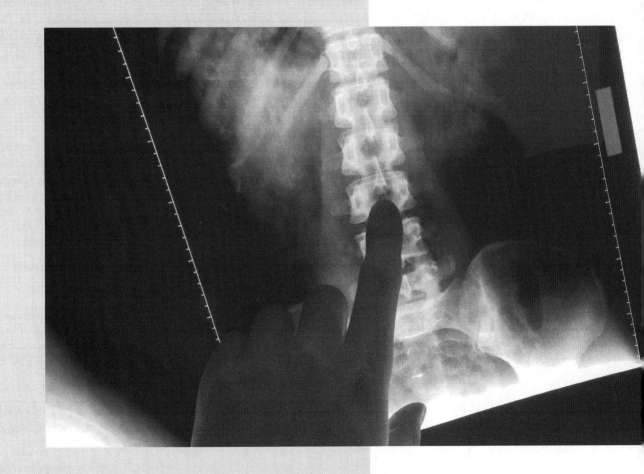

Question 1

A. Pulmonary valve
B. Aortic valve
C. Right ventricle
D. Left atrium
E. Right ventricular outflow tract

Question 2

A. Epiphyseal centre for left humeral trochlear
B. Epiphyseal centre for left humeral medial epicondyle
C. Left olecranon fossa
D. Epiphyseal centre for left humeral lateral epicondyle
E. Epiphyseal centre for left humeral capitellum

Question 3

A. Left common femoral vein
B. Left common femoral artery
C. Left sartorius muscle
D. Left iliopsoas muscle
E. Left tensor fasciae latae muscle

Question 4

A. Levator ani muscles
B. Right obturator externus
C. Right gracilis muscle
D. Left gluteus medius muscle
E. Left gluteus minimis muscle

Question 5

A. Bronchus intermedius
B. Left main bronchus
C. Lingula bronchus
D. Right lower lobe apical segment
E. Left upper lobe, apico-posterior segment

Question 6

A. Diaphysis of left femur
B. Left medial femoral condyle
C. Left lateral femoral epicondyle
D. Left medial tibial plateau
E. Neck of left fibula

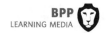

Question 7

A. Right psoas muscle
B. Right common iliac artery
C. Right iliacus muscle
D. Right gluteus medius muscle
E. Descending colon

Question 8

A. Bony nasal septum
B. Hard palate
C. Crista galli
D. Zygomaticofrontal suture
E. Concha bullosa

Question 9

A. Splenic vein and superior mesenteric vein
B. Pancreas (body)
C. Splenic vein
D. Superior mesenteric artery
E. Aorta

Question 10

A. Right brachiocephalic vein
B. Superior vena cava
C. Right atrium
D. Aortic valve
E. Main pulmonary artery

Question 11

A. Cerebrospinal fluid in spinal canal
B. Left kidney (cortex)
C. Cauda equina
D. Spinous process
E. Facet joint

Question 12

A. Head of fourth metatarsal
B. Lateral cuneiform
C. Sesamoid bones in flexor hallucis brevis muscle
D. Talus
E. Tibia

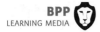

Question 13

A. Splenium of corpus callosum
B. Quadrigeminal plate of midbrain
C. Middle nasal turbinate
D. Fourth ventricle
E. Cervical spinal cord

Question 14

A. Frontal process of the right zygomatic bone
B. Temporal process of the right zygomatic bone
C. Right angle of the mandible
D. Left coronoid process of the mandible
E. Odontoid process of C2

Question 15

A. Optic chiasm
B. Left gyrus rectus
C. Midbrain
D. Superior sagittal sinus
E. Quadrigeminal cistern

Question 16

A. Gallbladder
B. Right lobe of liver
C. Ascending colon
D. Loops of jejunum
E. Descending colon

Question 17

A. Flexor digitorum brevis
B. Adductor hallucis muscle
C. Extensor digitorum brevis muscle
D. Fifth metatarsal
E. Abductor digiti minimi muscle

Question 18

A. Ribs
B. Aortic arch
C. Scapula
D. Pulmonary vessels
E. Diaphragm

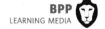

Question 19

A. Epiphyseal centre for first metacarpal
B. Epiphyseal centre for distal radius
C. Epiphyseal centre for fourth metacarpal
D. Hamate
E. Lunate

Question 20

A. Popliteal artery
B. Anterior tibial artery
C. Tibioperoneal trunk
D. Posterior tibial artery
E. Peroneal artery

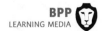

Paper 4

Question Bank

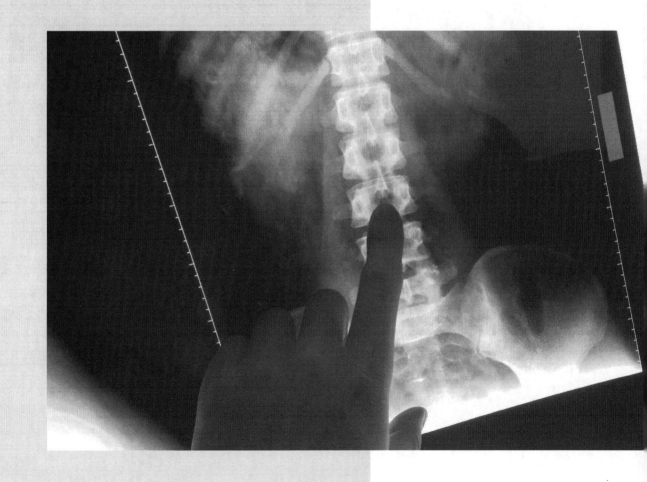

Question 1

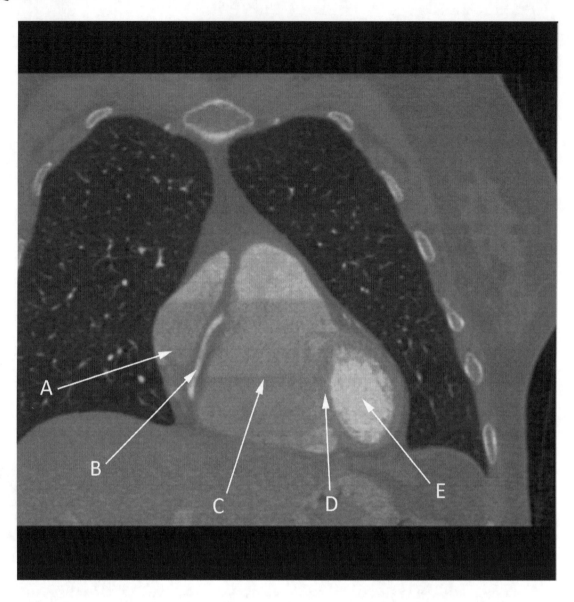

	QUESTION 1	WRITE YOUR ANSWER HERE
A	Name the structure labelled A	
B	Name the structure labelled B	
C	Name the structure labelled C	
D	Name the structure labelled D	
E	Name the structure labelled E	

Question 2

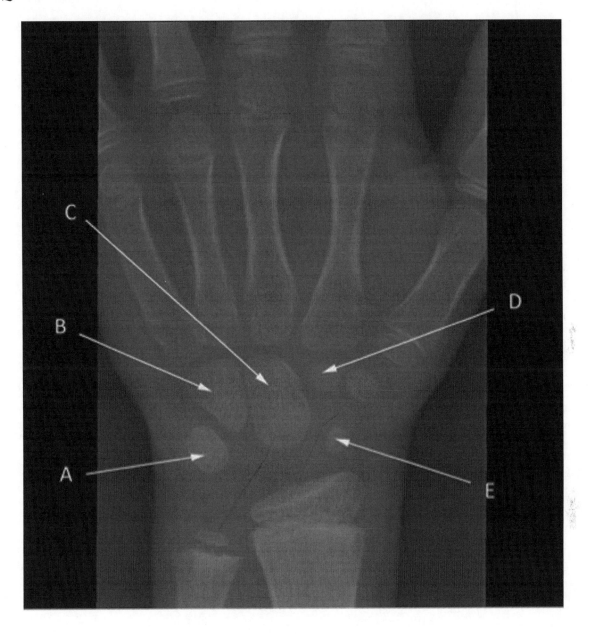

	QUESTION 2	WRITE YOUR ANSWER HERE
A	Name the structure labelled A	
B	Name the structure labelled B	
C	Name the structure labelled C	
D	Name the structure labelled D	
E	Name the structure labelled E	

Question 3

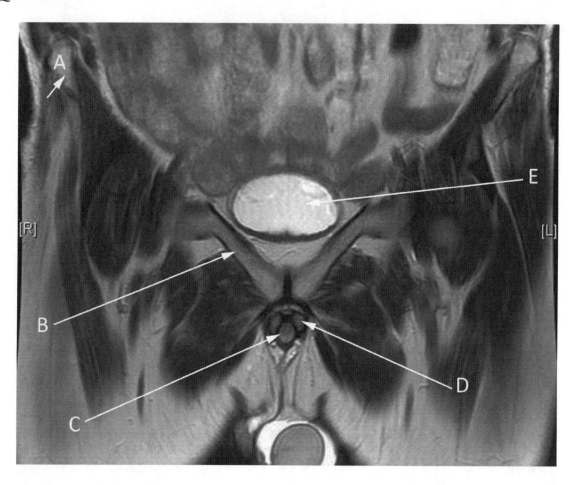

	QUESTION 3	WRITE YOUR ANSWER HERE
A	Name the structure labelled A	
B	Name the structure labelled B	
C	Name the structure labelled C	
D	Name the structure labelled D	
E	Name the structure labelled E	

Question 4

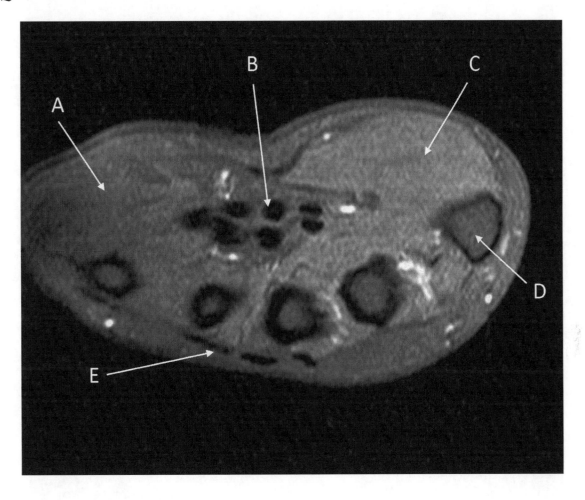

	QUESTION 4	WRITE YOUR ANSWER HERE
A	Name the structure labelled A	
B	Name the structure labelled B	
C	Name the structure labelled C	
D	Name the structure labelled D	
E	Name the structure labelled E	

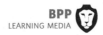

Question 5

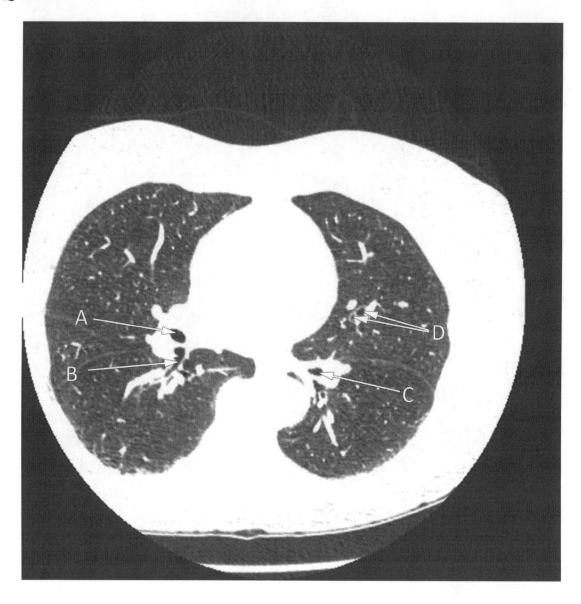

	QUESTION 5	WRITE YOUR ANSWER HERE
A	Name the lobar bronchus labelled A	
B	Name the segmental bronchus labelled B	
C	Name the lobar bronchus labelled C	
D	Which part of the lung is supplied by the segmental bronchi labelled D	
E	What segments will A bifurcate into?	

Question 6

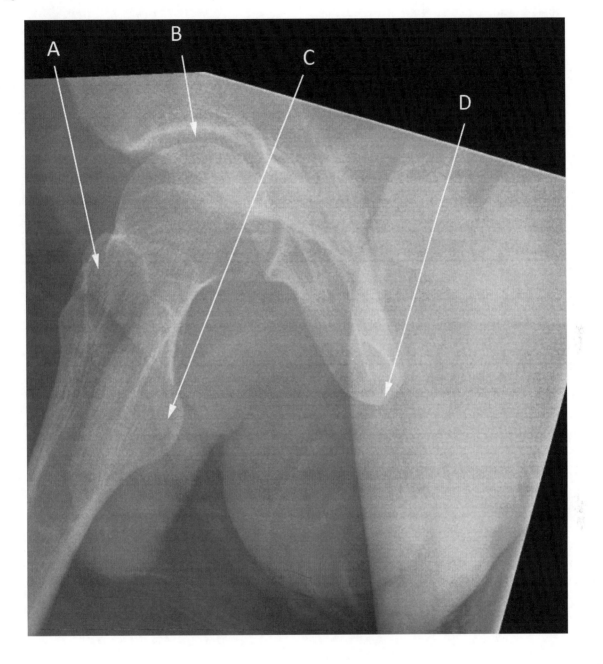

	QUESTION 6	WRITE YOUR ANSWER HERE
A	Name the structure labelled A	
B	Name the structure labelled B	
C	Name the structure labelled C	
D	Name the structure labelled D	
E	What attaches distally to C?	

Question 7

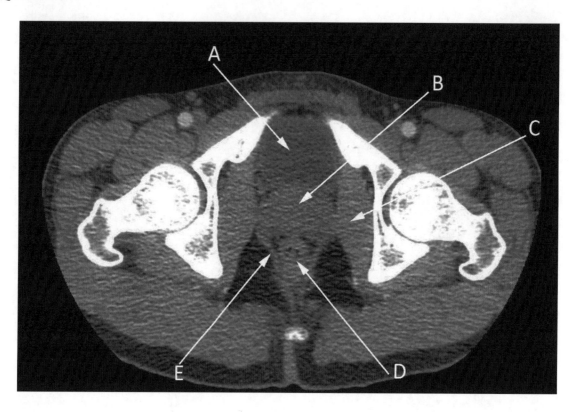

	QUESTION 7	WRITE YOUR ANSWER HERE
A	Name the structure labelled A	
B	Name the structure labelled B	
C	Name the structure labelled C	
D	Name the structure labelled D	
E	Name the structure labelled E	

Question 8

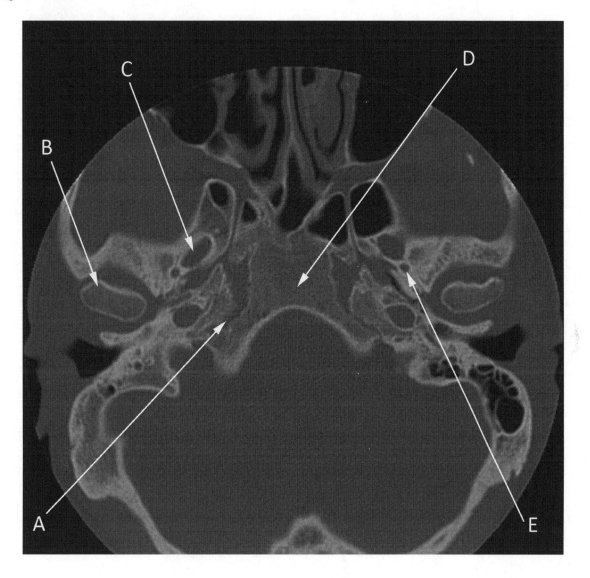

	QUESTION 8	WRITE YOUR ANSWER HERE
A	Name the structure labelled A	
B	Name the structure labelled B	
C	Name the structure labelled C	
D	Name the structure labelled D	
E	Which artery passes through E?	

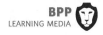

Question 9

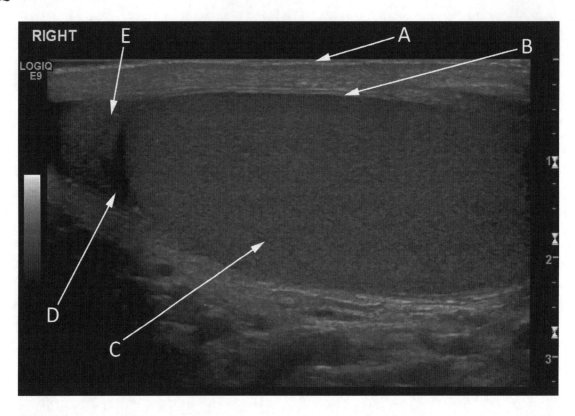

	QUESTION 9	WRITE YOUR ANSWER HERE
A	Name the structure labelled A	
B	Name the structure labelled B	
C	Name the structure labelled C	
D	Name the structure labelled D	
E	Name the structure labelled E	

Question 10

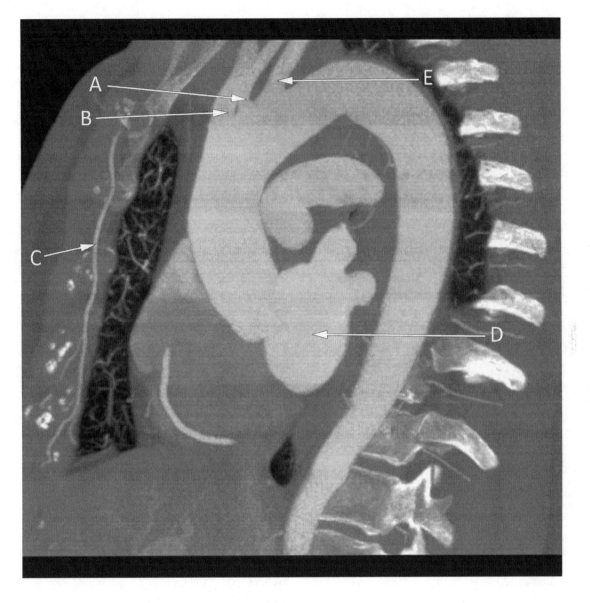

	QUESTION 10	WRITE YOUR ANSWER HERE
A	Name the structure labelled A	
B	Name the structure labelled B	
C	Name the structure labelled C	
D	Name the structure labelled D	
E	Name the structure labelled E	

Question 11

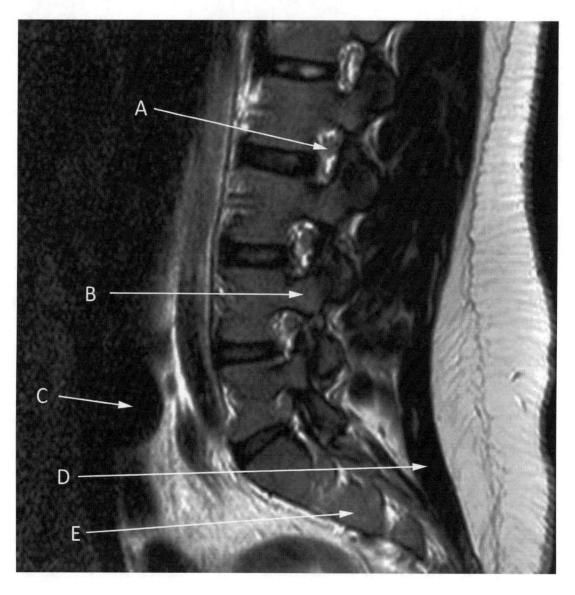

	QUESTION 11	WRITE YOUR ANSWER HERE
A	Name the structure labelled A	
B	Name the structure labelled B	
C	Name the structure labelled C	
D	Name the structure labelled D	
E	Name the structure labelled E	

Question 12

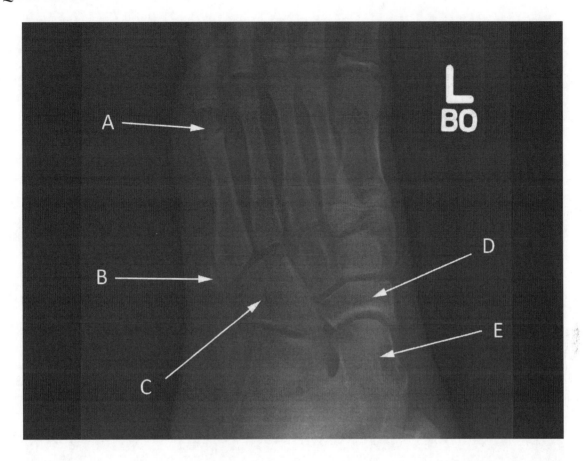

	QUESTION 12	WRITE YOUR ANSWER HERE
A	Name the structure labelled A	
B	Name the structure labelled B	
C	Name the structure labelled C	
D	Name the structure labelled D	
E	Name the structure labelled E	

Question 13

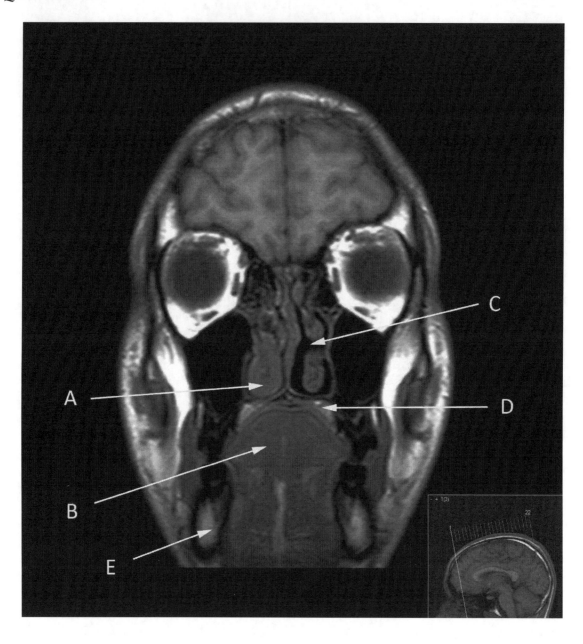

	QUESTION 13	WRITE YOUR ANSWER HERE
A	Name the structure labelled A	
B	Name the structure labelled B	
C	Name the structure labelled C	
D	Name the structure labelled D	
E	Name the structure labelled E	

Question 14

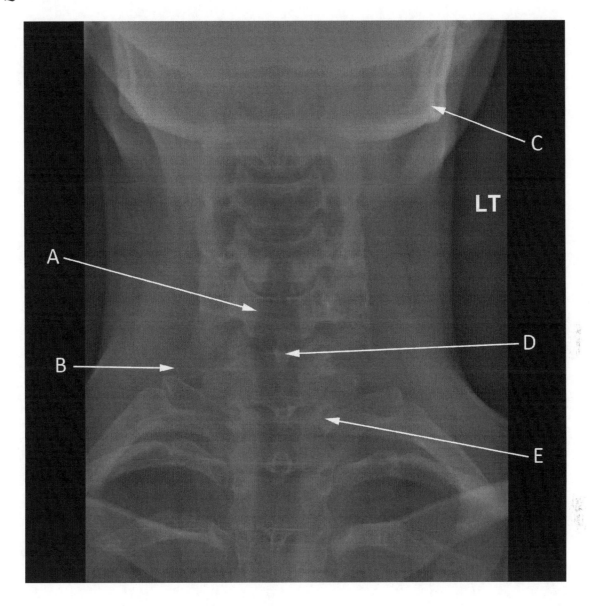

	QUESTION 14	WRITE YOUR ANSWER HERE
A	Name the structure labelled A	
B	Name the structure labelled B	
C	Name the structure labelled C	
D	Name the structure labelled D	
E	Name the structure labelled E	

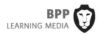

Question 15

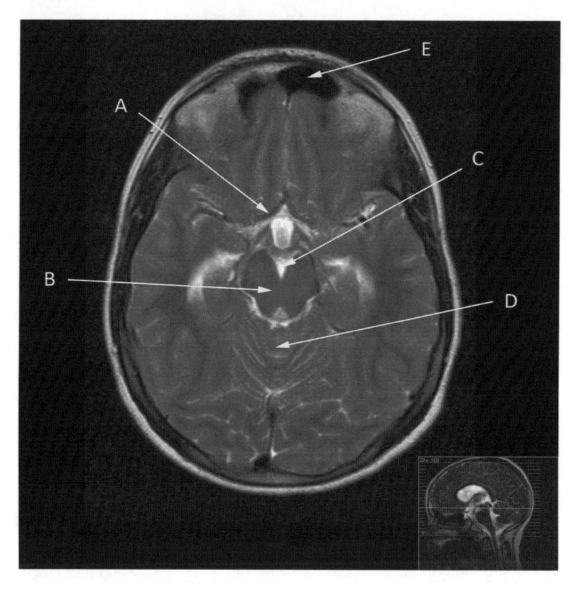

	QUESTION 15	WRITE YOUR ANSWER HERE
A	Name the structure labelled A	
B	Name the structure labelled B	
C	Name the structure labelled C	
D	Name the structure labelled D	
E	Name the structure labelled E	

Question 16

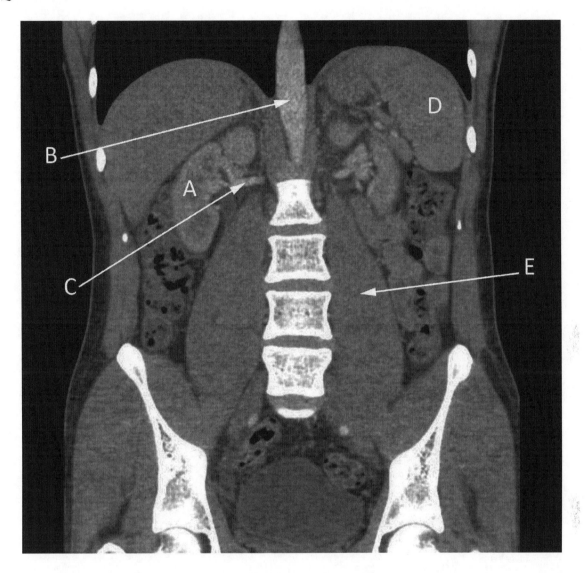

	QUESTION 16	WRITE YOUR ANSWER HERE
A	Name the structure labelled A	
B	Name the structure labelled B	
C	Name the structure labelled C	
D	Name the structure labelled D	
E	Name the structure labelled E	

BPP
LEARNING MEDIA

Question 17

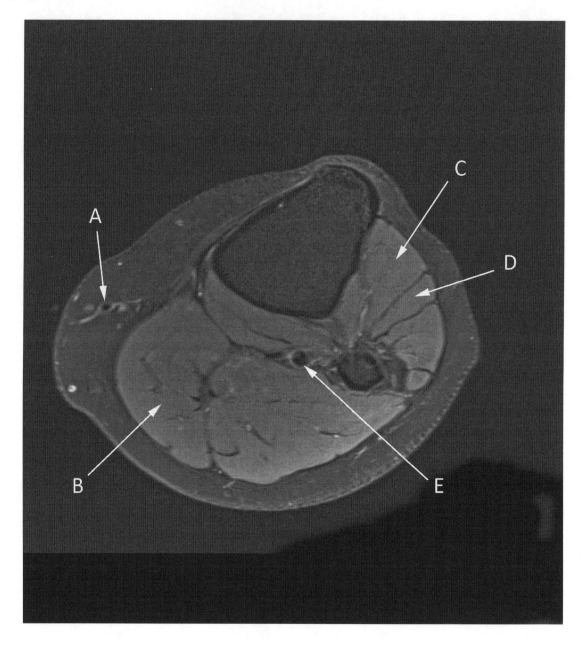

	QUESTION 17	WRITE YOUR ANSWER HERE
A	Name the structure labelled A	
B	Name the structure labelled B	
C	Name the structure labelled C	
D	Name the structure labelled D	
E	Name the structure labelled E	

Question 18

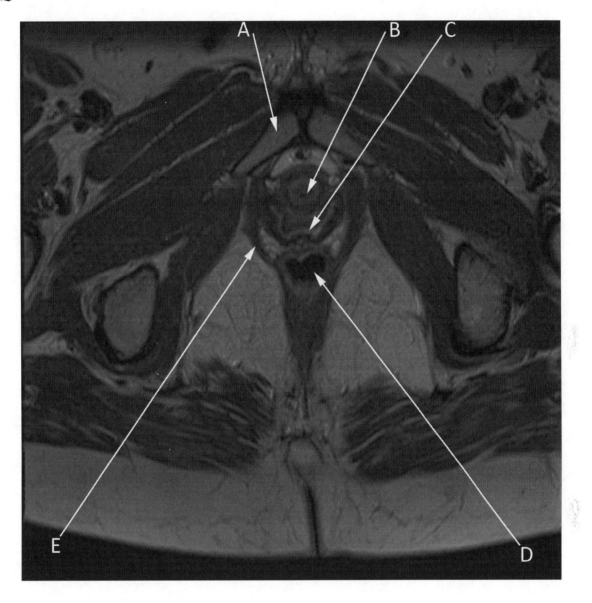

	QUESTION 18	WRITE YOUR ANSWER HERE
A	Name the structure labelled A	
B	Name the structure labelled B	
C	Name the structure labelled C	
D	Name the structure labelled D	
E	Name the structure labelled E	

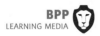

Question 19

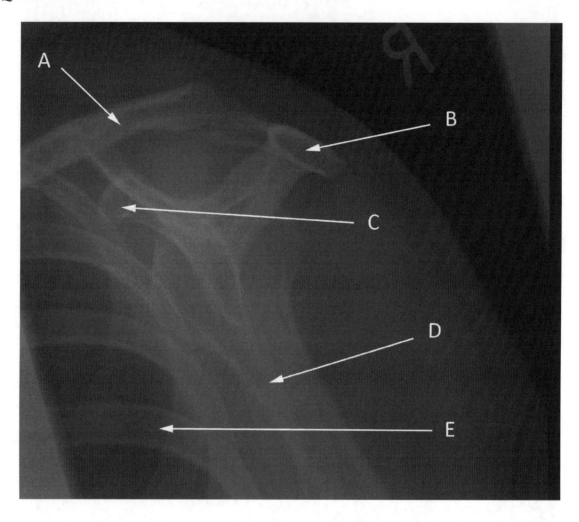

	QUESTION 19	WRITE YOUR ANSWER HERE
A	Name the structure labelled A	
B	Name the structure labelled B	
C	What attaches to C?	
D	Name the structure labelled D	
E	Name the structure labelled E	

Question 20

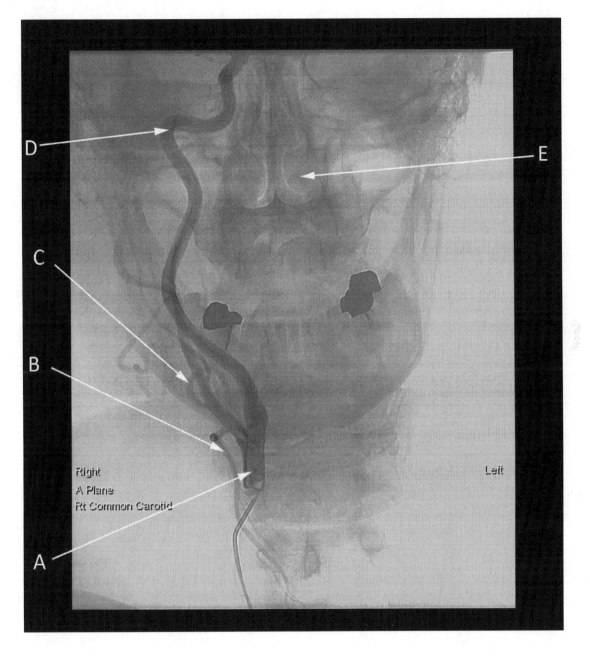

	QUESTION 20	WRITE YOUR ANSWER HERE
A	Name the structure labelled A	
B	Name the structure labelled B	
C	Name the structure labelled C	
D	Name the structure labelled D	
E	Name the structure labelled E	

Paper 4

Answers

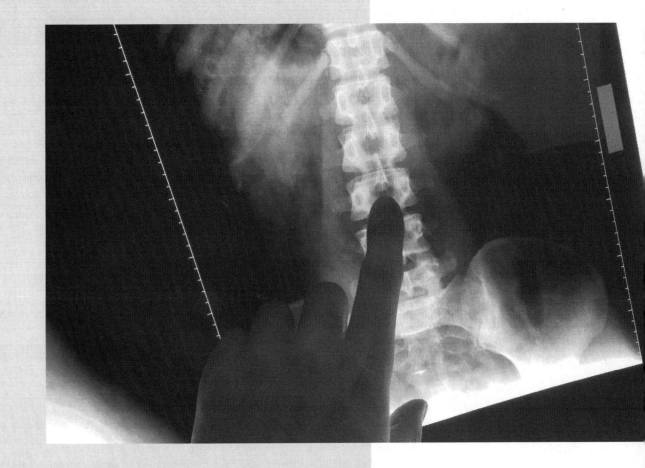

Question 1

A. Right atrium
B. Right coronary artery
C. Right ventricle
D. Interventricular septum
E. Left ventricle

Question 2

A. Left triquetral bone
B. Left hamate bone
C. Left capitate bone
D. Left trapezoid bone
E. Left scaphoid bone

Question 3

A. Right ilium
B. Right superior pubic ramus
C. Corpus spongiosum
D. Left corpus cavernosum
E. Urinary bladder

Question 4

A. Hypothenar muscles
B. Tendons of flexor digitorum superficialis
C. Thenar muscles
D. Base of first metacarpal
E. Tendons of extensor digitorum

Question 5

A. Middle lobe bronchus
B. Right lower lobe apical segment
C. Left lower lobe
D. Lingula
E. Medial and lateral segments of the middle lobe

Question 6

A. Greater trochanter of femur
B. Acetabulum
C. Lesser trochanter of femur
D. Ischial tuberosity
E. Iliopsoas

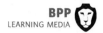

Question 7
A. Urinary bladder
B. Prostate
C. Left obturator internus muscle
D. Rectum
E. Levator ani muscle

Question 8
A. Right petro-occipital suture
B. Right condyle of mandible
C. Right foramen ovale
D. Clivus
E. Left middle meningeal artery

Question 9
A. Scrotal skin
B. Tunica albuginea
C. Right testis
D. Fluid
E. Right epididymis

Question 10
A. Left common carotid
B. Brachiocephalic artery
C. Internal mammary artery (right)
D. Left atrium
E. Left subclavian artery

Question 11
A. L2 nerve root
B. L4 pedicle
C. Loop of bowel
D. Erector spinae muscle
E. S2 vertebra

Question 12
A. Growth centre for left fifth metatarsal
B. Growth centre for tuberosity of base of left fifth metatarsal
C. Left cuboid bone
D. Left navicular bone
E. Left talus bone

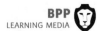

Question 13

A. Right inferior turbinate
B. Tongue
C. Left middle meatus
D. Hard palate
E. Mandible

Question 14

A. Tracheal outline projected over C6 vertebral body
B. Right transverse process of C7 vertebra
C. Mandible
D. Spinous process of C6 vertebra
E. Left pedicle of T1 vertebra

Question 15

A. Right anterior cerebral artery
B. Midbrain
C. Interpeduncular cistern
D. Superior cerebellar vermis
E. Left frontal sinus

Question 16

A. Right kidney
B. Aorta
C. Right renal artery
D. Spleen
E. Left psoas muscle

Question 17

A. Long saphenous vein
B. Medial head of gastrocnemius muscle
C. Tibialis anterior muscle
D. Extensor digitorum longus muscle
E. Posterior tibial artery

Question 18

A. Right pubic bone
B. Urethra (external sphincter)
C. Vagina
D. Anus
E. Levator ani

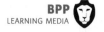

Question 19

A. Left clavicle
B. Left acromion of scapula
C. Left coracobrachialis / left short head of biceps
D. Spinous process of left scapula
E. Rib

Question 20

A. Right common carotid artery
B. Right superior thyroid artery
C. Right lingual artery
D. Petrous portion of right internal carotid artery
E. Left inferior turbinate

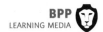

Paper 5

Question Bank

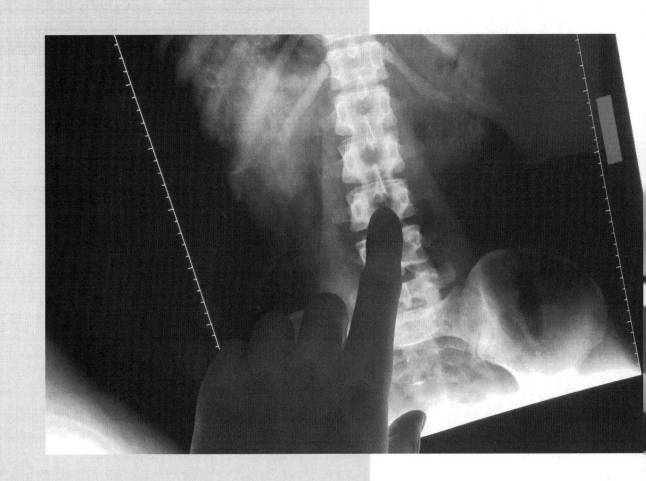

Question 1

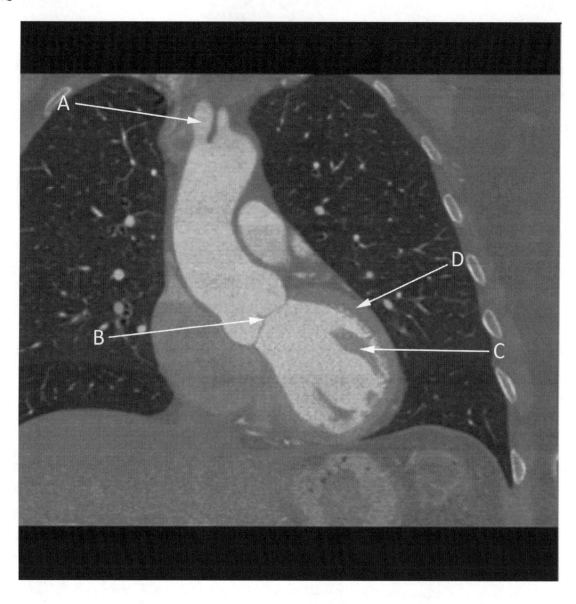

	QUESTION 1	WRITE YOUR ANSWER HERE
A	Name the structure labelled A	
B	Name the structure labelled B	
C	Name the structure labelled C	
D	Name the structure labelled D	
E	What structure does C attach to?	

Question 2

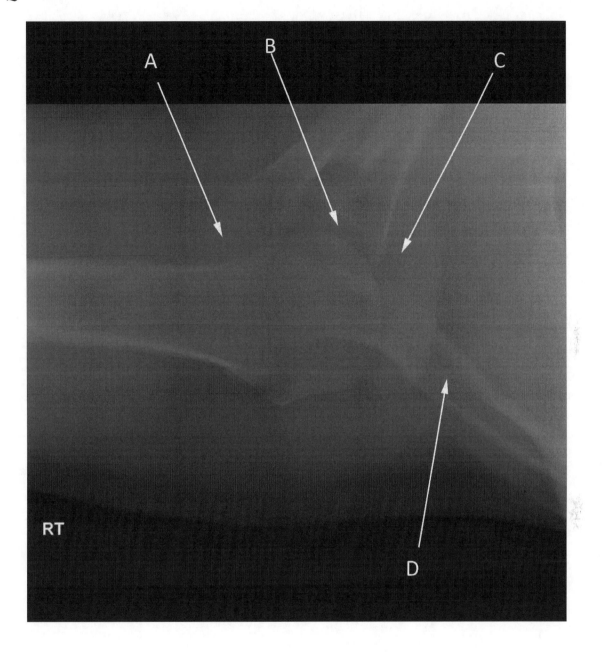

	QUESTION 2	WRITE YOUR ANSWER HERE
A	Name the structure labelled A	
B	Name the structure labelled B	
C	Name the structure labelled C	
D	Name the structure labelled D	
E	What attaches to C?	

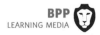

Question 3

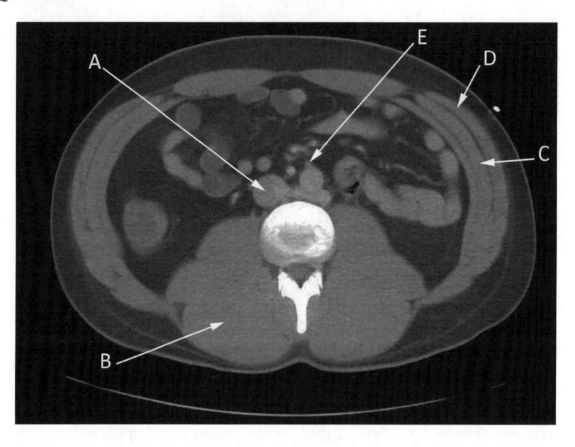

	QUESTION 3	WRITE YOUR ANSWER HERE
A	Name the structure labelled A	
B	Name the structure labelled B	
C	Name the structure labelled C	
D	Name the structure labelled D	
E	Name the structure labelled E	

Question 4

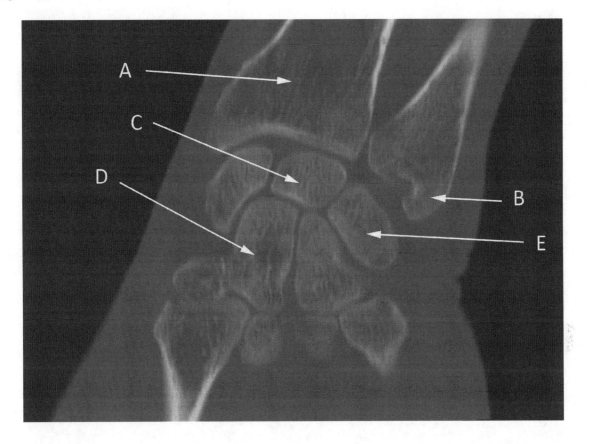

	QUESTION 4	WRITE YOUR ANSWER HERE
A	Name the structure labelled A	
B	Name the structure labelled B	
C	Name the structure labelled C	
D	Name the structure labelled D	
E	Name the structure labelled E	

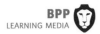

Question 5

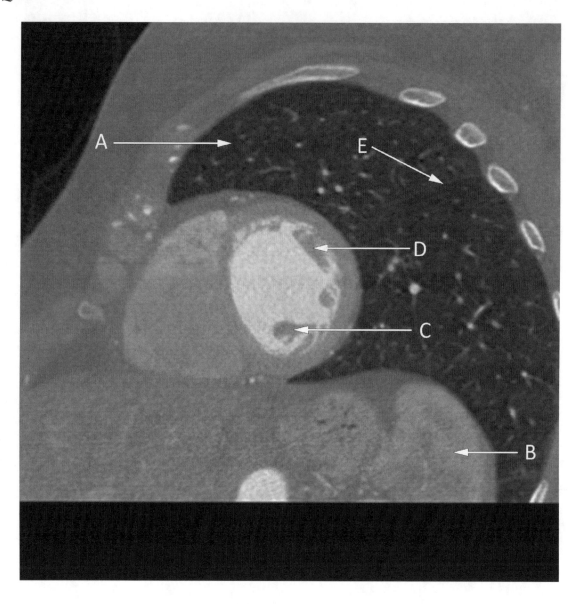

	QUESTION 5	WRITE YOUR ANSWER HERE
A	Name the lung segment labelled A	
B	Name the structure labelled B	
C	Name the structure labelled C	
D	Name the structure labelled D	
E	Name the structure labelled E	

Question 6

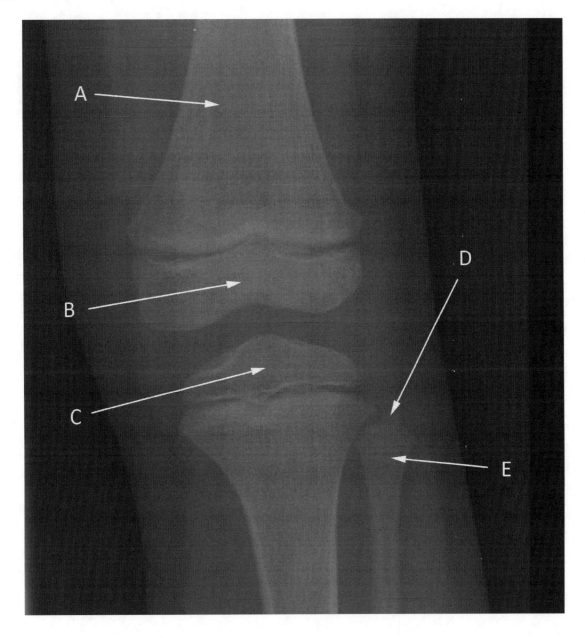

	QUESTION 6	WRITE YOUR ANSWER HERE
A	Name the structure labelled A	
B	Name the structure labelled B	
C	Name the structure labelled C	
D	Name the structure labelled D	
E	Name the structure labelled E	

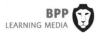

Question 7

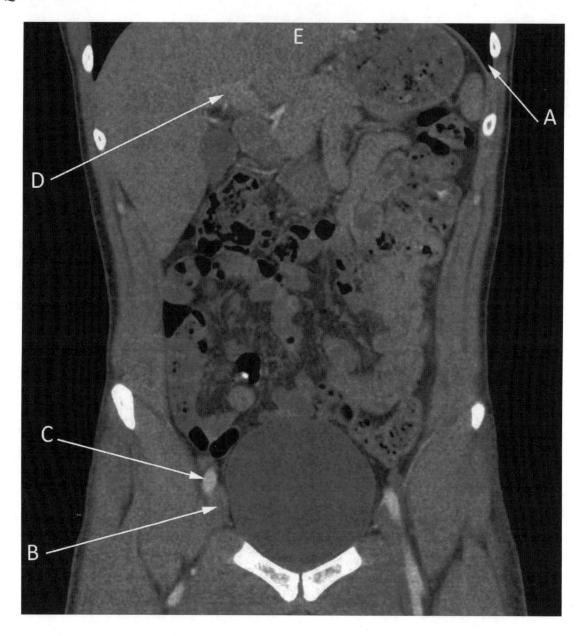

	QUESTION 7	WRITE YOUR ANSWER HERE
A	Name the structure labelled A	
B	Name the structure labelled B	
C	Name the structure labelled C	
D	Name the structure labelled D	
E	Name the structure labelled E	

Question 8

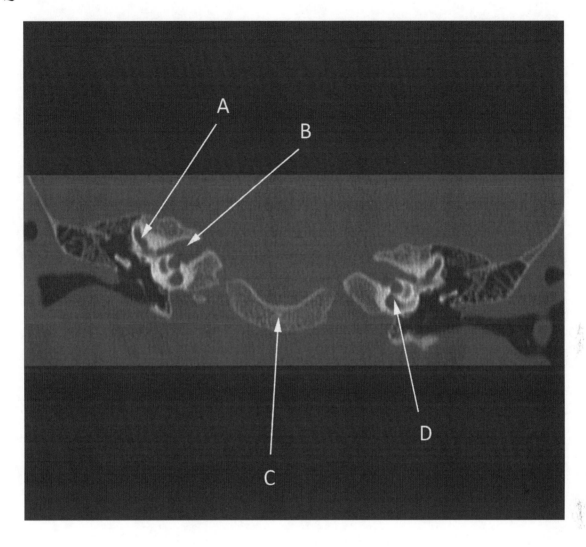

	QUESTION 8	WRITE YOUR ANSWER HERE
A	Name the structure labelled A	
B	Name the structure labelled B	
C	Name the structure labelled C	
D	Name the structure labelled D	
E	What passes through B?	

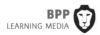

Question 9

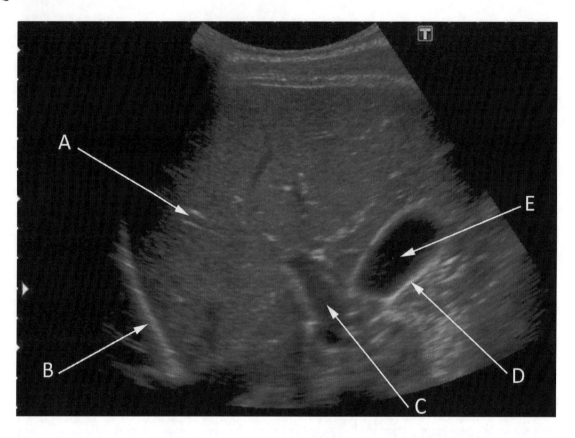

	QUESTION 9	WRITE YOUR ANSWER HERE
A	Name the structure labelled A	
B	Name the structure labelled B	
C	Name the structure labelled C	
D	What is the normal thickness of D?	
E	Name the structure labelled E	

Question 10

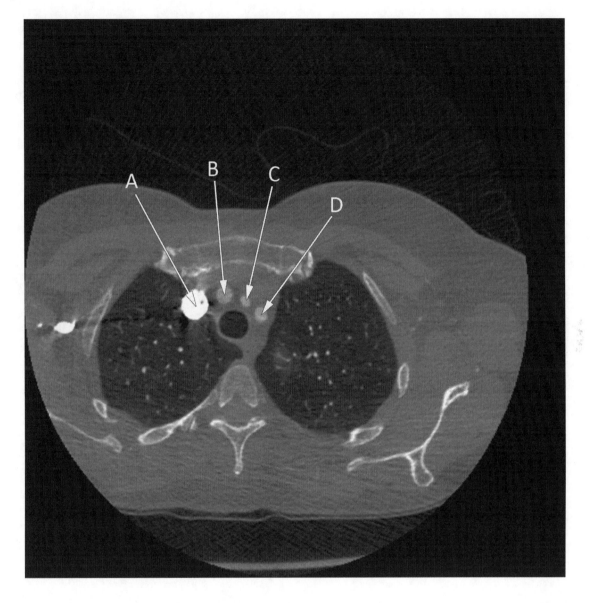

	QUESTION 10	WRITE YOUR ANSWER HERE
A	Name the structure labelled A	
B	Name the structure labelled B	
C	Name the structure labelled C	
D	Name the structure labelled D	
E	Which two vessels arise from B?	

BPP
LEARNING MEDIA

Question 11

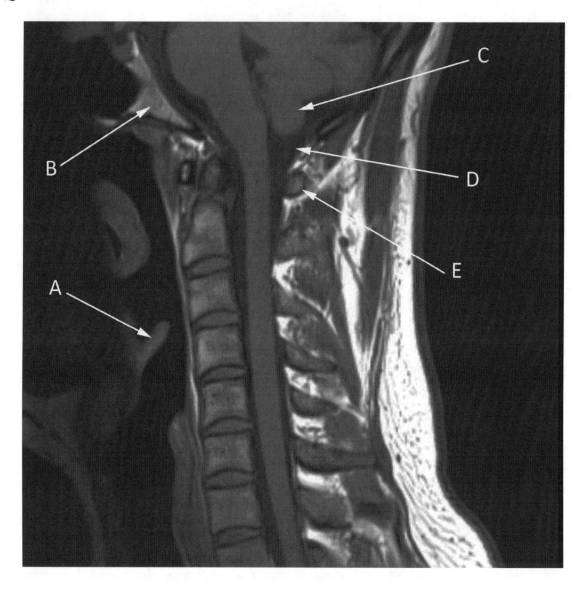

	QUESTION 11	WRITE YOUR ANSWER HERE
A	Name the structure labelled A	
B	Name the structure labelled B	
C	Name the structure labelled C	
D	Name the structure labelled D	
E	Name the structure labelled E	

Question 12

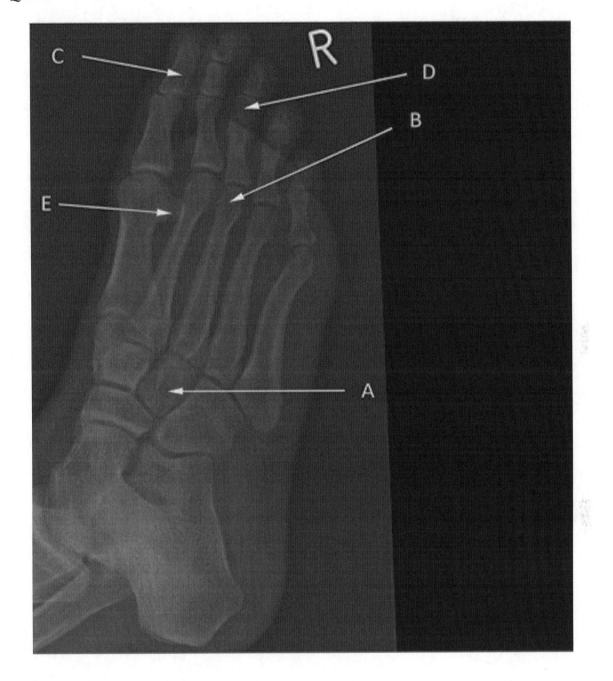

	QUESTION 12	WRITE YOUR ANSWER HERE
A	Name the structure labelled A	
B	Name the structure labelled B	
C	Name the structure labelled C	
D	Name the structure labelled D	
E	Name the structure labelled E	

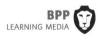

Question 13

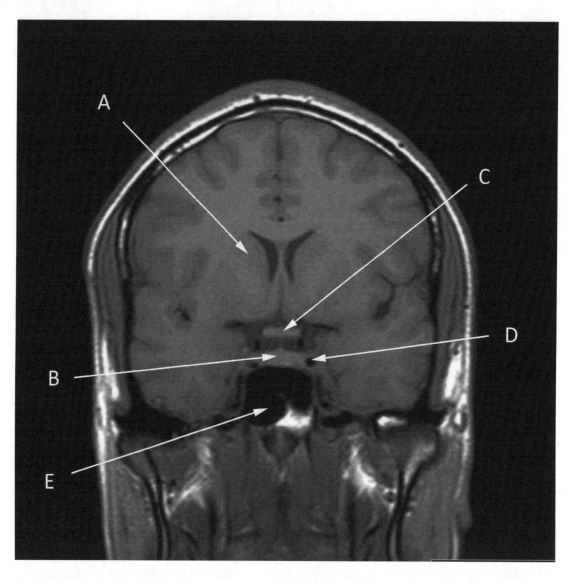

	QUESTION 13	WRITE YOUR ANSWER HERE
A	Name the structure labelled A	
B	Name the structure labelled B	
C	Name the structure labelled C	
D	Name the structure labelled D	
E	Name the structure labelled E	

Question 14

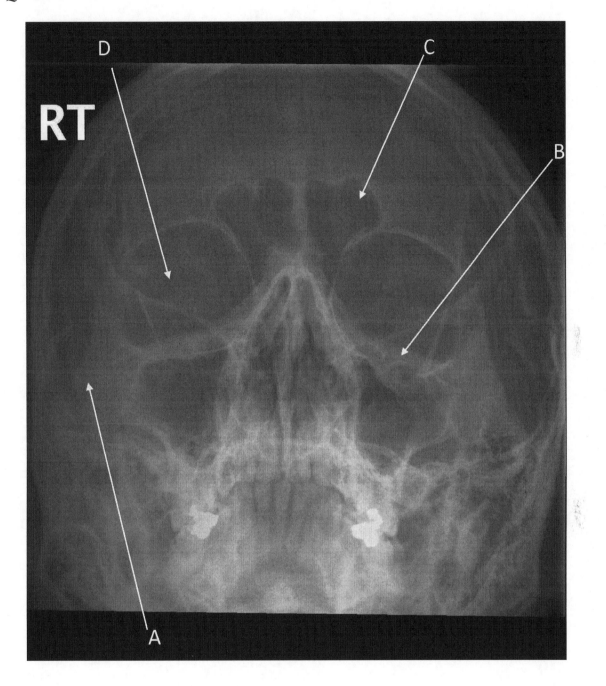

	QUESTION 14	WRITE YOUR ANSWER HERE
A	Name the structure labelled A	
B	Name the structure labelled B	
C	Name the structure labelled C	
D	Name the structure labelled D	
E	What nerves pass through D?	

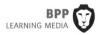

Question 15

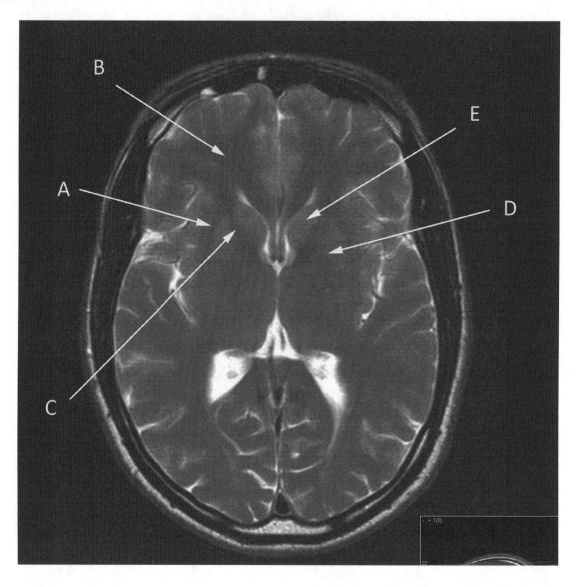

	QUESTION 15	WRITE YOUR ANSWER HERE
A	Name the structure labelled A	
B	Name the structure labelled B	
C	Name the structure labelled C	
D	Name the structure labelled D	
E	Name the structure labelled E	

Question 16

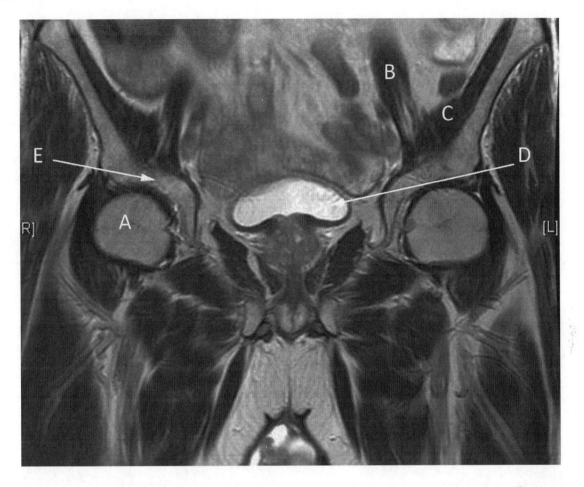

	QUESTION 16	WRITE YOUR ANSWER HERE
A	Name the structure labelled A	
B	Name the structure labelled B	
C	Name the structure labelled C	
D	Name the structure labelled D	
E	Name the structure labelled E	

Question 17

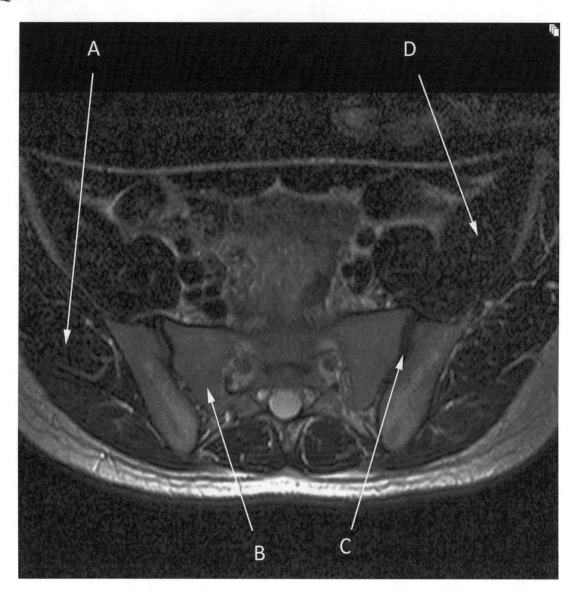

	QUESTION 17	WRITE YOUR ANSWER HERE
A	Name the structure labelled A	
B	Name the structure labelled B	
C	Name the structure labelled C	
D	Name the structure labelled D	
E	What is the distal attachment of D?	

Question 18

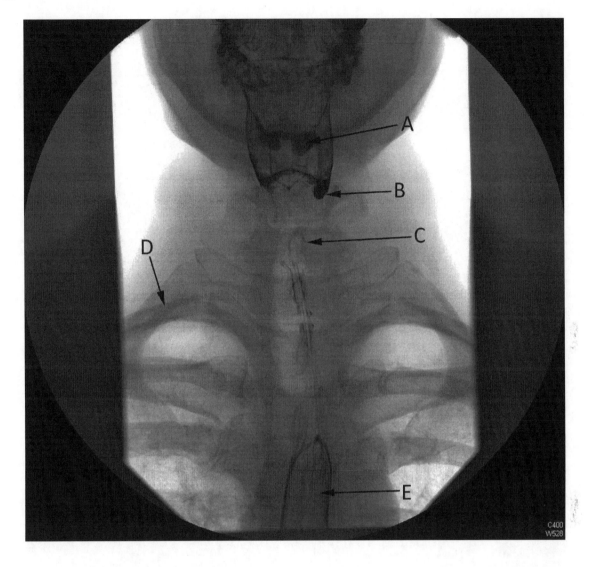

	QUESTION 18	WRITE YOUR ANSWER HERE
A	Name the structure labelled A	
B	Name the structure labelled B	
C	Name the structure labelled C	
D	Name the structure labelled D	
E	Name the structure labelled E	

Question 19

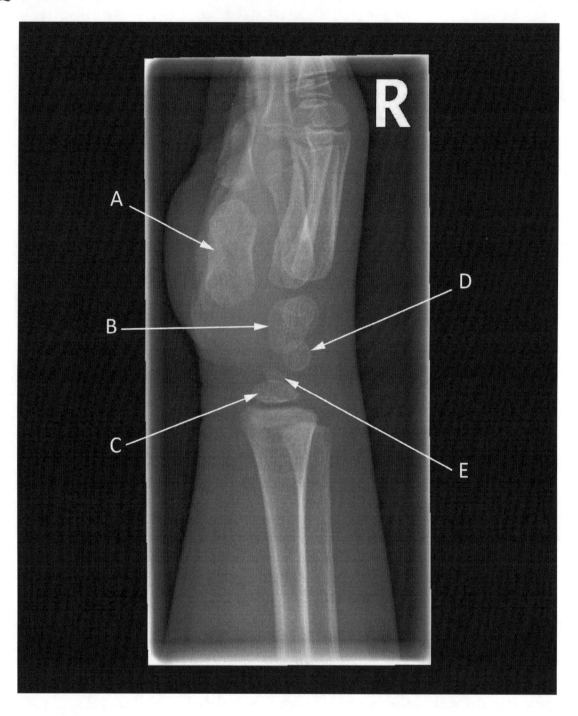

	QUESTION 19	WRITE YOUR ANSWER HERE
A	Name the structure labelled A	
B	Name the structure labelled B	
C	Name the structure labelled C	
D	Name the structure labelled D	
E	Name the structure labelled E	

Question 20

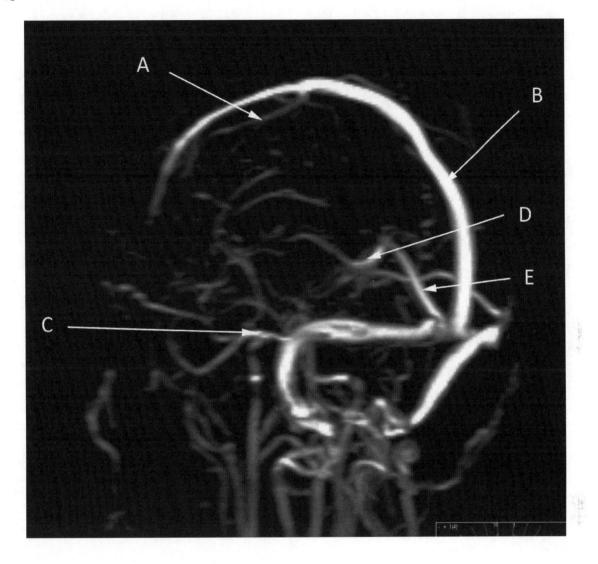

	QUESTION 20	WRITE YOUR ANSWER HERE
A	Name the structure labelled A	
B	Name the structure labelled B	
C	Name the structure labelled C	
D	Name the structure labelled D	
E	Name the structure labelled E	

Paper 5

Answers

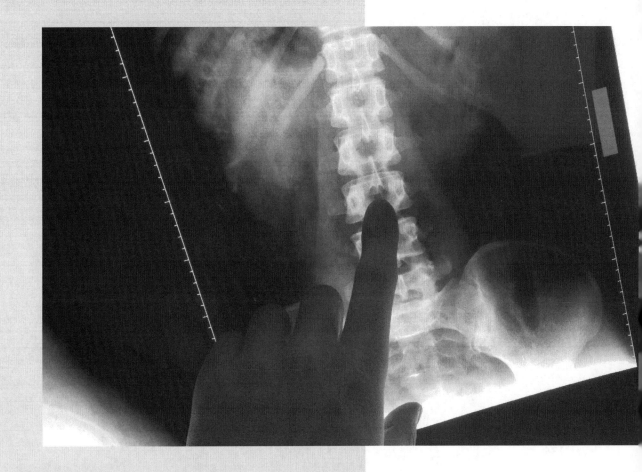

Question 1

A. Brachiocephalic artery
B. Aortic valve
C. Papillary muscle (anterior)
D. Left ventricular wall
E. Mitral valve (anterior leaflet)

Question 2

A. Acromion of right scapula
B. Glenoid fossa of right scapula
C. Coracoid process of right scapula
D. Right clavicle
E. Right coracobrachialis muscle / right short head of biceps muscle

Question 3

A. Inferior vena cava
B. Erector spinae muscle
C. Left internal oblique muscle
D. Left external oblique muscle
E. Origin of inferior mesenteric artery

Question 4

A. Radius
B. Ulna styloid
C. Lunate bone
D. Capitate bone
E. Triquetral bone

Question 5

A. Left upper lobe anterior
B. Spleen
C. Inferior / posterior papillary muscle
D. Superior / anterior papillary muscle
E. Left oblique fissure

Question 6

A. Femur
B. Distal epiphysis of femur
C. Proximal epiphysis of tibia
D. Proximal epiphysis of fibula
E. Neck of fibula

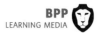

Question 7

A. Left costo-phrenic angle
B. Right external iliac vein
C. Right external iliac artery
D. Portal vein
E. Left lobe of liver

Question 8

A. Right superior semi-circular canal
B. Right internal acoustic canal
C. Basi-occiput / lower clivus
D. Left cochlear
E. Facial nerve / vestibulocochlear nerve / labyrinthine artery

Question 9

A. Branch of portal vein
B. Right crus of diaphragm
C. Portal vein
D. < 3mm
E. Gallbladder

Question 10

A. Right brachiocephalic vein
B. Brachiocephalic artery
C. Left common carotid artery
D. Left subclavian artery
E. Right common carotid and right subclavian artery

Question 11

A. Epiglottis
B. Clivus
C. Cerebellar tonsil
D. Cisterna magna
E. Posterior arch of atlas

Question 12

A. Right lateral cuneiform
B. Right head of third metatarsal
C. Distal phalanx of right first toe
D. Middle phalanx of right third toe
E. Sesamoid bone in right flexor hallucis brevis muscle

Question 13

A. Right caudate nucleus
B. Pituitary gland
C. Optic chiasm
D. Left internal carotid artery
E. Right sphenoid sinus

Question 14

A. Right zygomatic bone
B. Left inferior orbital margin
C. Left frontal sinus
D. Right superior orbital fissure
E. Cranial nerves III, IV, V and VI and sympathetic fibres

Question 15

A. Right external capsule
B. Right frontal lobe
C. Anterior limb of the right internal capsule
D. Left putamen
E. Head of left caudate nucleus

Question 16

A. Right femoral head
B. Left psoas muscle
C. Left iliacus muscle
D. Urinary bladder
E. Right acetabular roof

Question 17

A. Right gluteus medius muscle
B. Right sacral alum
C. Left sacroiliac joint
D. Left iliacus muscle
E. Lesser trochanter of left femur

Question 18

A. Vallecula
B. Piriform fossa
C. Vertebral process
D. Clavicle
E. Oesophagus

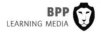

Question 19

A. Right first metacarpal
B. Right capitate bone
C. Distal epiphysis of right radius
D. Right triquetral bone
E. Right lunate bone

Question 20

A. Superficial cerebral veins
B. Superior sagittal sinus
C. Vein of Labbe
D. Vein of Galen
E. Straight sinus

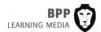

Paper 6

Question Bank

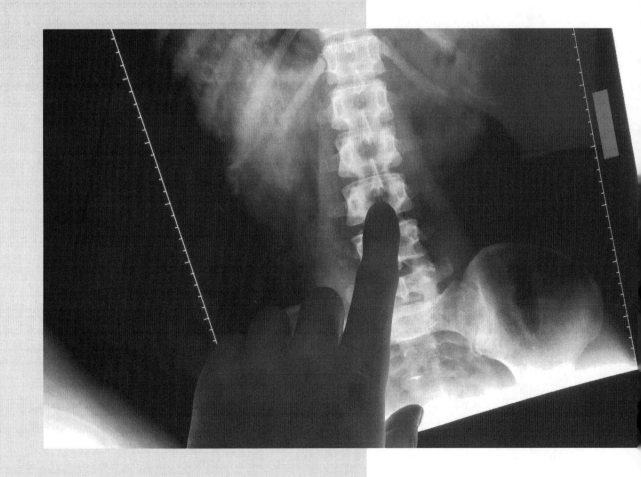

Question 1

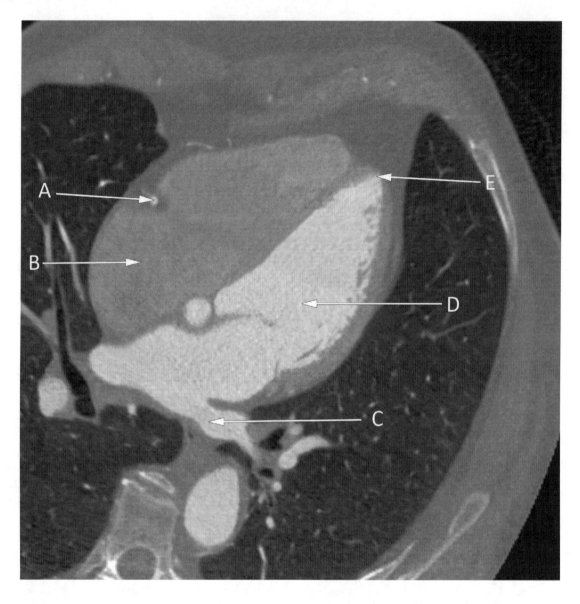

	QUESTION 1	WRITE YOUR ANSWER HERE
A	Name the structure labelled A	
B	Name the structure labelled B	
C	Name the structure labelled C	
D	Name the structure labelled D	
E	What anatomical region of D is labelled E?	

Question 2

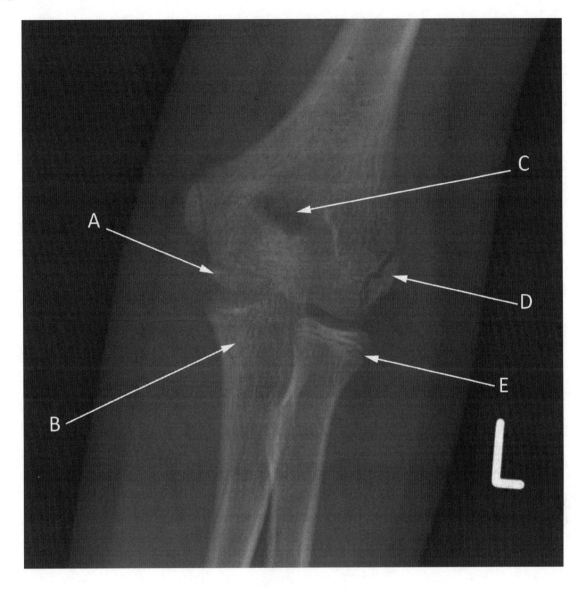

	QUESTION 2	WRITE YOUR ANSWER HERE
A	Name the structure labelled A	
B	Name the structure labelled B	
C	Name the structure labelled C	
D	Name the structure labelled D	
E	Name the structure labelled E	

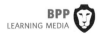

Question 3

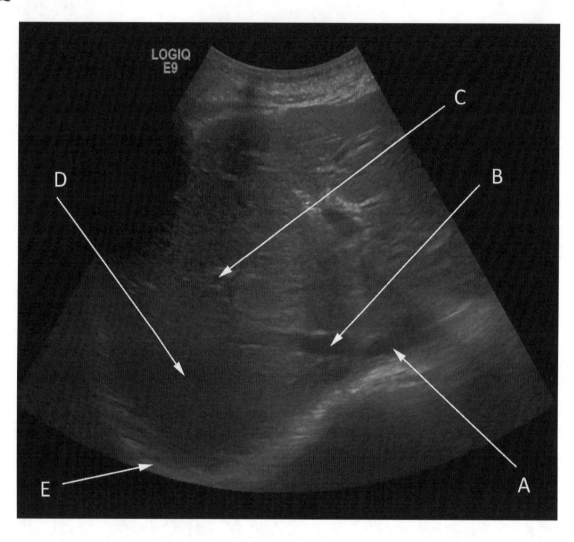

	QUESTION 3	WRITE YOUR ANSWER HERE
A	Name the structure labelled A	
B	Name the structure labelled B	
C	Name the structure labelled C	
D	Name the structure labelled D	
E	Name the structure labelled E	

Ques

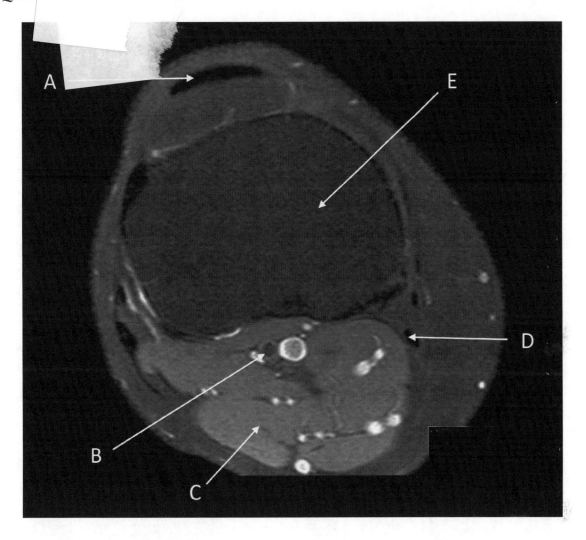

	QUESTION 4	WRITE YOUR ANSWER HERE
A	Name the structure labelled A	
B	Name the structure labelled B	
C	Name the structure labelled C	
D	Name the structure labelled D	
E	Name the structure labelled E	

Question 5

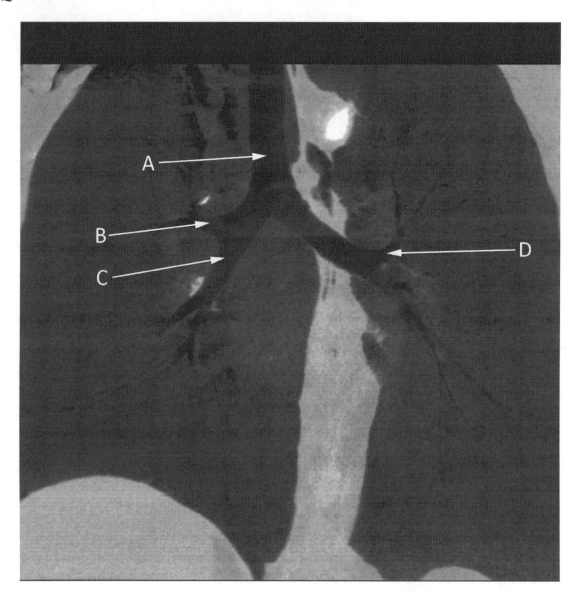

	QUESTION 5	WRITE YOUR ANSWER HERE
A	Name the structure labelled A	
B	Name the structure labelled B	
C	Name the structure labelled C	
D	Name the structure labelled D	
E	Which lobar segments arise from B?	

Question 6

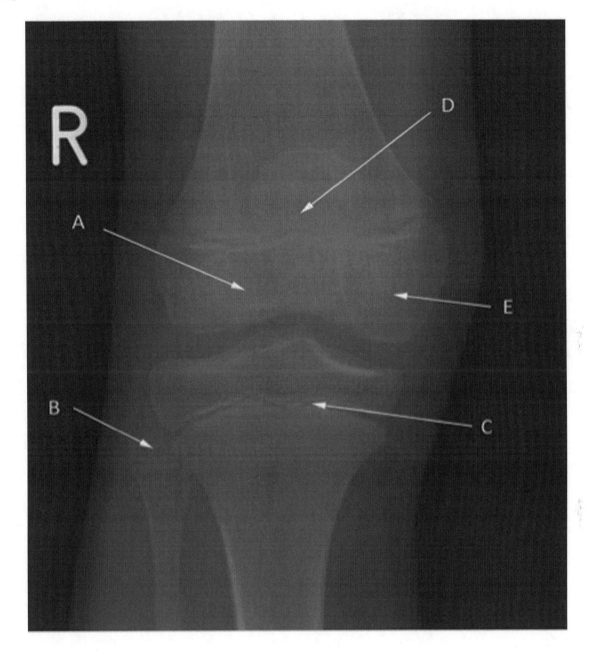

	QUESTION 6	WRITE YOUR ANSWER HERE
A	Name the structure labelled A	
B	Name the structure labelled B	
C	Name the structure labelled C	
D	Name the structure labelled D	
E	Name the structure labelled E	

Question 7

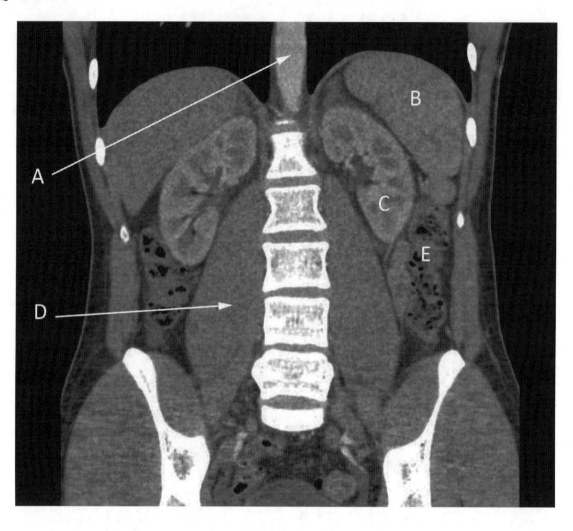

	QUESTION 7	WRITE YOUR ANSWER HERE
A	Name the structure labelled A	
B	Name the structure labelled B	
C	Name the structure labelled C	
D	Name the structure labelled D	
E	Name the structure labelled E	

Question 8

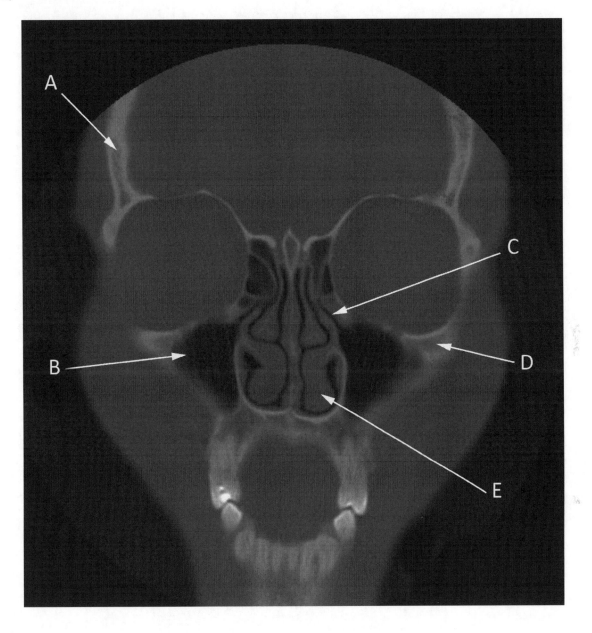

	QUESTION 8	WRITE YOUR ANSWER HERE
A	Name the structure labelled A	
B	Name the structure labelled B	
C	Name the structure labelled C	
D	Name the structure labelled D	
E	Name the structure labelled E	

Question 9

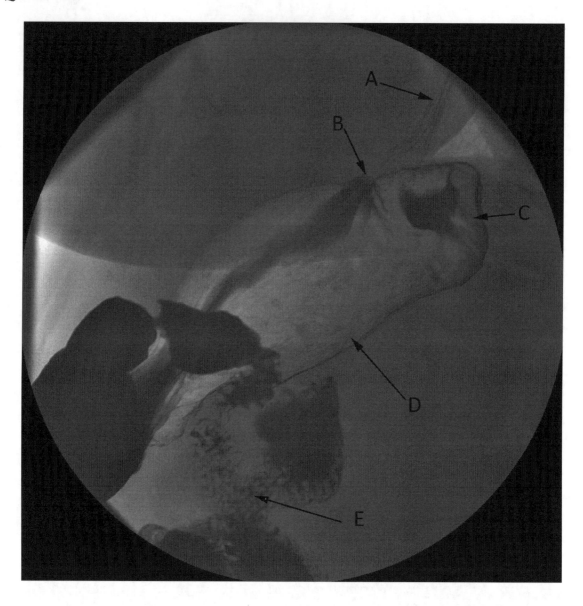

	QUESTION 9	WRITE YOUR ANSWERE HERE
A	Name the structure labelled A	
B	Name the structure labelled B	
C	Name the structure labelled C	
D	Name the structure labelled D	
E	Name the structure labelled E	

Question 10

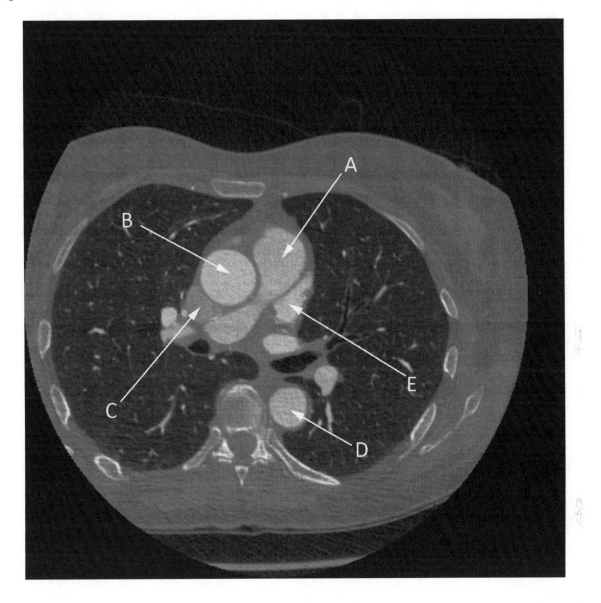

	QUESTION 10	WRITE YOUR ANSWER HERE
A	Name the structure labelled A	
B	Name the structure labelled B	
C	Name the structure labelled C	
D	Name the structure labelled D	
E	Name the structure labelled E	

Question 11

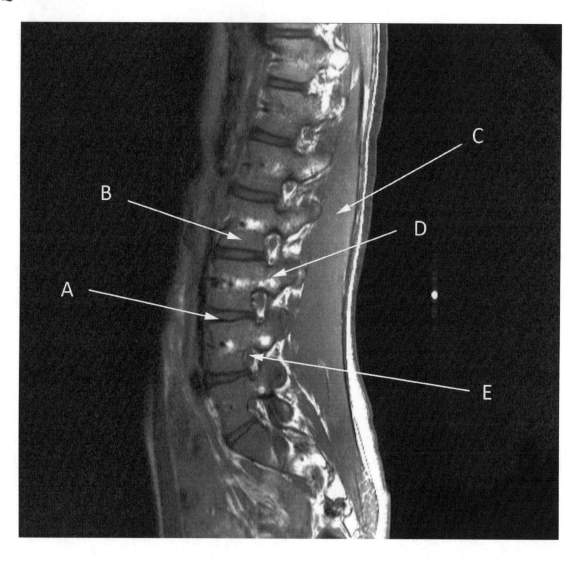

	QUESTION 11	WRITE YOUR ANSWER HERE
A	Name the structure labelled A	
B	Name the structure labelled B	
C	Name the structure labelled C	
D	Name the structure labelled D	
E	What exits at E?	

Question 12

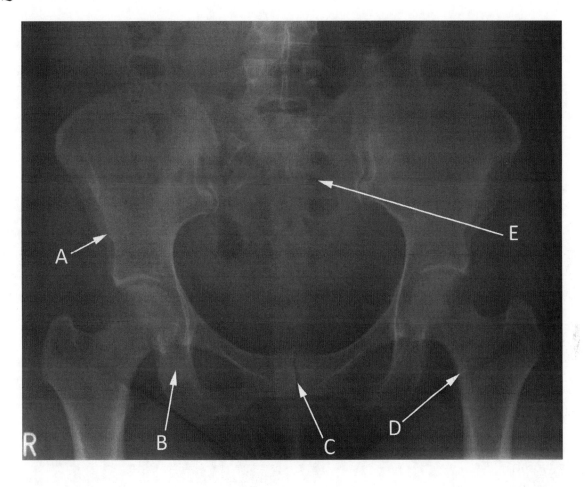

	QUESTION 12	WRITE YOUR ANSWER HERE
A	Name the structure labelled A	
B	Name the structure labelled B	
C	Name the structure labelled C	
D	Name the structure labelled D	
E	Name the structure labelled E	

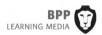

Question 13

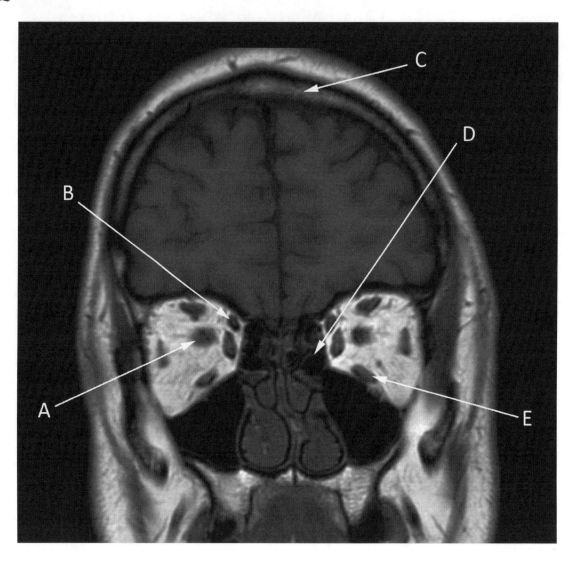

	QUESTION 13	WRITE YOUR ANSWER HERE
A	Name the structure labelled A	
B	Name the structure labelled B	
C	Name the structure labelled C	
D	Name the structure labelled D	
E	Name the structure labelled E	

Question 14

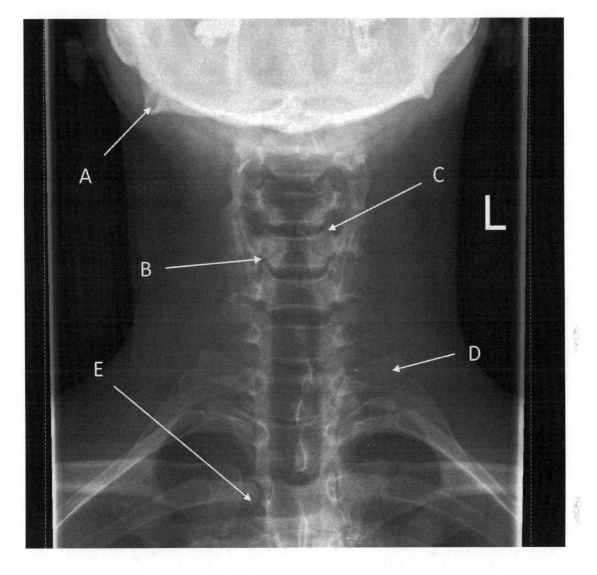

	QUESTION 14	WRITE YOUR ANSWER HERE
A	Name the structure labelled A	
B	Name the structure labelled B	
C	Name the structure labelled C	
D	Name the structure labelled D	
E	Name the structure labelled E	

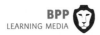

Question 15

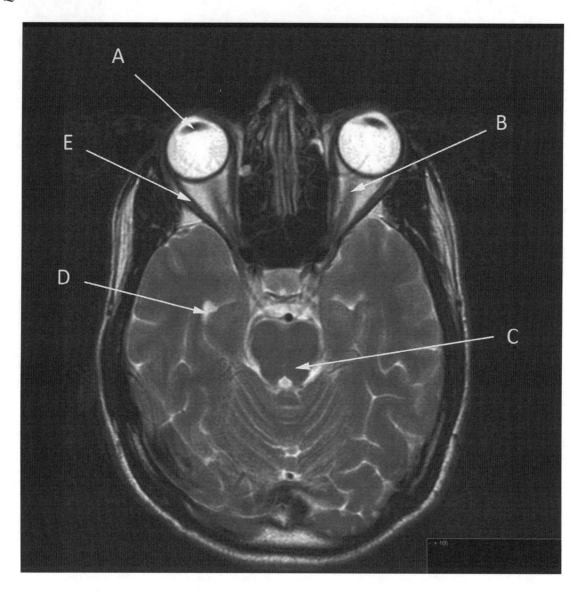

	QUESTION 15	WRITE YOUR ANSWER HERE
A	Name the structure labelled A	
B	Name the structure labelled B	
C	Name the structure labelled C	
D	Name the structure labelled D	
E	What innervates E?	

Question 16

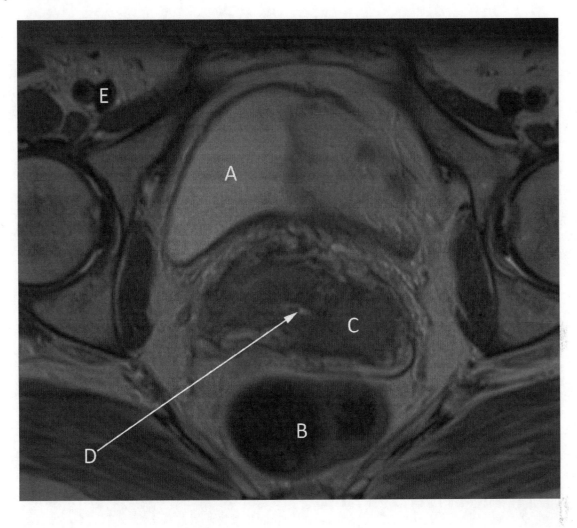

	QUESTION 16	WRITE YOUR ANSWER HERE
A	Name the structure labelled A	
B	Name the structure labelled B	
C	Name the structure labelled C	
D	Name the structure labelled D	
E	Name the structure labelled E	

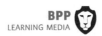

Question 17

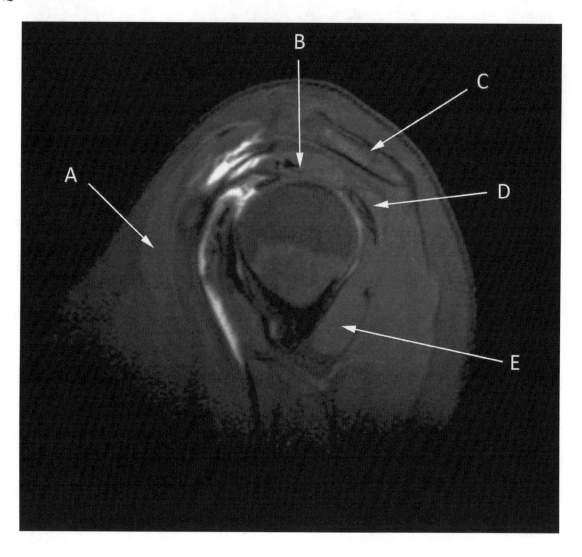

	QUESTION 17	WRITE YOUR ANSWER HERE
A	Name the structure labelled A	
B	Name the structure labelled B	
C	Name the structure labelled C	
D	Name the structure labelled D	
E	Name the structure labelled E	

Question 18

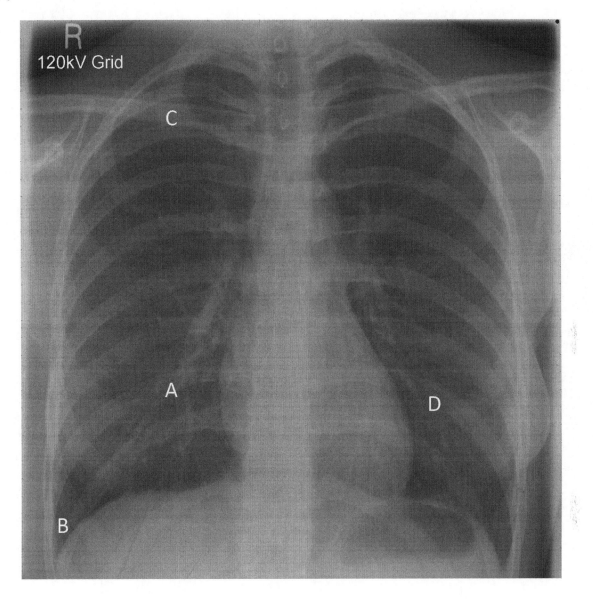

	QUESTION 18	WRITE YOUR ANSWER HERE
A	Name the segments of lobe A	
B	Name most superior segment of B	
C	How many segments does lobe C have?	
D	Name the segments of D	
E	Name the posterior anatomical boundary of D	

BPP
LEARNING MEDIA

Question 19

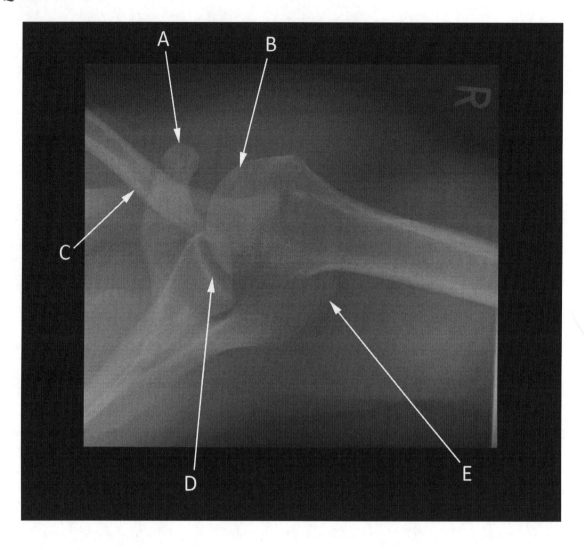

	QUESTION 19	WRITE YOUR ANSWER HERE
A	Name the structure labelled A	
B	Name the structure labelled B	
C	Name the structure labelled C	
D	Name the structure labelled D	
E	Name the structure labelled E	

Question 20

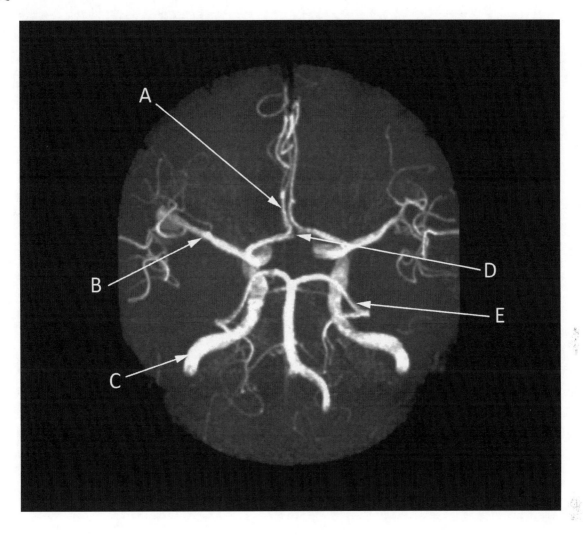

	QUESTION 20	WRITE YOUR ANSWER HERE
A	Name the structure labelled A	
B	Name the structure labelled B	
C	Name the structure labelled C	
D	Name the structure labelled D	
E	Name the origin of structure E	

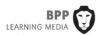

Paper 6

Answers

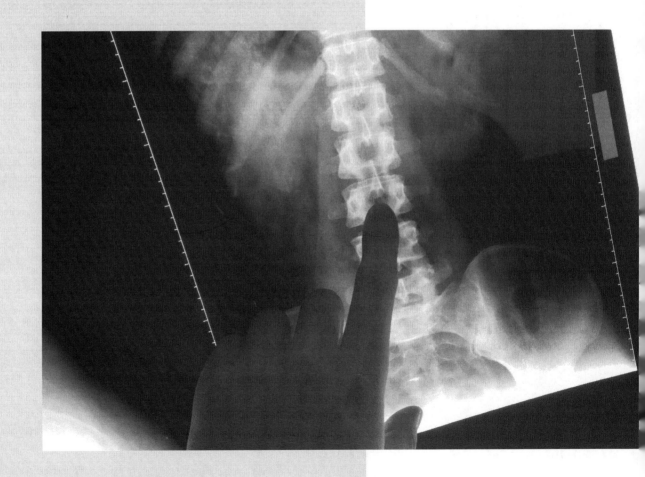

Question 1

A. Right coronary artery
B. Right atrium
C. Left inferior pulmonary vein
D. Left ventricle
E. Left ventricular apex

Question 2

A. Ossification centre for trochlea
B. Ulna
C. Olecranon fossa of humerus
D. Ossification centre for lateral epicondyle
E. Physis of proximal radius

Question 3

A. IVC
B. Hepatic vein
C. Branch of portal vein
D. Right lobe of liver
E. Diaphragm

Question 4

A. Patellar tendon
B. Popliteal artery
C. Lateral head of gastrocnemius
D. Semitendinosus tendon
E. Tibial plateau

Question 5

A. Trachea
B. Right upper lobe bronchus
C. Bronchus intermedius
D. Left upper lobe bronchus
E. Right upper lobe anterior, apical and posterior segments

Question 6

A. Right growth centre for distal femur
B. Right growth centre for proximal fibula
C. Proximal right tibial physis / epiphyseal line
D. Right patella
E. Medial condyle of right femur

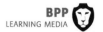

Question 7
A. Aorta
B. Spleen
C. Lower pole left kidney
D. Right psoas muscle
E. Descending colon

Question 8
A. Right frontal bone
B. Right maxillary sinus
C. Ostium of left maxillary antrum
D. Left zygomatic bone
E. Left inferior turbinate

Question 9
A. Oesophagus
B. Gastro-oesophageal junction
C. Gastric fundus
D. Gastric body
E. Jejunum

Question 10
A. Main pulmonary artery
B. Ascending aorta
C. Superior vena cava
D. Descending aorta
E. Left atrial appendage

Question 11
A. L3/L4 intervertebral disc
B. L2 vertebral body
C. Erector spinae muscle
D. L3 pedicle
E. L4 nerve root

Question 12
A. Anterior inferior iliac spine
B. Ramus of right ischium
C. Symphysis pubis
D. Intertrochanteric line of left femur
E. Sacral foramen

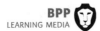

Question 13

A. Right optic nerve
B. Right superior oblique muscle
C. Diploë
D. Left ethmoidal air cells
E. Left inferior rectus muscle

Question 14

A. Right angle of the mandible
B. Uncovertebral joint of C5/6
C. Uncus (posterolateral lip) of C5
D. Left transverse process of T1
E. Right sternoclavicular joint

Question 15

A. Lens of right eye
B. Left optic nerve
C. Pons
D. Temporal horn of right lateral ventricle
E. Left abducens nerve (cranial nerve VI)

Question 16

A. Bladder
B. Rectum
C. Myometrium
D. Endometrial cavity
E. Right external iliac vein

Question 17

A. Deltoid muscle
B. Supraspinatus muscle
C. Acromion
D. Infraspinatus muscle
E. Teres minor muscle

Question 18

A. Medial and lateral segments
B. Apical segment
C. 3 (anterior, apical, posterior)
D. Superior and inferior lingular segments
E. Left oblique fissure

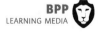

Question 19

A. Coracoid process of scapula
B. Head of humerus
C. Clavicle
D. Glenoid fossa of scapula
E. Acromion of scapula

Question 20

A. Right anterior cerebral artery
B. Right middle cerebral artery
C. Right internal carotid artery
D. Anterior communicating artery
E. Left posterior cerebral artery

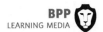

Paper 7

Question Bank

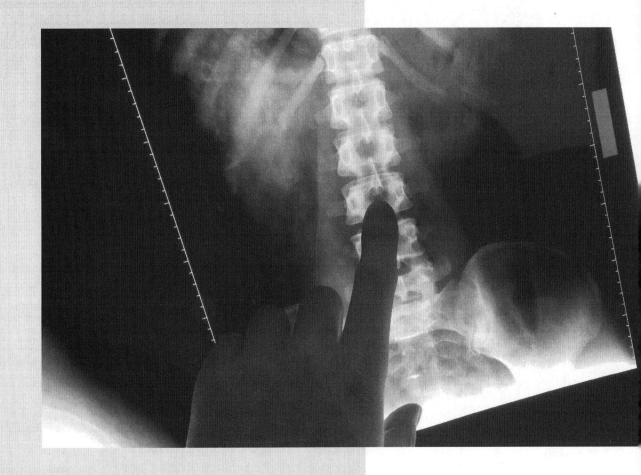

Question 1

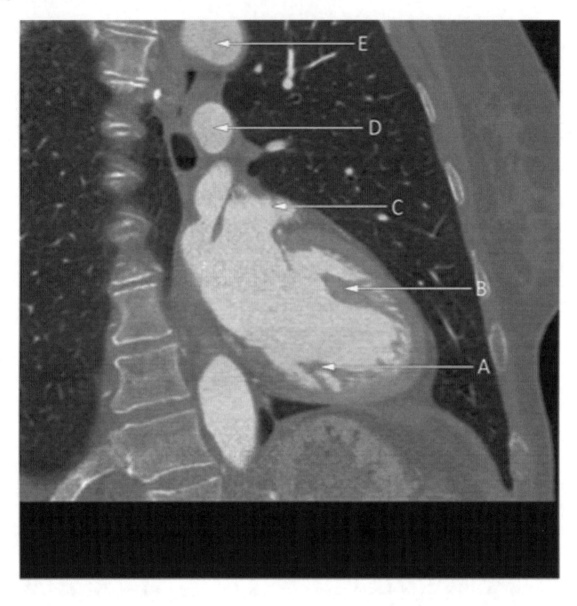

	QUESTION 1	WRITE YOUR ANSWER HERE
A	Name the structure labelled A	
B	Name the structure labelled B	
C	Name the structure labelled C	
D	Name the structure labelled D	
E	Name the structure labelled E	

Question 2

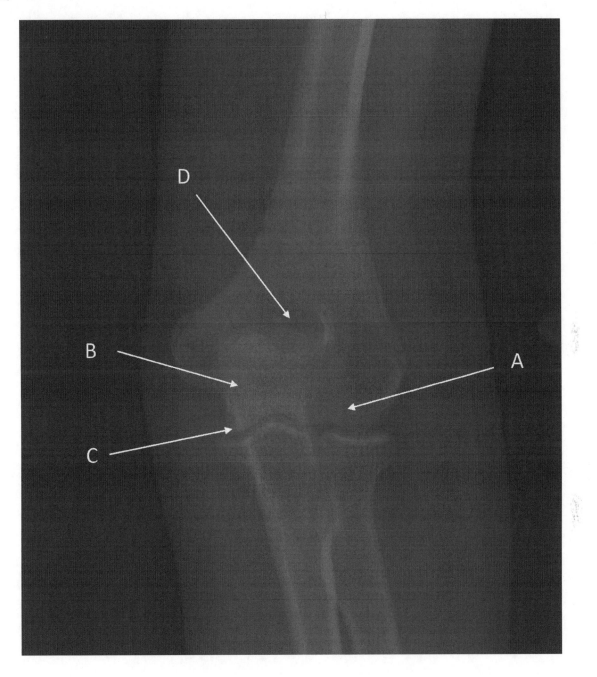

	QUESTION 2	WRITE YOUR ANSWER HERE
A	Name the structure labelled A	
B	Name the structure labelled B	
C	Name the structure labelled C	
D	Name the structure labelled D	
E	What attaches to C?	

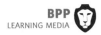

Question 3

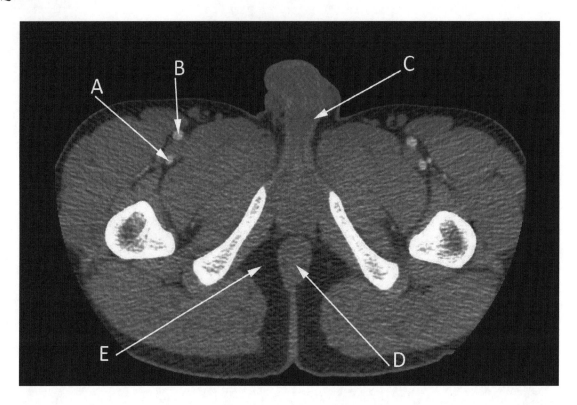

	QUESTION 3	WRITE YOUR ANSWER HERE
A	Name the structure labelled A	
B	Name the structure labelled B	
C	Name the structure labelled C	
D	Name the structure labelled D	
E	Name the structure labelled E	

Question 4

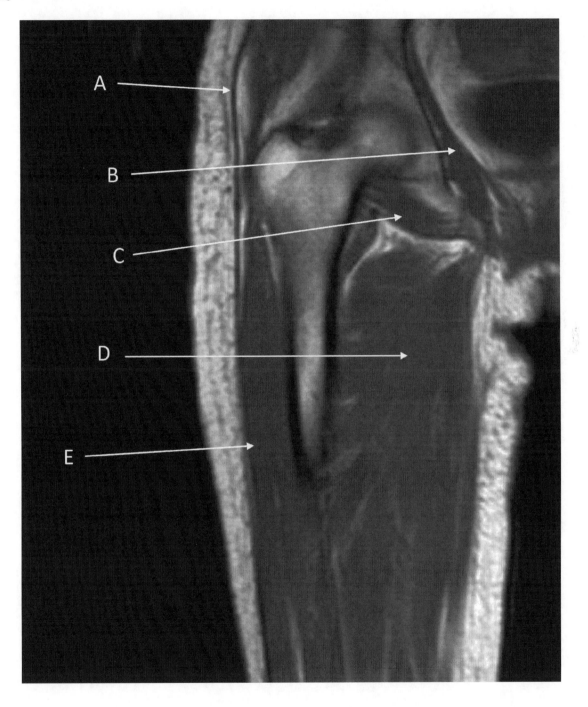

	QUESTION 4	WRITE YOUR ANSWER HERE
A	Name the structure labelled A	
B	Name the structure labelled B	
C	Name the structure labelled C	
D	Name the structure labelled D	
E	Name the structure labelled E	

Question 5

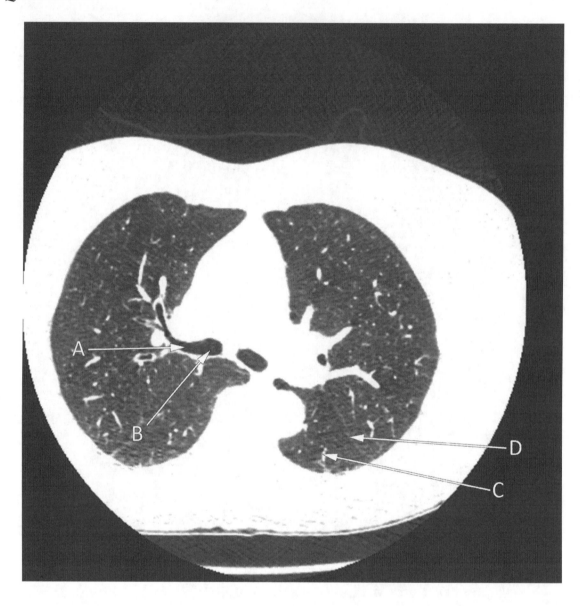

	QUESTION 5	WRITE YOUR ANSWER HERE
A	Name the structure labelled A	
B	Name the structure labelled B	
C	Name the lobar segment labelled C	
D	Name the linear structure labelled D	
E	What lobar segments will be aerated by A?	

Question 6

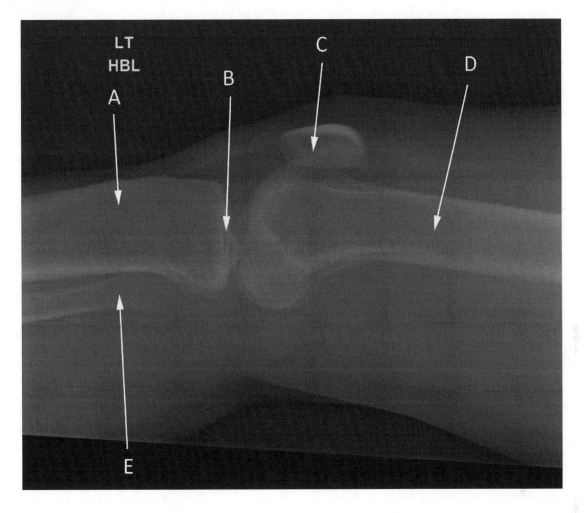

	QUESTION 6	WRITE YOUR ANSWER HERE
A	Name the structure labelled A	
B	Name the structure labelled B	
C	Name the structure labelled C	
D	Name the structure labelled D	
E	Name the structure labelled E	

BPP
LEARNING MEDIA

Question 7

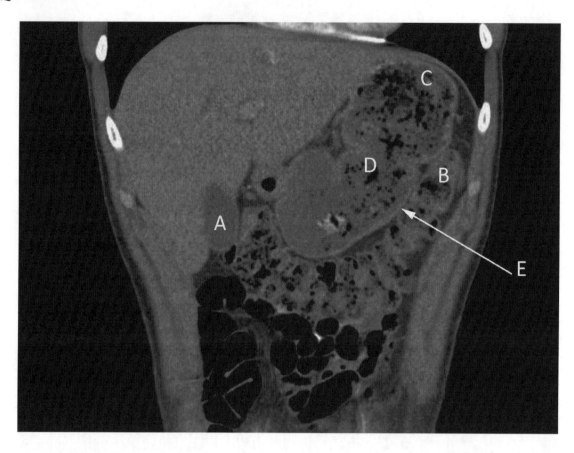

	QUESTION 7	WRITE YOUR ANSWER HERE
A	Name the structure labelled A	
B	Name the structure labelled B	
C	Name the structure labelled C	
D	Name the structure labelled D	
E	Name the structure labelled E	

Question 8

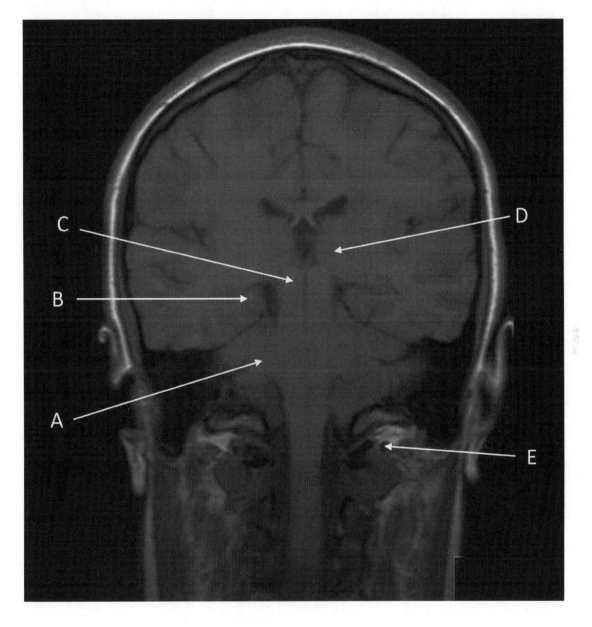

	QUESTION 8	WRITE YOUR ANSWER HERE
A	Name the structure labelled A	
B	Name the structure labelled B	
C	Name the structure labelled C	
D	Name the structure labelled D	
E	Name the structure labelled E	

Question 9

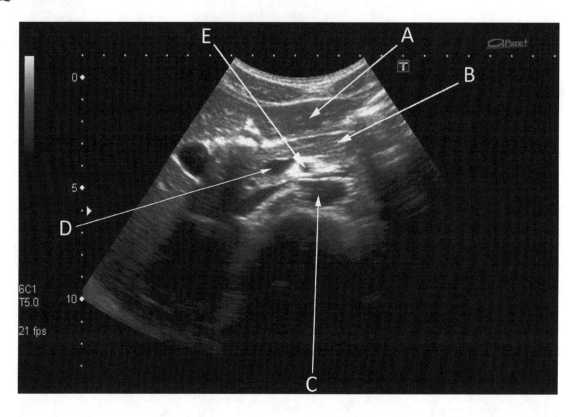

	QUESTION 9	WRITE YOUR ANSWER HERE
A	Name the structure labelled A	
B	Name the structure labelled B	
C	Name the structure labelled C	
D	Name the structure labelled D	
E	Name the structure labelled E	

Question 10

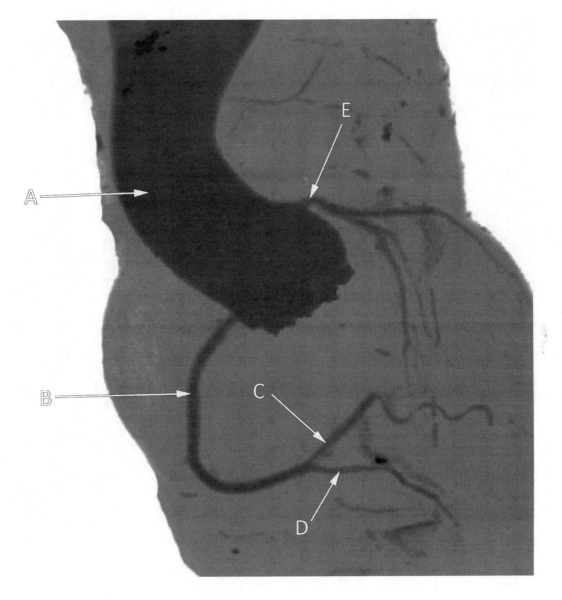

	QUESTION 10	WRITE YOUR ANSWER HERE
A	Name the structure labelled A	
B	Name the structure labelled B	
C	Name the structure labelled C	
D	Name the structure labelled D	
E	Name the structure labelled E	

Question 11

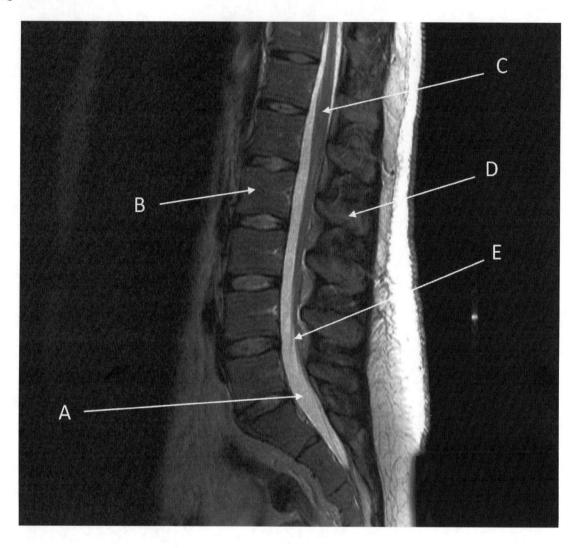

	QUESTION 11	WRITE YOUR ANSWER HERE
A	Name the structure labelled A	
B	Name the structure labelled B	
C	Name the structure labelled C	
D	Name the structure labelled D	
E	Name the structure labelled E	

Question 12

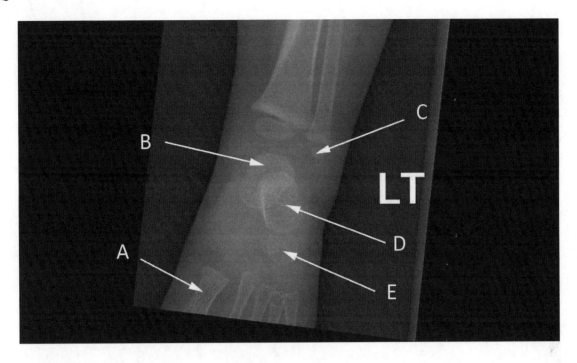

	QUESTION 12	WRITE YOUR ANSWER HERE
A	Name the structure labelled A	
B	Name the structure labelled B	
C	Name the structure labelled C	
D	Name the structure labelled D	
E	Name the structure labelled E	

BPP
LEARNING MEDIA

Question 13

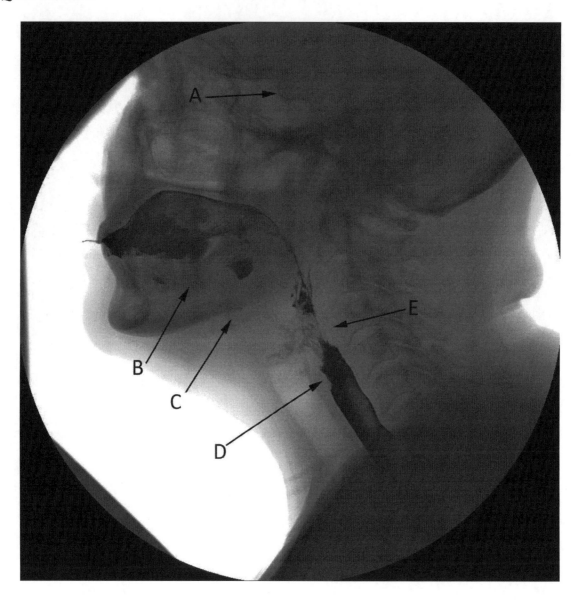

	QUESTION 13	WRITE YOUR ANSWER HERE
A	Name the structure labelled A	
B	Name the structure labelled B	
C	Name the structure labelled C	
D	Name the structure causing the impression labelled D	
E	Name the structure causing the impression labelled E	

Question 14

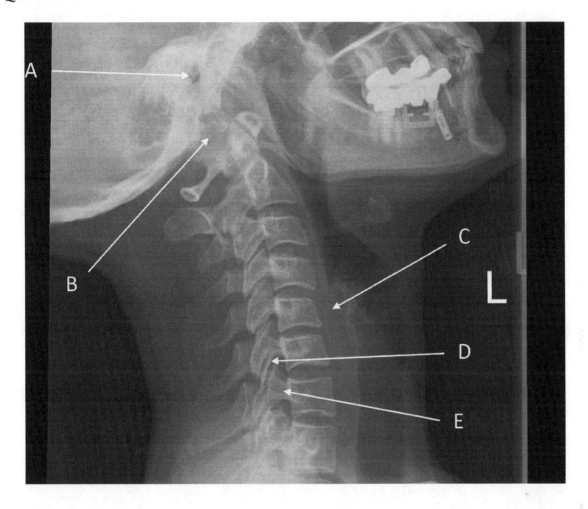

	QUESTION 14	WRITE YOUR ANSWER HERE
A	Name the structure labelled A	
B	Name the structure labelled B	
C	Name the structure labelled C	
D	Name the structure labelled D	
E	Name the structure labelled E	

Question 15

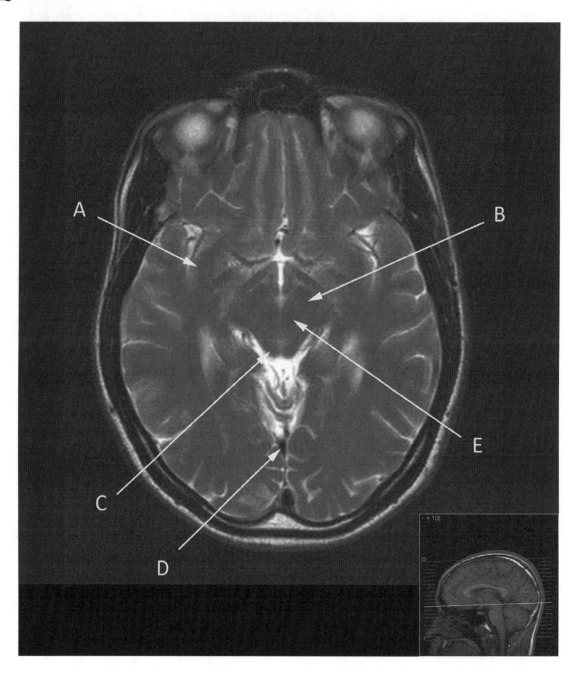

	QUESTION 15	WRITE YOUR ANSWER HERE
A	Name the structure labelled A	
B	Name the structure labelled B	
C	Name the structure labelled C	
D	Name the structure labelled D	
E	Name the structure labelled E	

Question 16

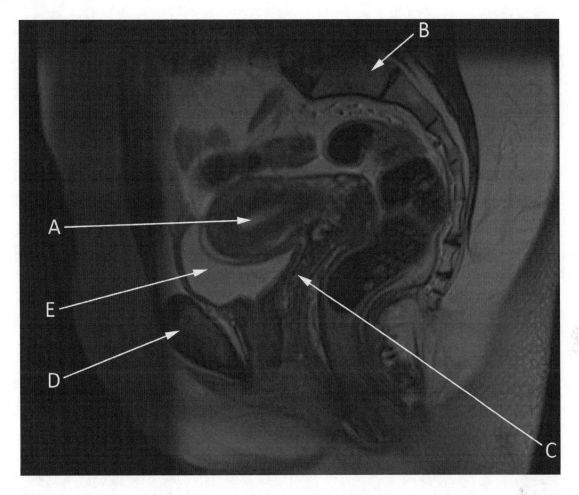

	QUESTION 16	WRITE YOUR ANSWER HERE
A	Name the structure labelled A	
B	Name the structure labelled B	
C	Name the structure labelled C	
D	Name the structure labelled D	
E	Name the structure labelled E	

Question 17

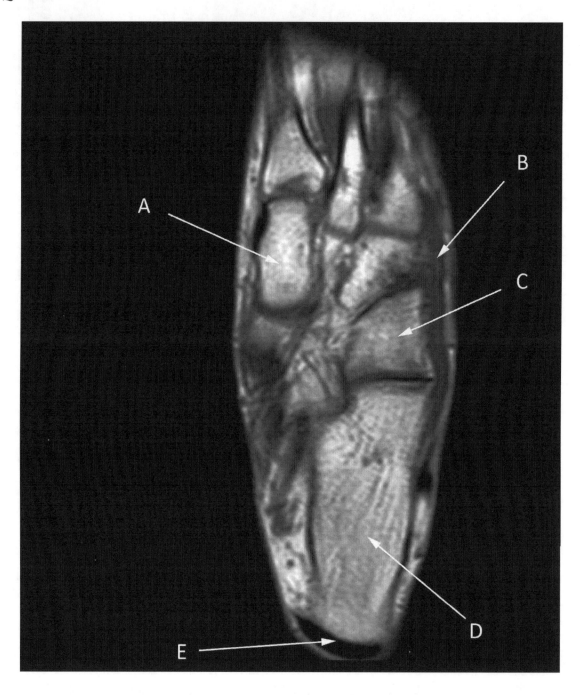

	QUESTION 17	WRITE YOUR ANSWER HERE
A	Name the structure labelled A	
B	Name the structure labelled B	
C	Name the structure labelled C	
D	Name the structure labelled D	
E	Name the structure labelled E	

Question 18

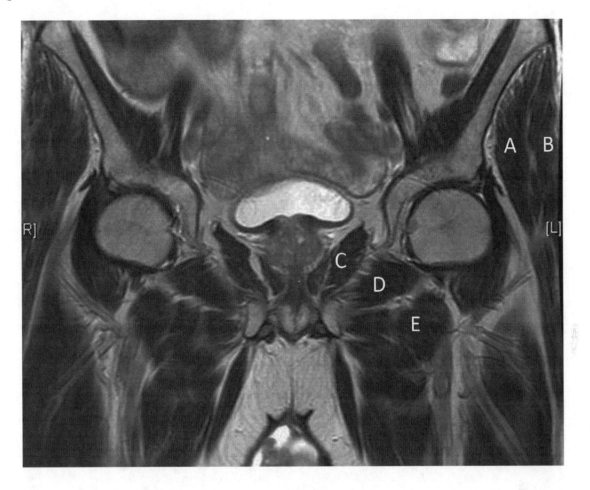

	QUESTION 18	WRITE YOUR ANSWER HERE
A	Name the structure labelled A	
B	Name the structure labelled B	
C	Name the structure labelled C	
D	Name the structure labelled D	
E	Name the structure labelled E	

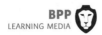

Question 19

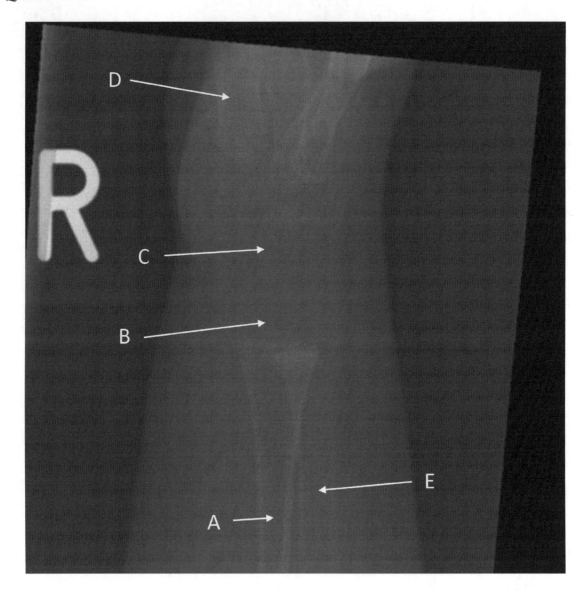

	QUESTION 19	WRITE YOUR ANSWER HERE
A	Name the structure labelled A	
B	Name the structure labelled B	
C	Name the structure labelled C	
D	Name the structure labelled D	
E	Name the structure labelled E	

Question 20

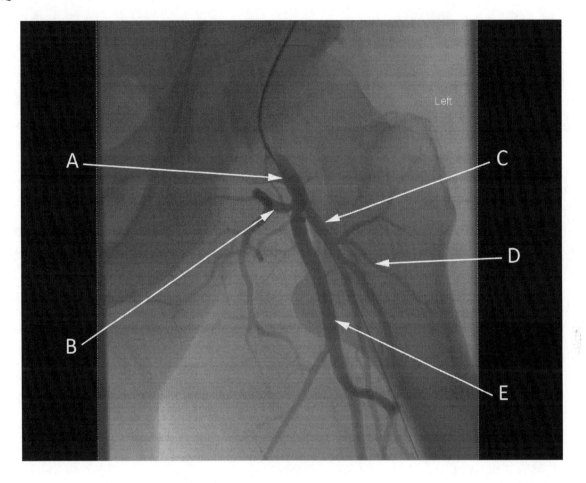

	QUESTION 20	WRITE YOUR ANSWER HERE
A	Name the structure labelled A	
B	Name the structure labelled B	
C	Name the structure labelled C	
D	Name the structure labelled D	
E	Name the structure labelled E	

Paper 7

Answers

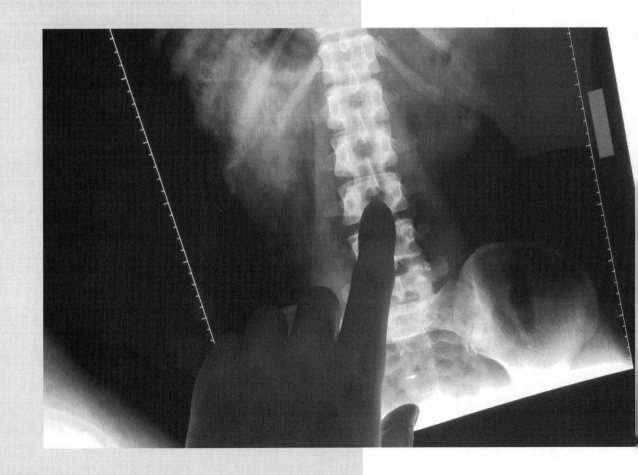

Question 1

A. Inferior / posterior papillary muscle
B. Superior / anterior papillary muscle
C. Left atrial appendage
D. Left pulmonary artery
E. Aortic arch (transverse)

Question 2

A. Capitellum of humerus
B. Olecranon
C. Coronoid process of the ulna
D. Olecranon fossa
E. Brachialis muscle

Question 3

A. Right profunda femoris artery
B. Right superficial femoral artery
C. Corpus cavernosum
D. Anal canal
E. Ischio-anal fossa

Question 4

A. Right iliotibial tract
B. Right obturator internus muscle
C. Right gemellus muscle
D. Right adductor magnus
E. Right vastus lateralis

Question 5

A. Right upper lobe bronchus
B. Right main bronchus
C. Apical segment of the left lower lobe
D. Left oblique fissure
E. Right upper lobe anterior segment / right upper lobe apical segment / right upper lobe posterior segment

Question 6

A. Left proximal tibia
B. Left tibial plateau
C. Left patella
D. Left distal femur
E. Neck of left fibula

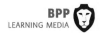

Question 7

A. Gallbladder
B. Splenic flexure
C. Fundus of stomach
D. Body of stomach
E. Greater curve of stomach

Question 8

A. Right middle cerebellar peduncle
B. Right parahippocampal gyrus
C. Quadrigeminal plate (tectum) of midbrain
D. Left thalamus
E. Left vertebral artery

Question 9

A. Left lobe of liver
B. Body of pancreas
C. Abdominal aorta
D. Splenic vein
E. Superior mesenteric artery

Question 10

A. Ascending aorta
B. Right coronary artery (RCA)
C. Postero-lateral branch of the RCA
D. Posterior descending artery
E. Left coronary artery / left main stem

Question 11

A. Thecal sac
B. L2 vertebral body
C. Conus medullaris
D. Spinous process of L2
E. Cauda equina

Question 12

A. Left first metatarsal
B. Left talus
C. Distal epiphysis of left fibula
D. Left calcaneus
E. Left cuboid bone

Question 13

A. Sphenoid sinus
B. Inferior alveolar ridge
C. Hyoid
D. Cricoid cartilage
E. Cricopharyngeus

Question 14

A. Right external auditory meatus
B. Occipital condyle
C. Prevertebral soft tissue
D. C6/7 facet joint
E. Pedicle of C7

Question 15

A. Right insular cortex
B. Left cerebral peduncle
C. Right superior colliculus
D. Straight sinus
E. Left red nucleus

Question 16

A. Uterine endometrium
B. Sacral vertebral body
C. Vagina
D. Pubic bone
E. Urinary bladder

Question 17

A. Medial cuneiform
B. Extensor digitorum brevis muscle
C. Cuboid
D. Calcaneus
E. Tendo calcaneus / Achilles' tendon

Question 18

A. Left gluteus minimus muscle
B. Left gluteus medius muscle
C. Left obturator internus muscle
D. Left obturator externus muscle
E. Left pectineus muscle

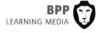

Question 19

A. Right radius
B. Distal epiphysis of right radius
C. Capitate
D. Right first metacarpal
E. Right ulna

Question 20

A. Left common femoral artery
B. Left lateral circumflex femoral artery
C. Left profunda femoris artery
D. Perforating artery
E. Left superficial femoral artery

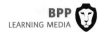

Paper 8

Question Bank

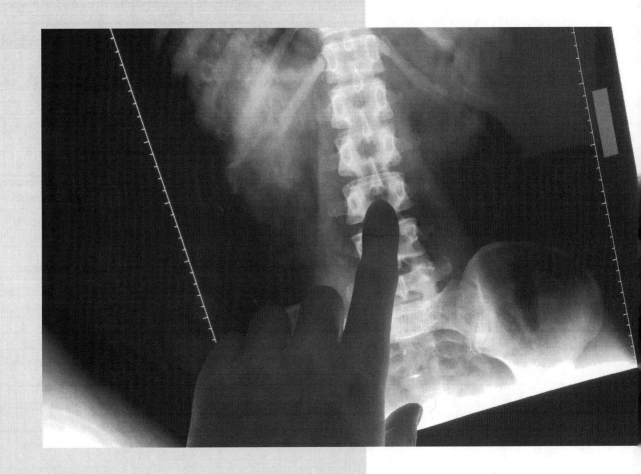

Question 1

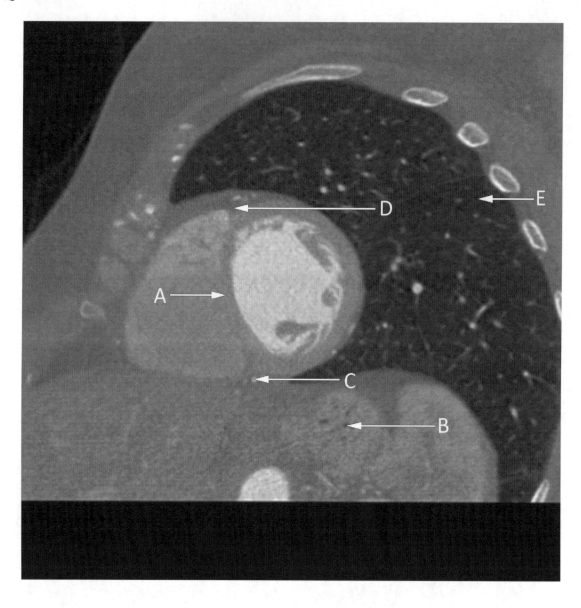

	QUESTION 1	WRITE YOUR ANSWER HERE
A	Name the structure labelled A	
B	Name the structure labelled B	
C	Name the vessel labelled C	
D	What artery runs in groove D?	
E	Name the lung segment labelled E	

Question 2

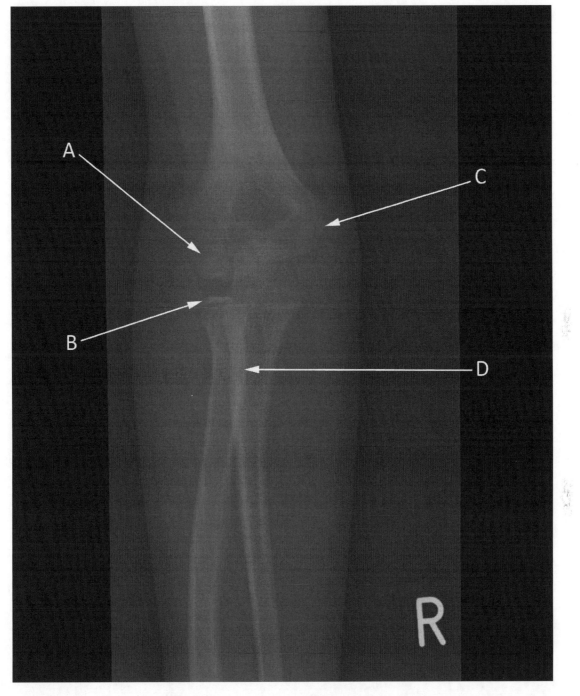

	QUESTION 2	WRITE YOUR ANSWER HERE
A	Name the structure labelled A	
B	Name the structure labelled B	
C	Name the structure labelled C	
D	Name the structure labelled D	
E	In normal development, which ossification centre should appear next?	

Question 3

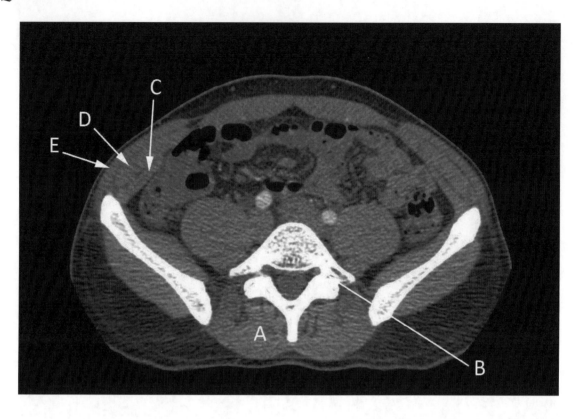

	QUESTION 3	WRITE YOUR ANSWER HERE
A	Name the structure labelled A	
B	Name the structure labelled B	
C	Name the structure labelled C	
D	Name the structure labelled D	
E	Name the structure labelled E	

Question 4

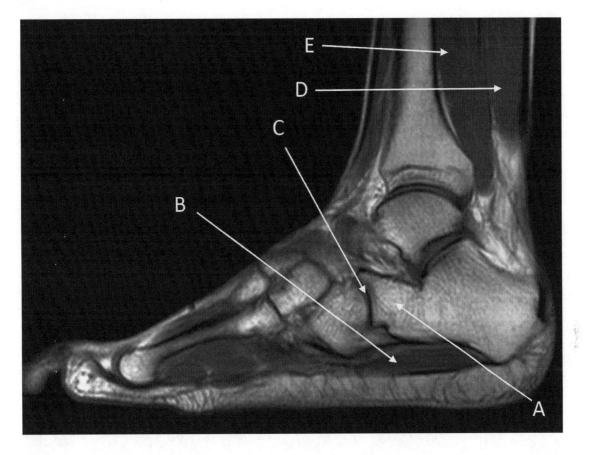

	QUESTION 4	WRITE YOUR ANSWER HERE
A	Name the structure labelled A	
B	Name the structure labelled B	
C	Name the structure labelled C	
D	Name the structure labelled D	
E	Name the structure labelled E	

Question 5

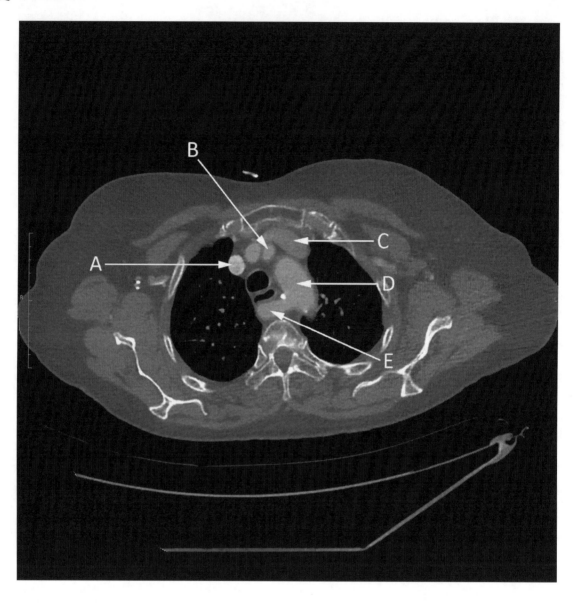

	QUESTION 5	WRITE YOUR ANSWER HERE
A	Name the structure labelled A	
B	Name the structure labelled B	
C	Name the structure labelled C	
D	Name the structure labelled D	
E	Name the variant labelled E	

Question 6

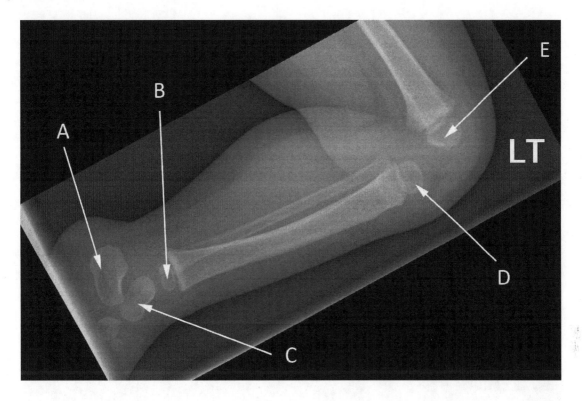

	QUESTION 6	WRITE YOUR ANSWER HERE
A	Name the structure labelled A	
B	Name the structure labelled B	
C	Name the structure labelled C	
D	Name the structure labelled D	
E	Name the structure labelled E	

Question 7

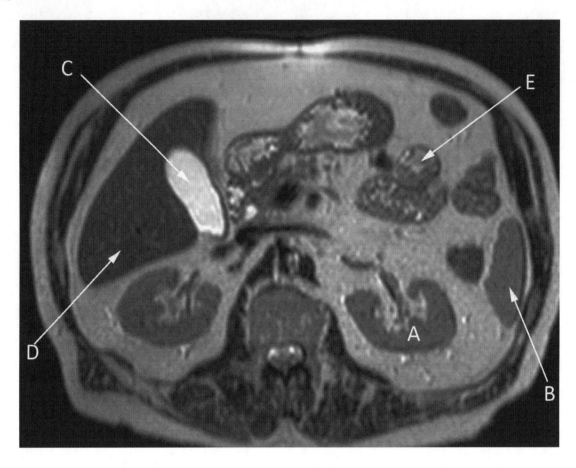

	QUESTION 7	WRITE YOUR ANSWER HERE
A	Name the structure labelled A	
B	Name the structure labelled B	
C	Name the structure labelled C	
D	Name the structure labelled D	
E	Name the structure labelled E	

Question 8

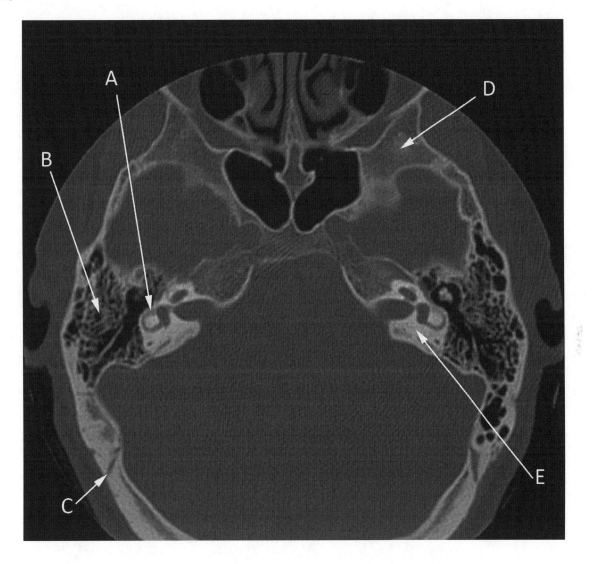

	QUESTION 8	WRITE YOUR ANSWER HERE
A	Name the structure labelled A	
B	Name the structure labelled B	
C	Name the structure labelled C	
D	Name the structure labelled D	
E	Name the structure labelled E	

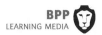

Question 9

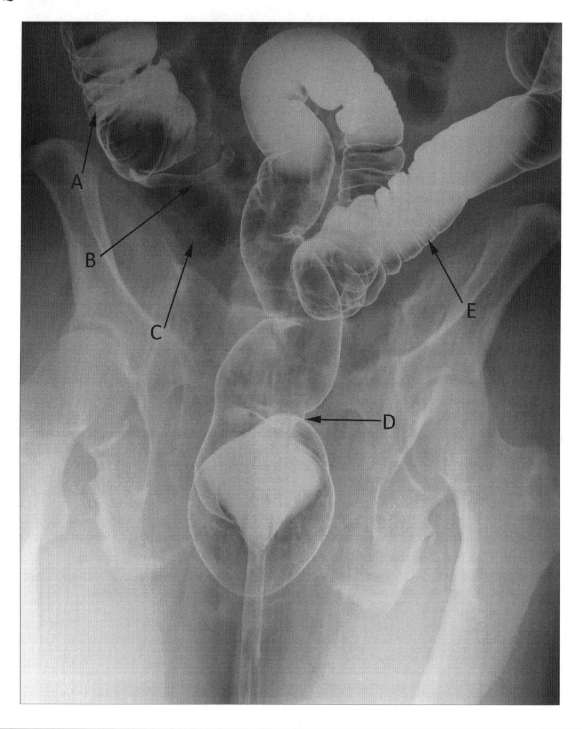

	QUESTION 9	WRITE YOUR ANSWER HERE
A	Name the structure labelled A	
B	Name the structure labelled B	
C	Name the structure labelled C	
D	Name the structure labelled D	
E	Name the structure labelled E	

Question 10

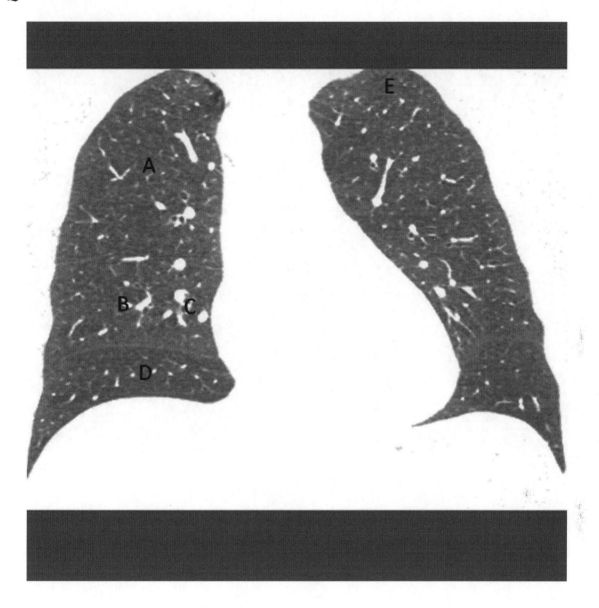

	QUESTION 10	WRITE YOUR ANSWER HERE
A	Name lung lobe labelled A	
B	Name the lobar segment labelled B	
C	Name the lobar segment labelled C	
D	Name the lung lobe labelled D	
E	Name the lobar segment labelled E	

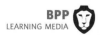

Question 11

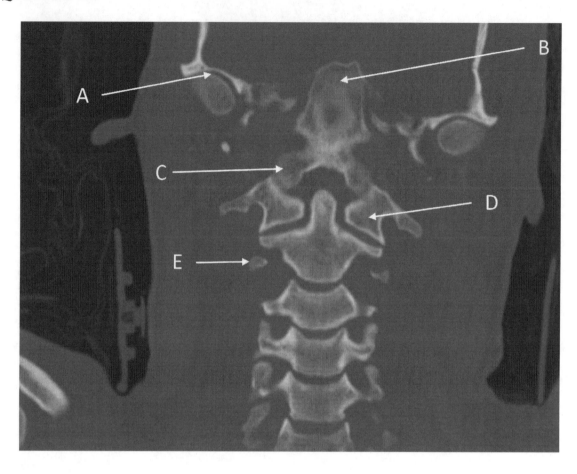

	QUESTION 11	WRITE YOUR ANSWER HERE
A	Name the structure labelled A	
B	Name the structure labelled B	
C	Name the structure labelled C	
D	Name the structure labelled D	
E	Name the structure labelled E	

Question 12

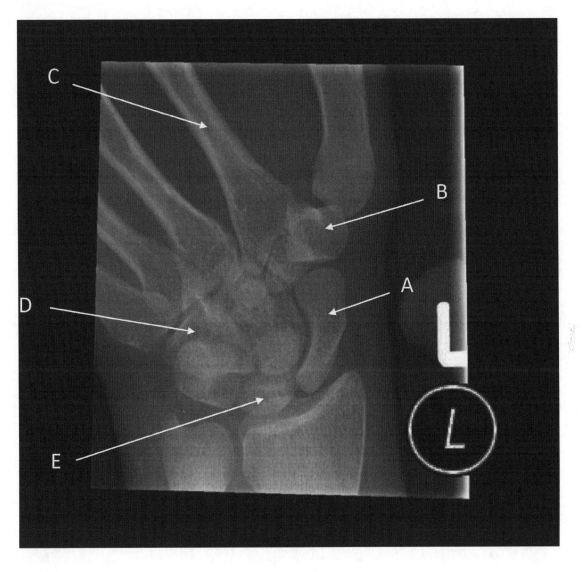

	QUESTION 12	WRITE YOUR ANSWER HERE
A	Name the structure labelled A	
B	Name the structure labelled B	
C	Name the structure labelled C	
D	Name the structure labelled D	
E	Name the structure labelled E	

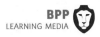

Question 13

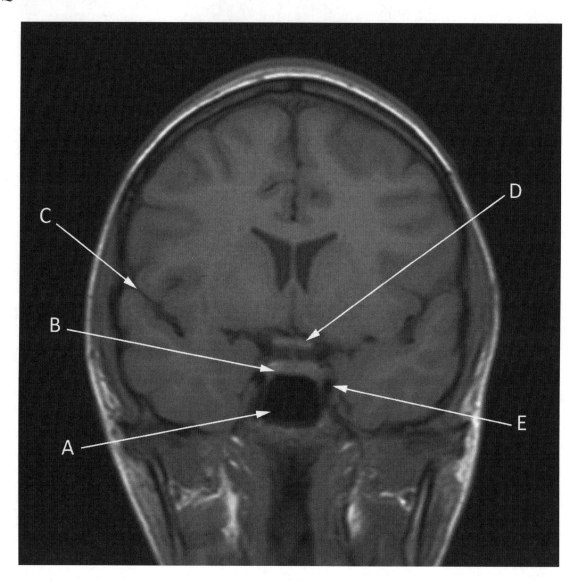

	QUESTION 13	WRITE YOUR ANSWER HERE
A	Name the structure labelled A	
B	Name the structure labelled B	
C	Name the structure labelled C	
D	Name the structure labelled D	
E	Name the structure labelled E	

Question 14

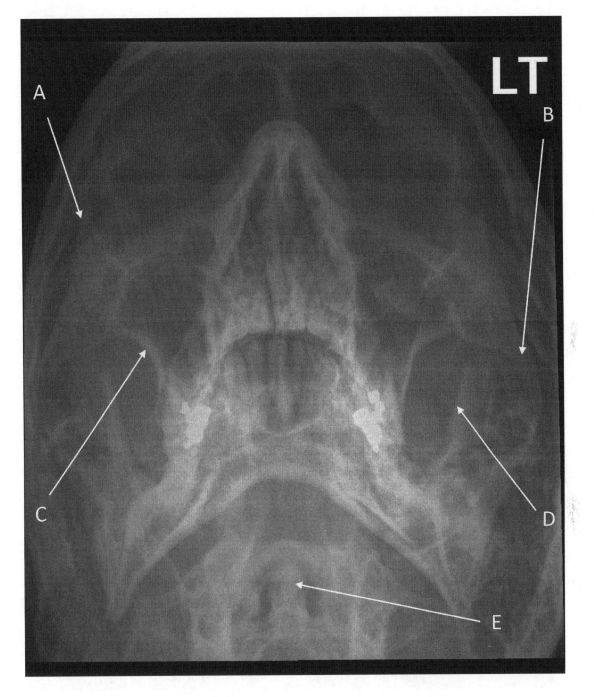

	QUESTION 14	WRITE YOUR ANSWER HERE
A	Name the structure labelled A	
B	Name the structure labelled B	
C	Name the structure labelled C	
D	Name the structure labelled D	
E	Name the structure labelled E	

Question 15

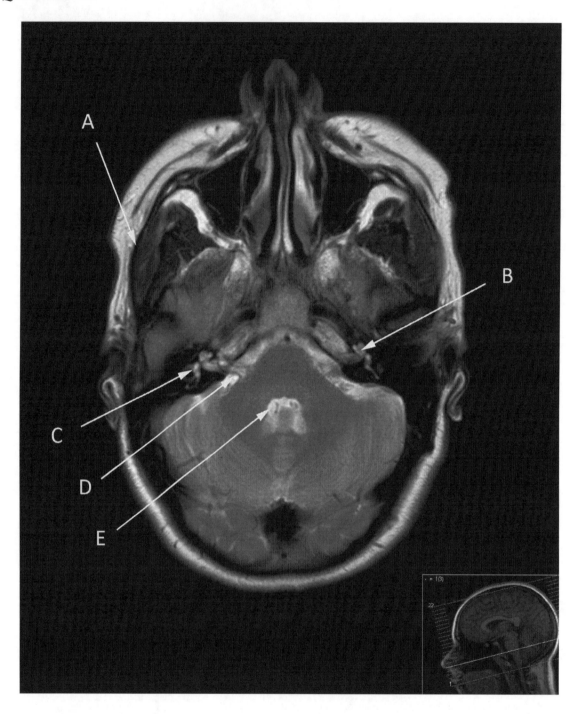

	QUESTION 15	WRITE YOUR ANSWER HERE
A	Name the structure labelled A	
B	Name the structure labelled B	
C	Name the structure labelled C	
D	Name the structure labelled D	
E	Name the structure labelled E	

Question 16

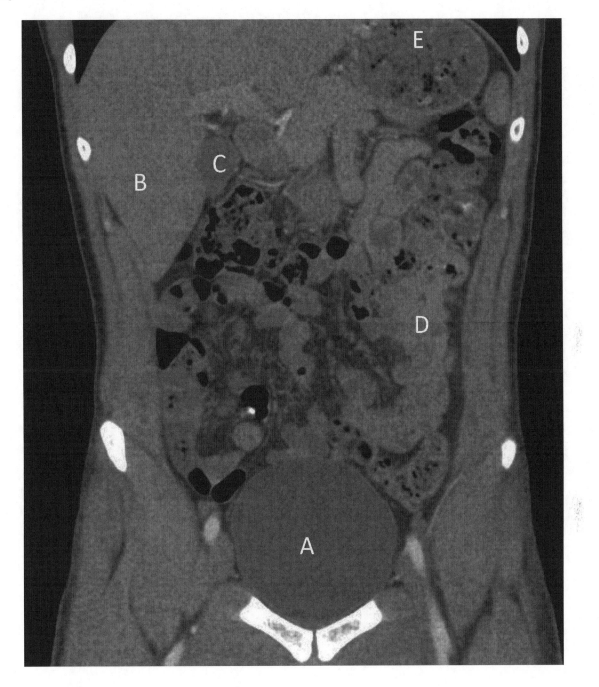

	QUESTION 16	WRITE YOUR ANSWER HERE
A	Name the structure labelled A	
B	Name the structure labelled B	
C	Name the structure labelled C	
D	Name the structure labelled D	
E	Name the structure labelled E	

Question 17

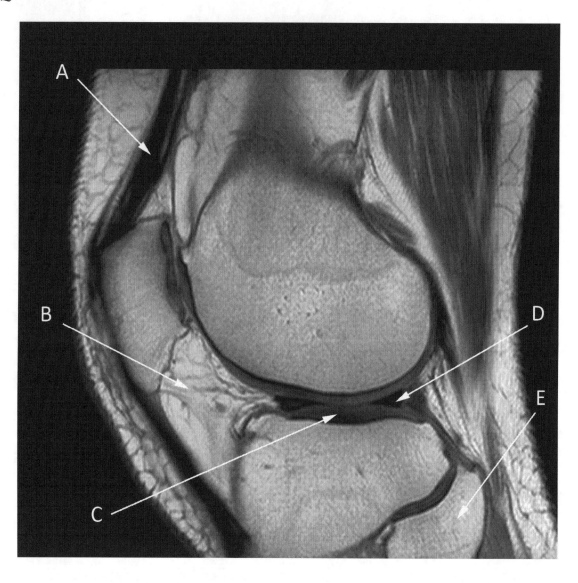

	QUESTION 17	WRITE YOUR ANSWER HERE
A	Name the structure labelled A	
B	Name the structure labelled B	
C	Name the structure labelled C	
D	Name the structure labelled D	
E	Name the structure labelled E	

Question 18

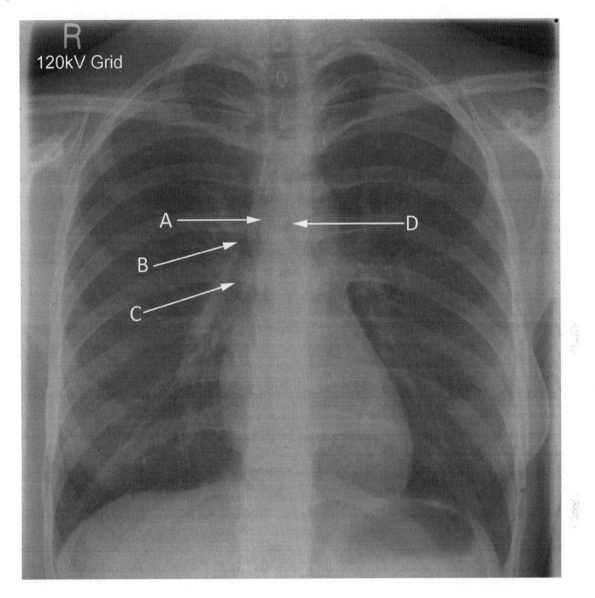

	QUESTION 18	WRITE YOUR ANSWER HERE
A	Name the airway labelled A	
B	Name the airway labelled B	
C	Name the airway labelled C	
D	Name the airway labelled D	
E	What is the first lobar branch of C?	

Question 19

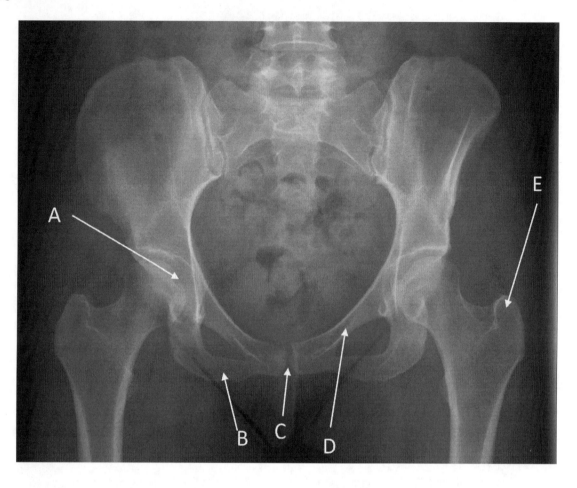

	QUESTION 19	WRITE YOUR ANSWER HERE
A	Name the structure labelled A	
B	Name the structure labelled B	
C	Name the structure labelled C	
D	Name the structure labelled D	
E	Name a muscle that attaches to E	

Question 20

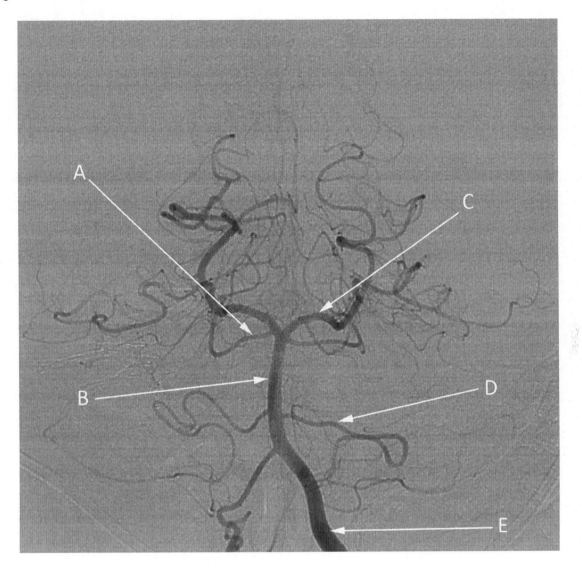

	QUESTION 20	WRITE YOUR ANSWER HERE
A	Name the structure labelled A	
B	Name the structure labelled B	
C	Name the structure labelled C	
D	Name the structure labelled D	
E	Name the structure labelled E	

Paper 8

Answers

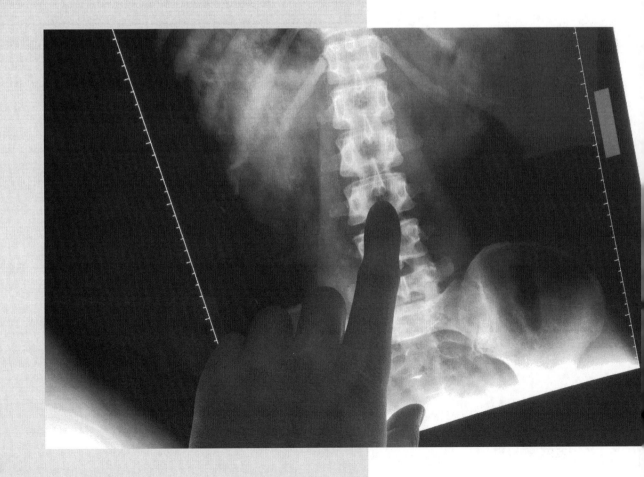

Question 1

A. Interventricular septum
B. Stomach
C. Posterior descending artery
D. Left anterior descending
E. Left lower lobe apical segment

Question 2

A. Ossification centre for capitellum
B. Ossification centre for radial head
C. Ossification centre for medial epicondyle
D. Radial tuberosity
E. Trochlea

Question 3

A. Right erector spinae muscle
B. Pedicle of lumbar vertebra
C. Right transversus abdominis muscle
D. Right internal oblique muscle
E. Right external oblique muscle

Question 4

A. Head of calcaneus
B. Abductor digiti minimi muscle
C. Calcaneocuboid joint
D. Soleus muscle
E. Flexor digitorum longus muscle

Question 5

A. Right brachiocephalic vein
B. Left common carotid
C. Left brachiocephalic vein
D. Aortic arch
E. Aberrant right subclavian artery

Question 6

A. Left calcaneus
B. Growth centre for distal left tibia
C. Left talus
D. Growth centre for proximal left tibia
E. Growth centre for distal left femur

Question 7

A. Left kidney
B. Spleen
C. Gallbladder
D. Right lobe of liver
E. Jejunum

Question 8

A. Right lateral semicircular canal
B. Right mastoid air cells
C. Lambdoid suture (right)
D. Greater wing of sphenoid bone (left)
E. Petrous temporal bone (left)

Question 9

A. Caecal pole
B. Appendix
C. Ileum
D. Rectum
E. Sigmoid colon

Question 10

A. Right upper lobe
B. Middle lobe (right) lateral segment
C. Middle lobe (right) medial segment
D. Right lower lobe
E. Left upper lobe apico-posterior segment

Question 11

A. Right temperomandibular joint
B. Clivus bone
C. Right occipital condyle
D. Left lateral mass of C1
E. Right transverse process of C2

Question 12

A. Left scaphoid
B. Left trapezium
C. Shaft of left second metacarpal
D. Left hamate
E. Left lunate

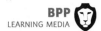

Question 13

A. Sphenoid sinus
B. Pituitary gland
C. Right Sylvian fissure
D. Optic chiasm
E. Left internal carotid artery

Question 14

A. Frontal process of right zygoma
B. Temporal process of left zygoma
C. Lateral wall of right maxillary antrum
D. Left coronoid process of the mandible
E. Odontoid peg

Question 15

A. Right temporalis muscle
B. Left cochlear
C. Right semicircular canal
D. Right vestibulocochlear nerve
E. Fourth ventricle

Question 16

A. Bladder
B. Right lobe of liver
C. Gallbladder
D. Descending colon
E. Stomach

Question 17

A. Quadriceps tendon
B. Infrapatellar fat pad
C. Articular cartilage of tibial plateau
D. Posterior horn of lateral meniscus
E. Head of fibula

Question 18

A. Right main bronchus
B. Right upper lobe bronchus
C. Bronchus intermedius
D. Left main bronchus
E. Middle lobe bronchus

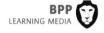

Question 19

A. Right fovea
B. Right inferior pubic ramus
C. Pubic symphysis
D. Left superior pubic ramus
E. Gluteal muscles (gluteus medius and minimus, piriformis, obturator internus, superior and inferior gemelli), vastus lateralis

Question 20

A. Right superior cerebellar artery
B. Basilar artery
C. Left posterior cerebral artery
D. Left anterior inferior cerebellar artery
E. Left vertebral artery

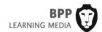

Paper 9

Question Bank

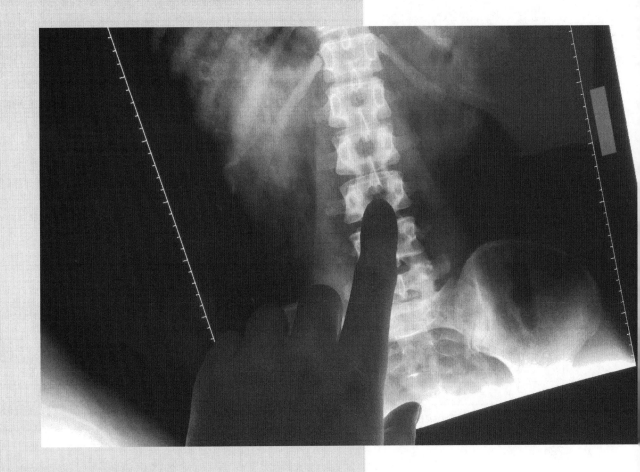

Question 1

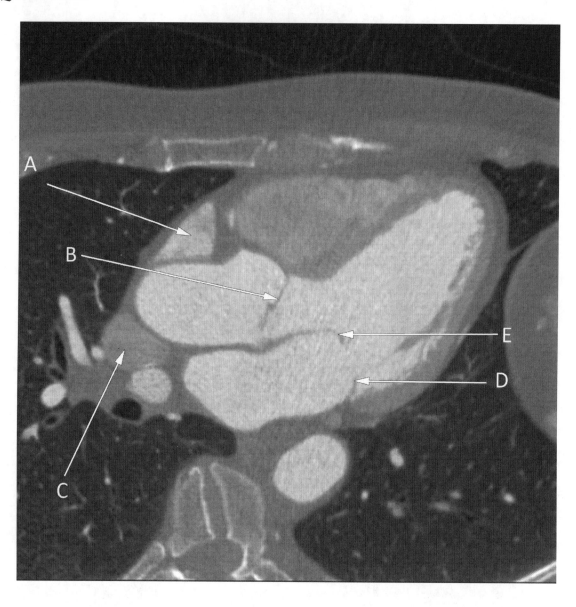

	QUESTION 1	WRITE YOUR ANSWER HERE
A	Name the structure labelled A	
B	Name the structure labelled B	
C	Name the structure labelled C	
D	Name the structure labelled D	
E	Name the structure labelled E	

Question 2

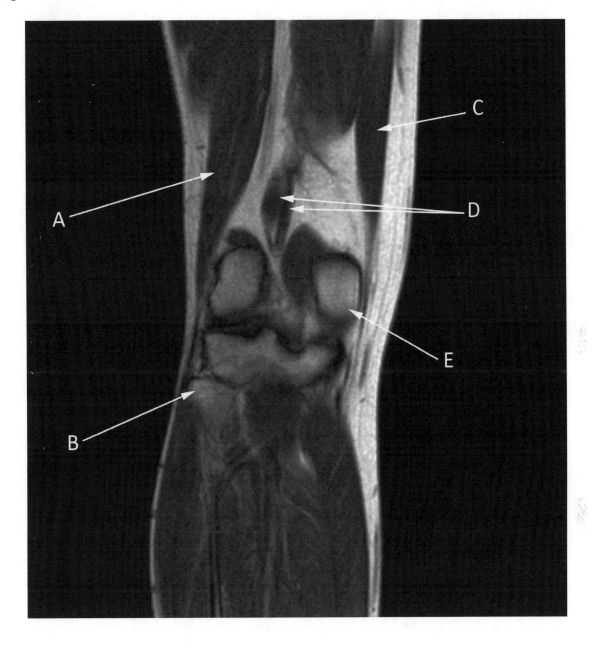

	QUESTION 2	WRITE YOUR ANSWER HERE
A	Name the structure labelled A	
B	Name the structure labelled B	
C	Name the structure labelled C	
D	Name the structure labelled D	
E	Name the structure labelled E	

BPP
LEARNING MEDIA

Question 3

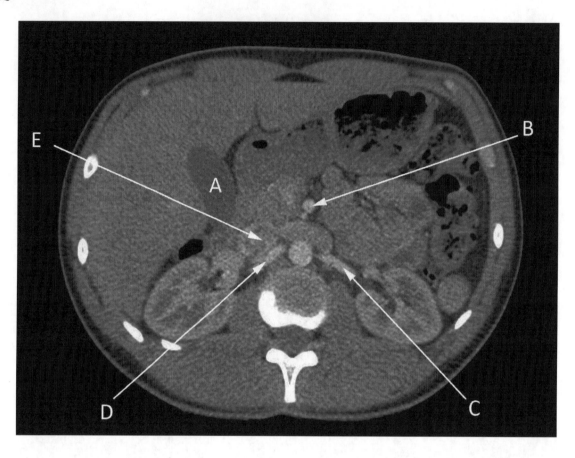

	QUESTION 3	WRITE YOUR ANSWER HERE
A	Name the structure labelled A	
B	Name the structure labelled B	
C	Name the structure labelled C	
D	Name the structure labelled D	
E	Name the structure labelled E	

Question 4

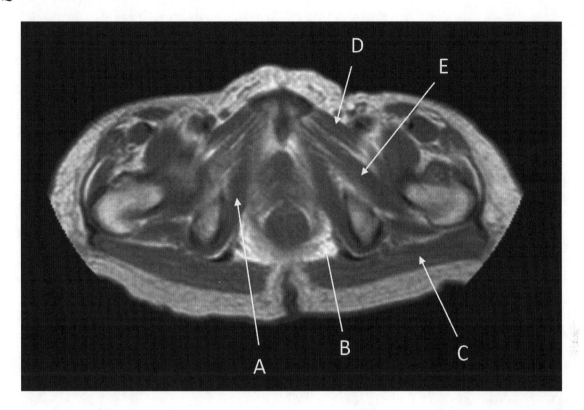

	QUESTION 4	WRITE YOUR ANSWER HERE
A	Name the structure labelled A	
B	Name the structure labelled B	
C	Name the structure labelled C	
D	Name the structure labelled D	
E	Name the structure labelled E	

Question 5

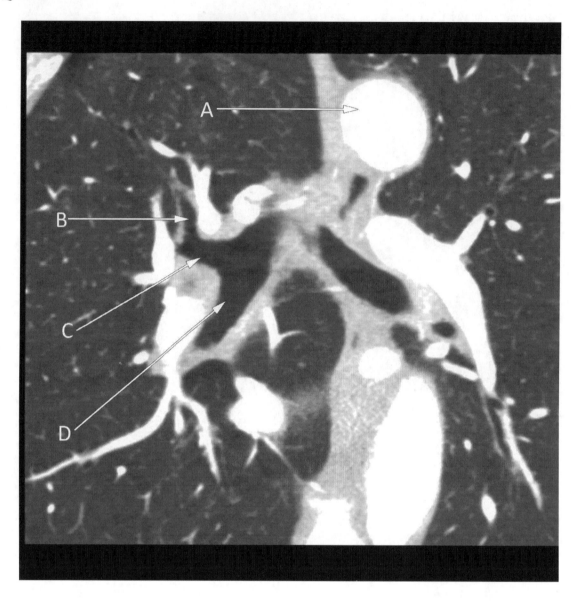

	QUESTION 5	WRITE YOUR ANSWER HERE
A	Name the structure labelled A	
B	Name the structure labelled B	
C	Name the structure labelled C	
D	Name the structure labelled D	
E	Which other structures arise from C?	

Question 6

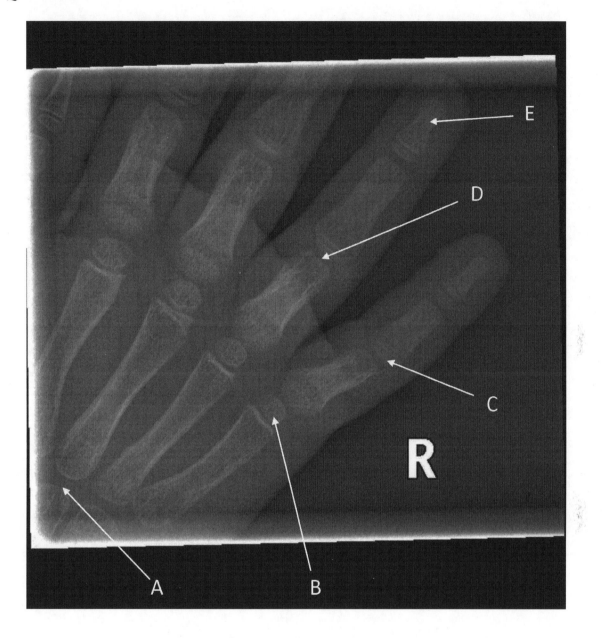

	QUESTION 6	WRITE YOUR ANSWER HERE
A	Name the structure labelled A	
B	Name the structure labelled B	
C	Name the structure labelled C	
D	Name the structure labelled D	
E	Name the structure labelled E	

Question 7

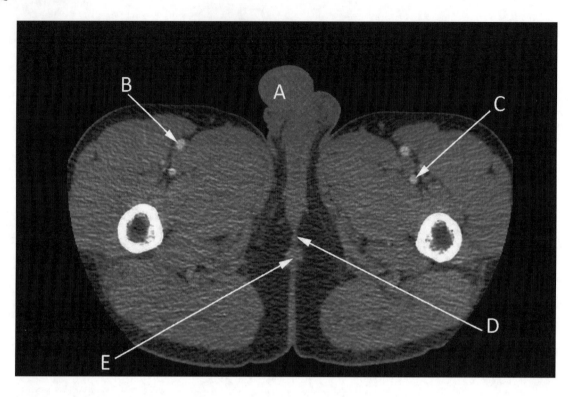

	QUESTION 7	WRITE YOUR ANSWER HERE
A	Name the structure labelled A	
B	Name the structure labelled B	
C	Name the structure labelled C	
D	Name the structure labelled D	
E	Name the structure labelled E	

Question 8

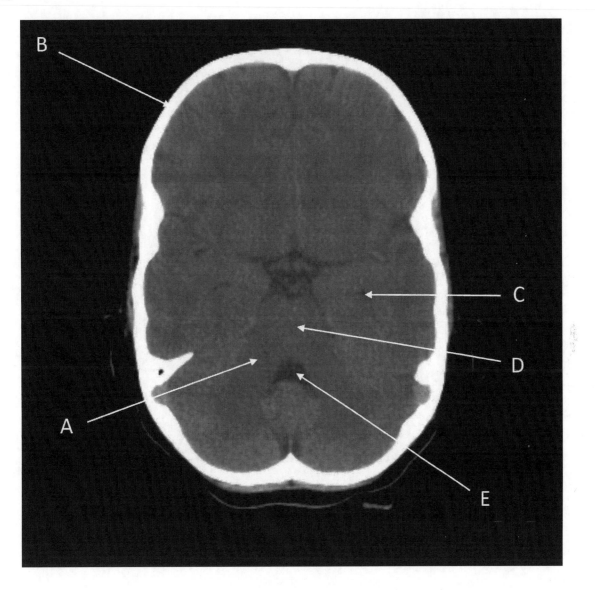

	QUESTION 8	WRITE YOUR ANSWER HERE
A	Name the structure labelled A	
B	Name the structure labelled B	
C	Name the structure labelled C	
D	Name the structure labelled D	
E	What connects this with the third ventricle?	

Question 9

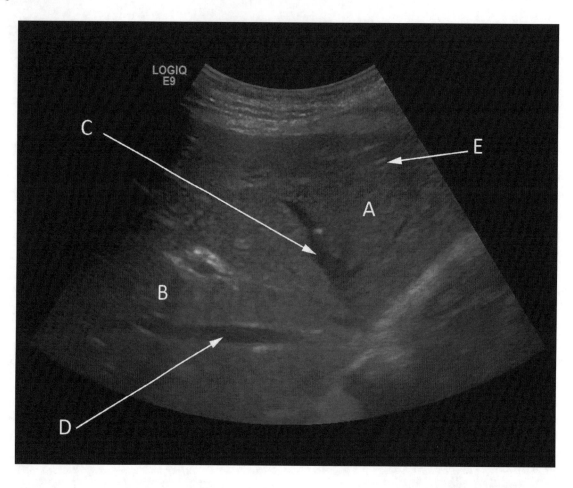

	QUESTION 9	WRITE YOUR ANSWER HERE
A	Name the structure labelled A	
B	Name the structure labelled B	
C	Name the structure labelled C	
D	Name the structure labelled D	
E	Name the structure labelled E	

Question 10

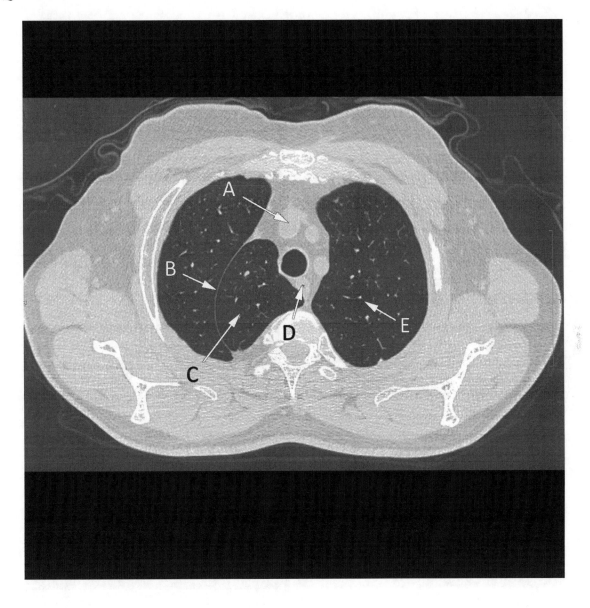

	QUESTION 10	WRITE YOUR ANSWER HERE
A	Name the structure labelled A	
B	Name the structure labelled B	
C	Name the structure labelled C	
D	Name the structure labelled D	
E	Name the structure labelled E	

Question 11

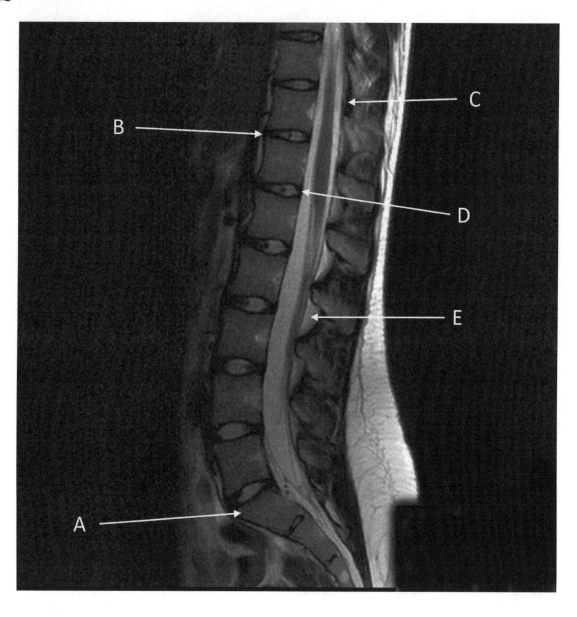

	QUESTION 11	WRITE YOUR ANSWER HERE
A	Name the structure labelled A	
B	Name the structure labelled B	
C	Name the structure labelled C	
D	Name the structure labelled D	
E	Name the structure labelled E	

Question 12

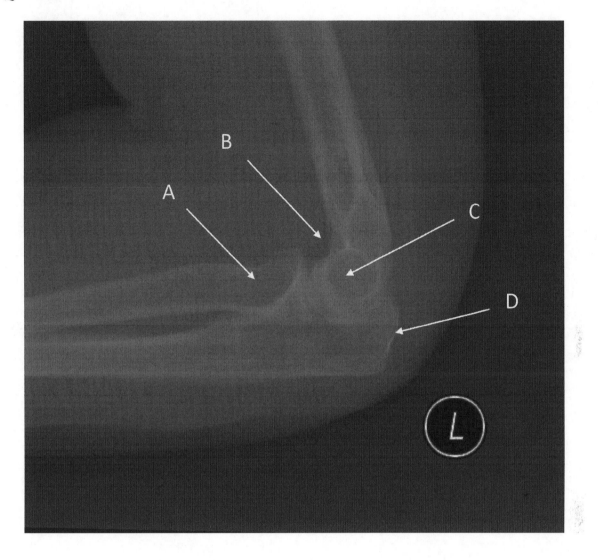

	QUESTION 12	WRITE YOUR ANSWER HERE
A	Name the structure labelled A	
B	Name the structure labelled B	
C	Name the structure labelled C	
D	Name the structure labelled D	
E	What attaches to D?	

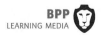

Question 13

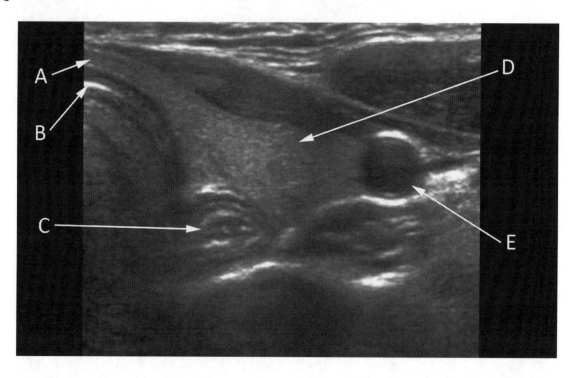

	QUESTION 13	WRITE YOUR ANSWER HERE
A	Name the structure labelled A	
B	Name the structure labelled B	
C	Name the structure labelled C	
D	Name the structure labelled D	
E	Name the structure labelled E	

Question 14

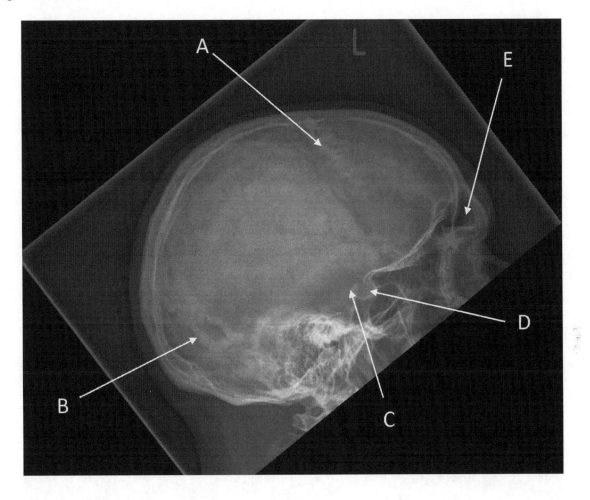

	QUESTION 14	WRITE YOUR ANSWER HERE
A	Name the structure labelled A	
B	Name the structure labelled B	
C	Name the structure labelled C	
D	Name the structure labelled D	
E	Name the structure labelled E	

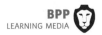

Question 15

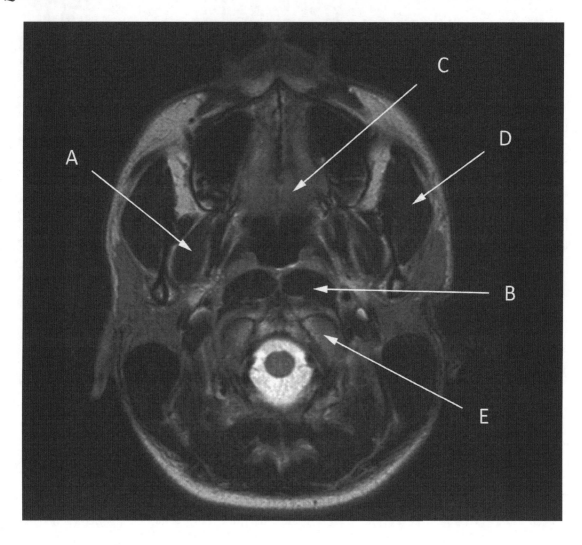

	QUESTION 15	WRITE YOUR ANSWER HERE
A	Name the structure labelled A	
B	Name the structure labelled B	
C	Name the structure labelled C	
D	Name the structure labelled D	
E	Name the structure labelled E	

Question 16

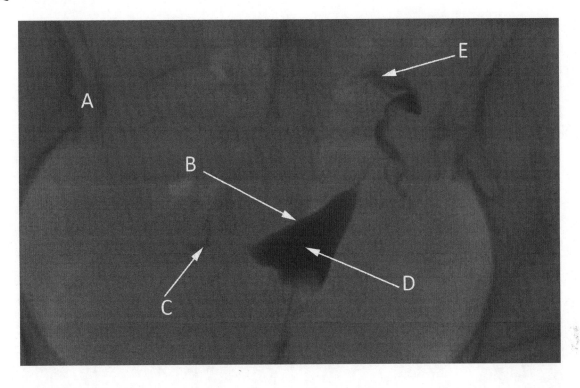

	QUESTION 16	WRITE YOUR ANSWER HERE
A	Name the structure labelled A	
B	Name the structure labelled B	
C	Name the structure labelled C	
D	Name the structure labelled D	
E	What compartment does the contrast E lie in?	

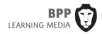

Question 17

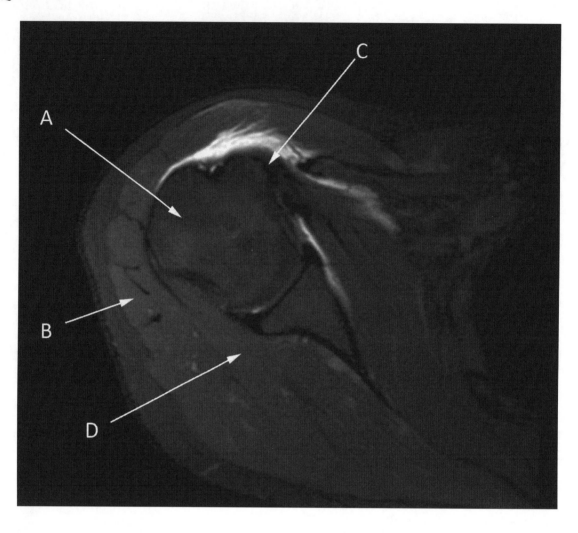

	QUESTION 17	WRITE YOUR ANSWER HERE
A	Name the structure labelled A	
B	Name the structure labelled B	
C	Name the structure labelled C	
D	Name the structure labelled D	
E	What is the distal attachment of D?	

Question 18

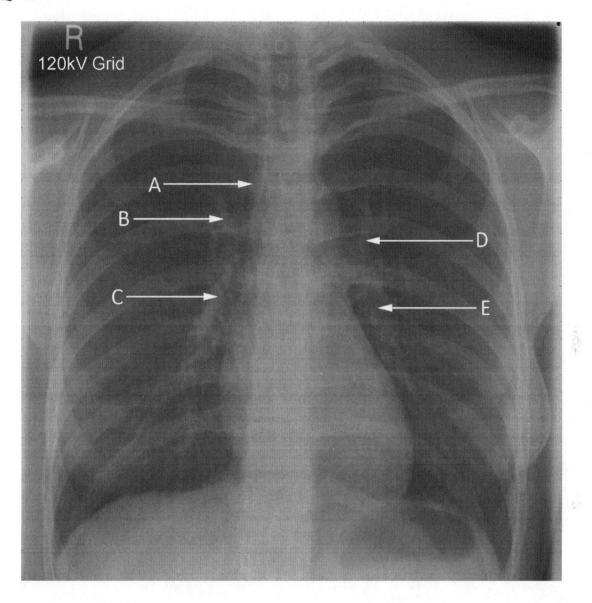

	QUESTION 18	WRITE YOUR ANSWER HERE
A	Name the structure labelled A	
B	Name the structure labelled B	
C	Name the structure labelled C	
D	Name the structure labelled D	
E	Name the structure labelled E	

Question 19

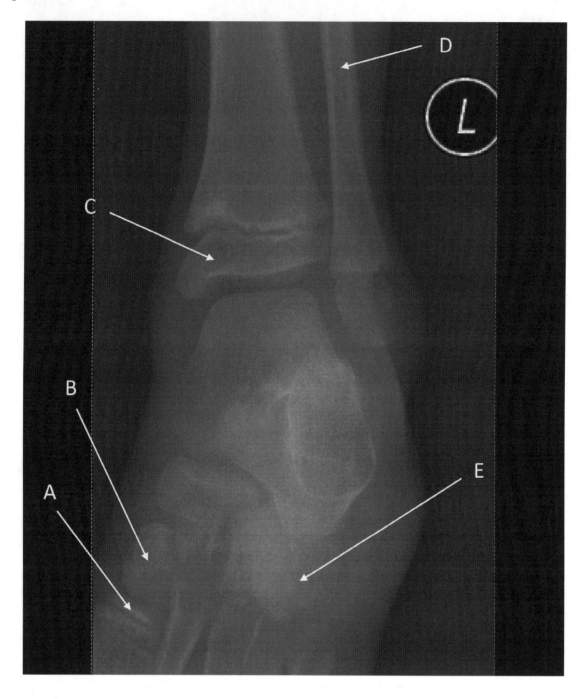

	QUESTION 19	WRITE YOUR ANSWER HERE
A	Name the structure labelled A	
B	Name the structure labelled B	
C	Name the structure labelled C	
D	Name the structure labelled D	
E	Name the structure labelled E	

Question 20

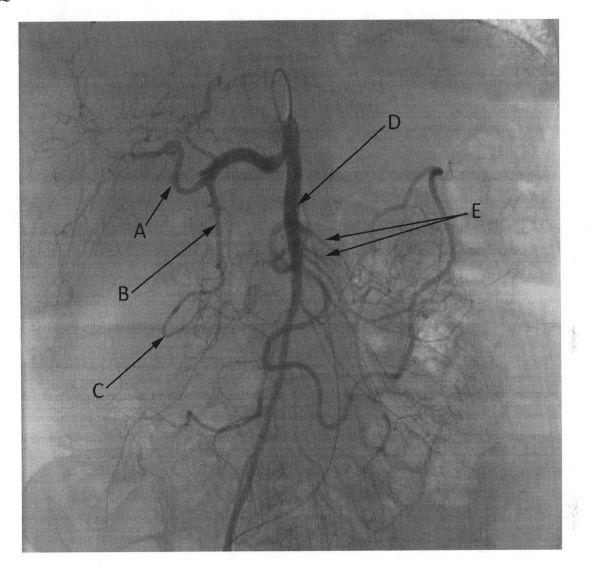

	QUESTION 20	WRITE YOUR ANSWER HERE
A	Name the structure labelled A	
B	Name the structure labelled B	
C	Name the structure labelled C	
D	Name the structure labelled D	
E	Name the structure labelled E	

Paper 9

Answers

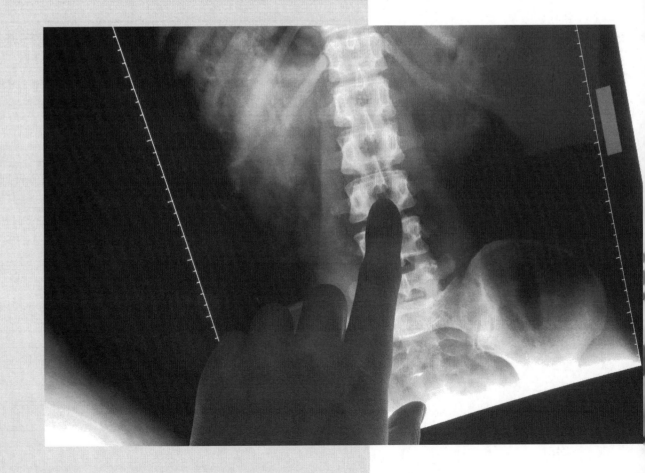

Question 1

A. Right atrial appendage
B. Aortic valve
C. Superior vena cava
D. Mitral valve posterior leaflet
E. Mitral valve anterior leaflet

Question 2

A. Biceps femoris muscle
B. Head of fibula
C. Sartorius muscle
D. Popliteal artery and vein
E. Medial femoral condyle

Question 3

A. Gallbladder
B. Superior mesenteric artery
C. Left renal artery
D. Right renal artery
E. Inferior vena cava

Question 4

A. Right obturator internus muscle
B. Left ischio-anal fossa
C. Left gluteus maximus muscle
D. Left pectineus muscle
E. Left obturator externus muscle

Question 5

A. Aortic arch
B. Right upper lobe apical segmental bronchus
C. Right upper lobe bronchus
D. Bronchus intermedius
E. Anterior and posterior segmental bronchi

Question 6

A. Right third carpometacarpal joint
B. Epiphysis of right fifth metacarpal
C. Epiphysis of middle phalanx of right little finger
D. Proximal interphalangeal joint of the right ring finger
E. Distal phalanx of the right ring finger

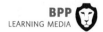

Question 7

A. Right testis
B. Right superficial femoral artery
C. Left profunda femoris artery
D. Anal canal
E. External anal sphincter

Question 8

A. Right middle cerebellar peduncle
B. Right frontal bone
C. Temporal horn of the left lateral ventricle
D. Pons
E. Fourth ventricle

Question 9

A. Left lobe of liver
B. Right lobe of liver
C. Middle hepatic vein
D. Right hepatic vein
E. Branch of portal vein

Question 10

A. Brachiocephalic artery
B. Accessory (Azygous) fissure
C. Accessory (Azygous) lobe
D. Oesophagus
E. Left upper lobe apico-posterior segment

Question 11

A. Sacral promontory
B. Anterior longitudinal ligament
C. Ligamentum flavum
D. Posterior longitudinal ligament
E. Epidural space

Question 12

A. Left radial neck
B. Left anterior fat pad
C. Left capitellum
D. Left olecranon
E. Left triceps brachii muscle

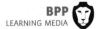

Question 13

A. Isthmus of thyroid gland
B. Tracheal cartilage
C. Oesophagus
D. Left lobe of thyroid gland
E. Left common carotid artery

Question 14

A. Coronal suture
B. Lambdoid suture
C. Posterior clinoid process
D. Sella turcica / pituitary fossa
E. Frontal sinus

Question 15

A. Right medial pterygoid muscle
B. Left longus capitis muscle
C. Hard palate
D. Left masseter muscle
E. Left occipital condyle

Question 16

A. Right sacro-iliac joint
B. Fundus of uterus
C. Ampulla of right uterine tube / Fallopian tube
D. Body of uterus
E. Peritoneal cavity

Question 17

A. Humeral head
B. Deltoid muscle
C. Subscapularis tendon
D. Infraspinatus muscle
E. Greater tubercle of humerus

Question 18

A. Superior vena cava
B. Right upper lobe pulmonary vein
C. Interlobar artery
D. Left upper lobe pulmonary vein
E. Left lower lobe pulmonary artery

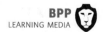

Question 19

A. Epiphysis of left first metatarsal
B. Left medial cuneiform
C. Distal epiphysis of left tibia
D. Left fibula
E. Left cuboid

Question 20

A. Right hepatic artery
B. Gastroduodenal artery
C. Right gastroepiploic artery
D. Superior mesenteric artery
E. Jejunal branches

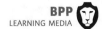

Paper 10

Question Bank

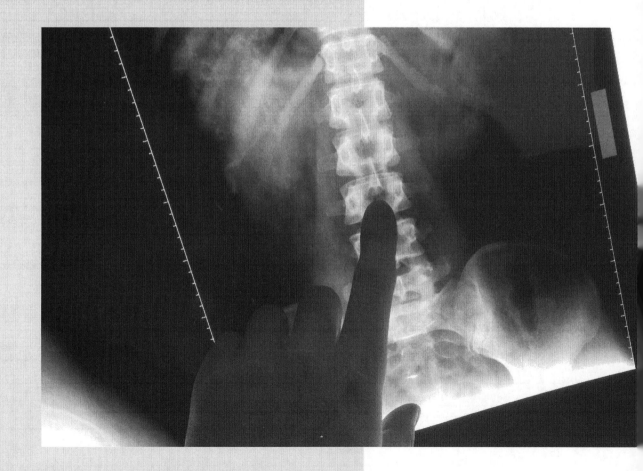

Question 1

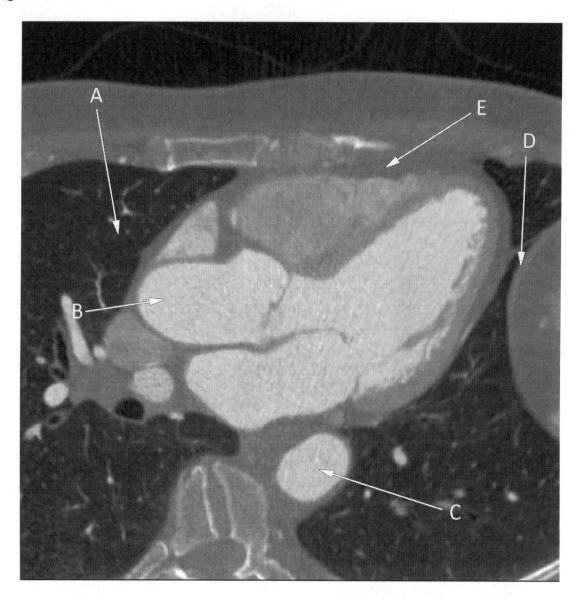

	QUESTION 1	WRITE YOUR ANSWER HERE
A	Name the lobe and segment labelled A	
B	Name the structure labelled B	
C	Name the structure labelled C	
D	Name the structure labelled D	
E	Name the layer labelled E	

Question 2

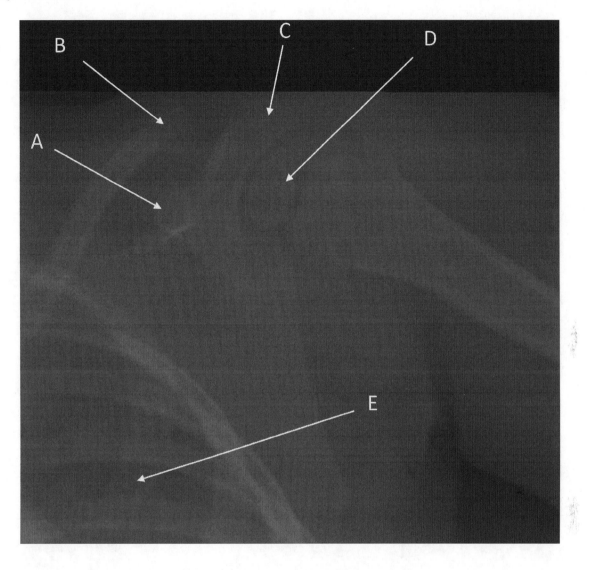

	QUESTION 2	WRITE YOUR ANSWER HERE
A	Name the structure labelled A	
B	Name the structure labelled B	
C	Name the structure labelled C	
D	Name the structure labelled D	
E	Name the structure labelled E	

Question 3

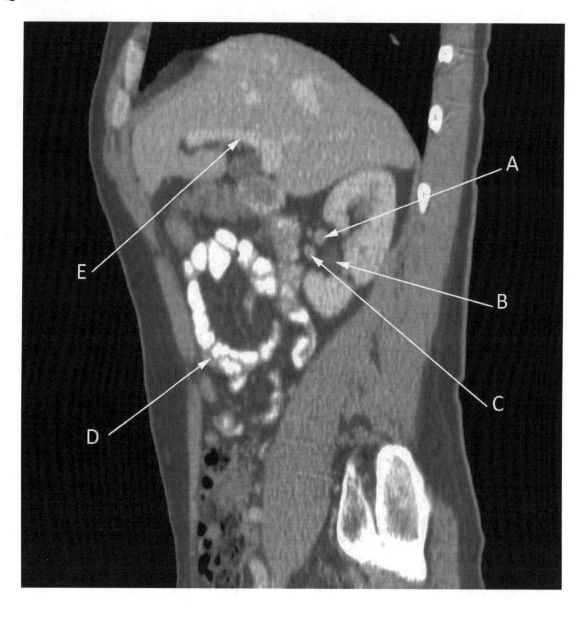

	QUESTION 3	WRITE YOUR ANSWER HERE
A	Name the structure labelled A	
B	Name the structure labelled B	
C	Name the structure labelled C	
D	Name the structure labelled D	
E	Name the structure labelled E	

Question 4

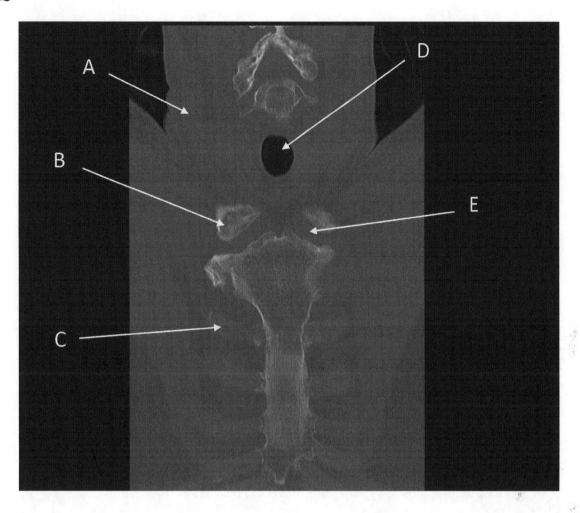

	QUESTION 4	WRITE YOUR ANSWER HERE
A	Name the structure labelled A	
B	Name the structure labelled B	
C	Name the structure labelled C	
D	Name the structure labelled D	
E	Name the structure labelled E	

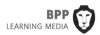

Question 5

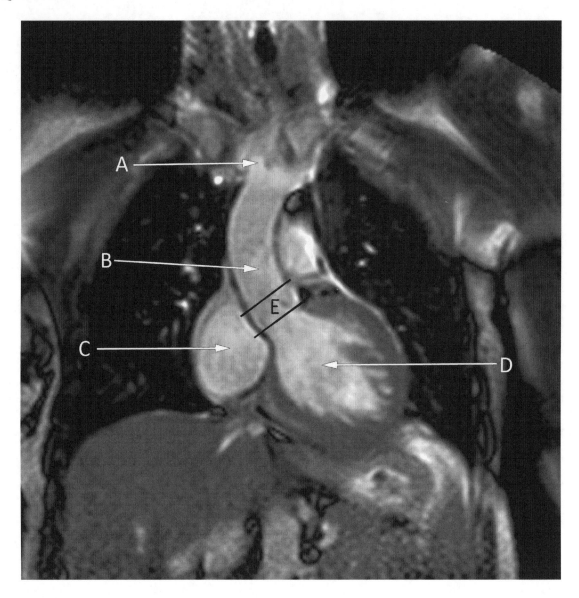

	QUESTION 5	WRITE YOUR ANSWER HERE
A	Name the structure labelled A	
B	Name the structure labelled B	
C	Name the structure labelled C	
D	Name the structure labelled D	
E	Which vessels originate from this anatomical region (E)?	

Question 6

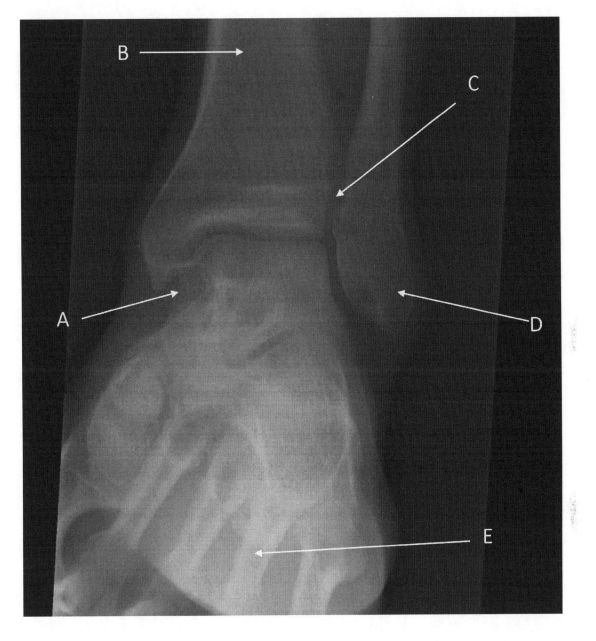

	QUESTION 6	WRITE YOUR ANSWER HERE
A	Name the structure labelled A	
B	Name the structure labelled B	
C	Name the structure labelled C	
D	Name the structure labelled D	
E	Name the structure labelled E	

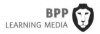

Question 7

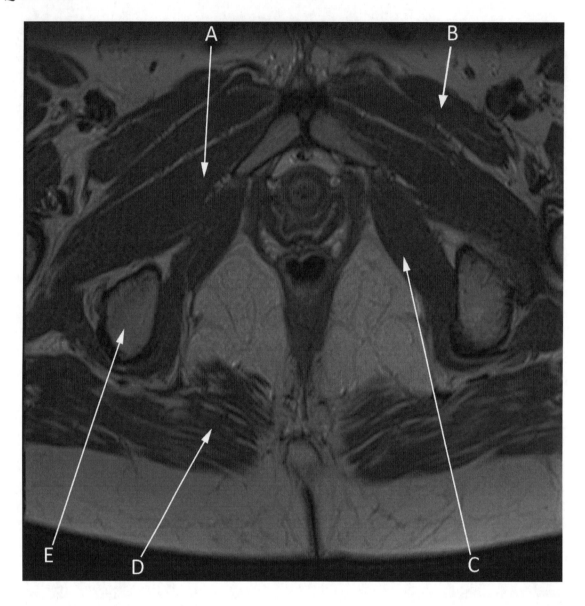

	QUESTION 7	WRITE YOUR ANSWER HERE
A	Name the structure labelled A	
B	Name the structure labelled B	
C	Name the structure labelled C	
D	Name the structure labelled D	
E	Name the structure labelled E	

Question 8

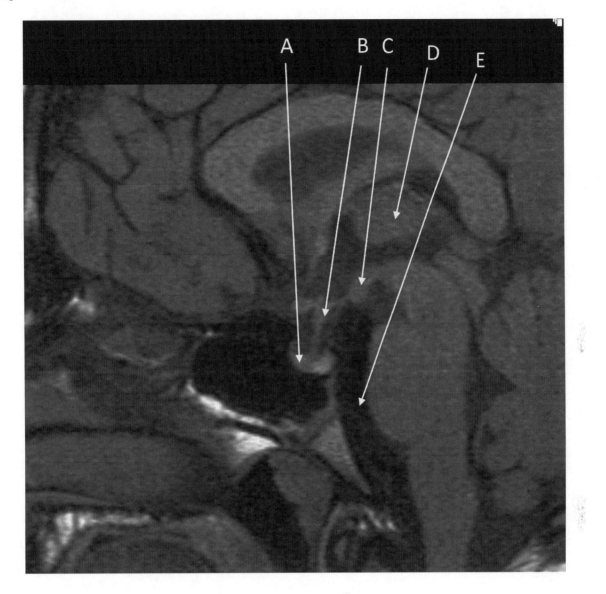

	QUESTION 8	WRITE YOUR ANSWER HERE
A	Name the structure labelled A	
B	Name the structure labelled B	
C	Name the structure labelled C	
D	Name the structure labelled D	
E	Name the structure labelled E	

Question 9

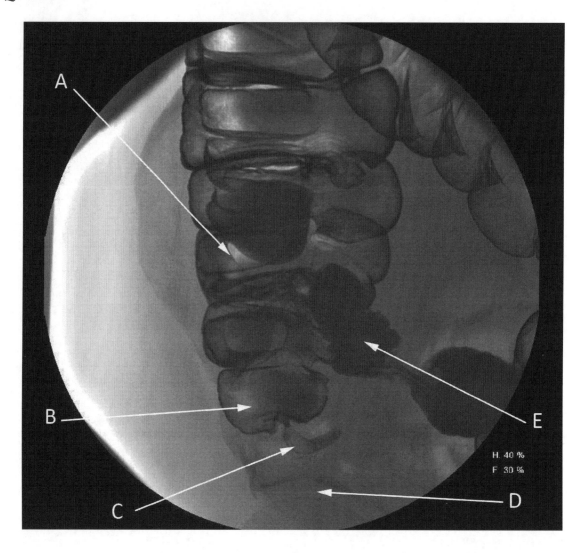

	QUESTION 9	WRITE YOUR ANSWER HERE
A	Name the structure labelled A	
B	Name the structure labelled B	
C	Name the structure labelled C	
D	Name the structure labelled D	
E	Name the structure labelled E	

Question 10

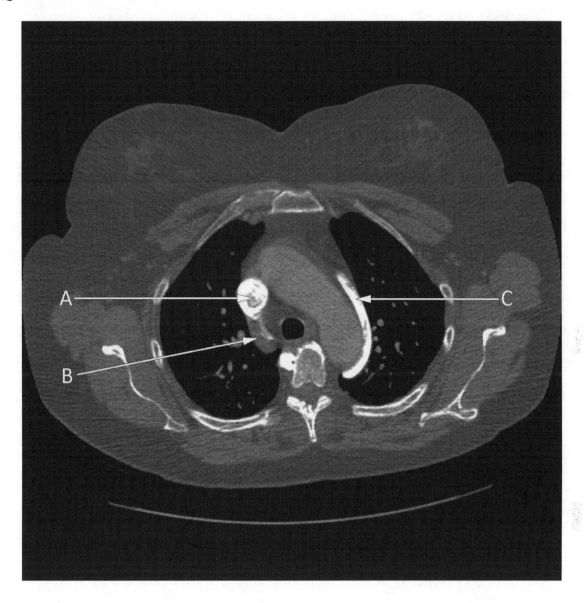

	QUESTION 10	WRITE YOUR ANSWER HERE
A	Name the structure labelled A	
B	Name the structure labelled B	
C	Name the structure labelled C	
D	Which two vessels can C communicate with?	
E	What structure does B arch over?	

Question 11

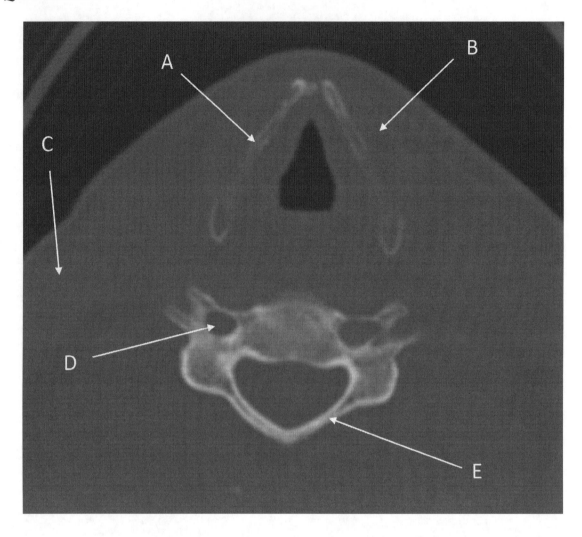

	QUESTION 11	WRITE YOUR ANSWER HERE
A	Name the structure labelled A	
B	Name the structure labelled B	
C	Name the structure labelled C	
D	Name the structure labelled D	
E	Name the structure labelled E	

Question 12

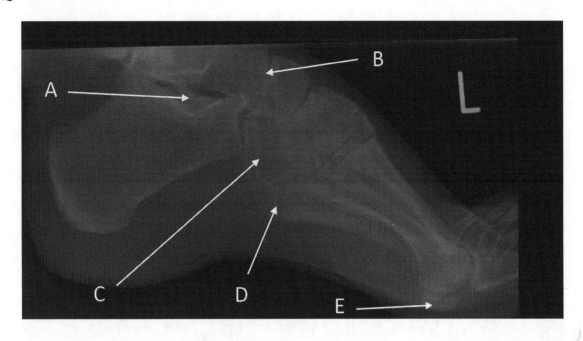

	QUESTION 12	WRITE YOUR ANSWER HERE
A	Name the structure labelled A	
B	Name the structure labelled B	
C	Name the structure labelled C	
D	Name the structure labelled D	
E	Name the structure labelled E	

BPP
LEARNING MEDIA

Question 13

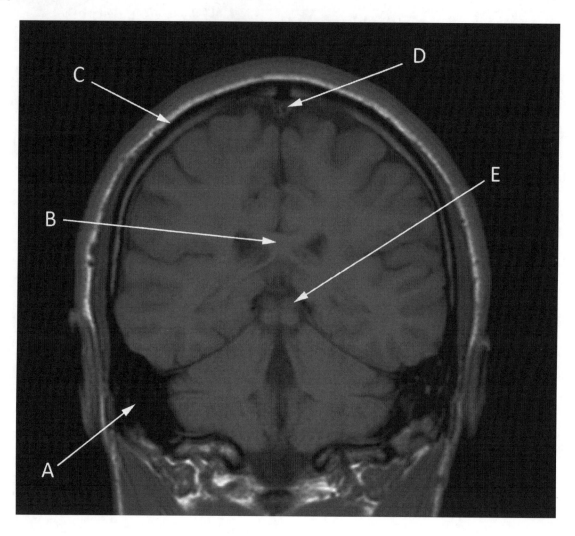

	QUESTION 13	WRITE YOUR ANSWER HERE
A	Name the structure labelled A	
B	Name the structure labelled B	
C	Name the structure labelled C	
D	Name the structure labelled D	
E	Name the structure labelled E	

Question 14

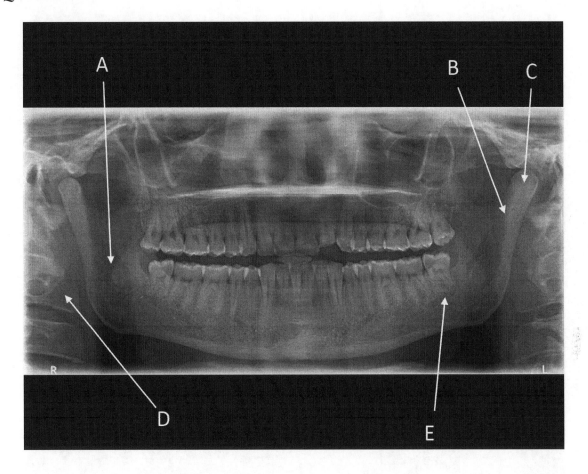

	QUESTION 14	WRITE YOUR ANSWER HERE
A	Name the structure labelled A	
B	Name the structure labelled B	
C	Name the structure labelled C	
D	Name the structure labelled D	
E	Name the structure labelled E	

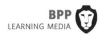

Question 15

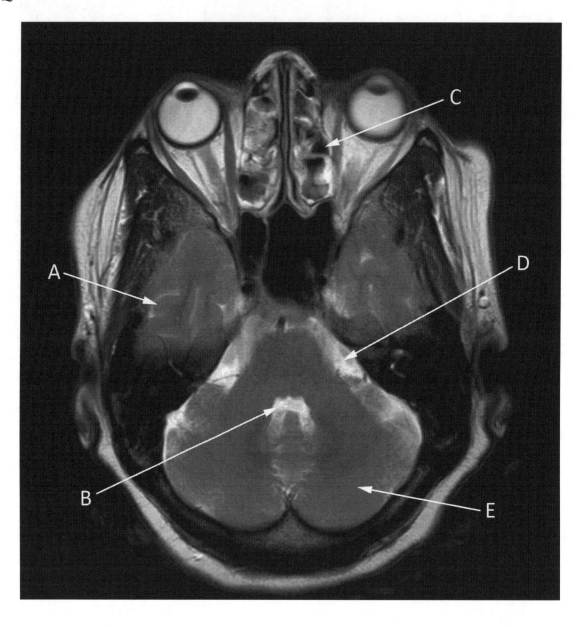

	QUESTION 15	WRITE YOUR ANSWER HERE
A	Name the structure labelled A	
B	Name the structure labelled B	
C	Name the structure labelled C	
D	Name the structure labelled D	
E	Name the structure labelled E	

Question 16

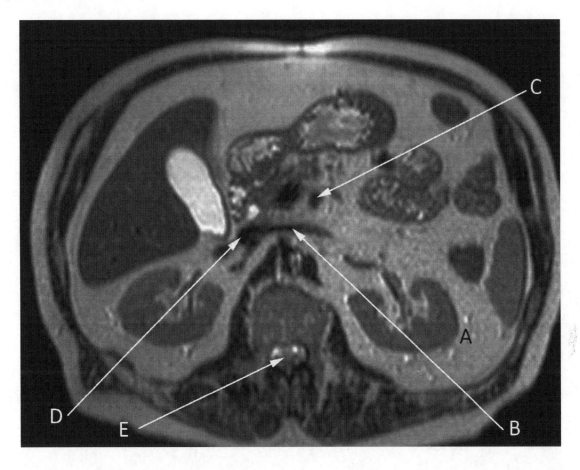

	QUESTION 16	WRITE YOUR ANSWER HERE
A	Name the structure labelled A	
B	Name the structure labelled B	
C	Name the structure labelled C	
D	Name the structure labelled D	
E	Name the structure labelled E	

Question 17

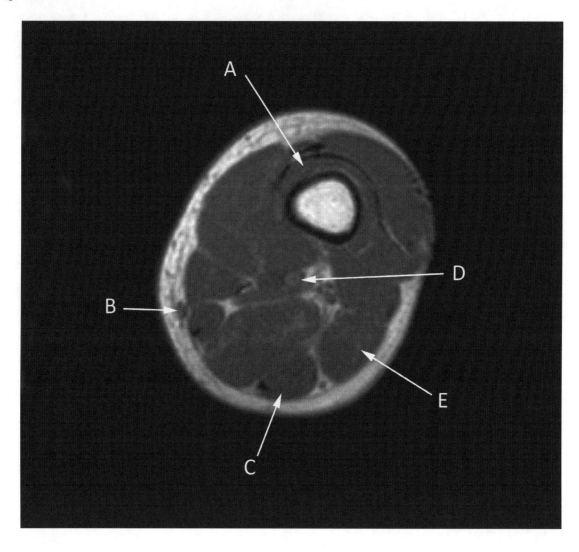

	QUESTION 17	WRITE YOUR ANSWER HERE
A	Name the structure labelled A	
B	Name the structure labelled B	
C	Name the structure labelled C	
D	Name the structure labelled D	
E	Name the structure labelled E	

Question 18

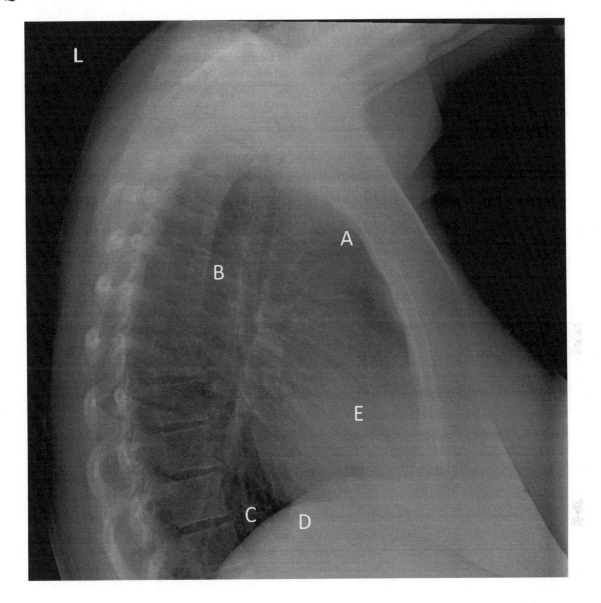

	QUESTION 18	WRITE YOUR ANSWER HERE
A	Name the right lung lobe overlying A	
B	Name the vessel labelled B	
C	Name the right lung lobe overlying C	
D	Name the structure labelled D	
E	Name the right lung lobe overlying E	

Question 19

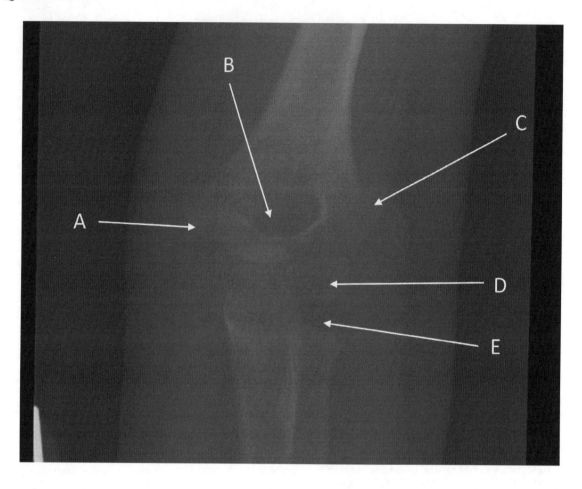

	QUESTION 19	WRITE YOUR ANSWER HERE
A	Name the structure labelled A	
B	Name the structure labelled B	
C	Name the structure labelled C	
D	Name the structure labelled D	
E	Name the structure labelled E	

Question 20

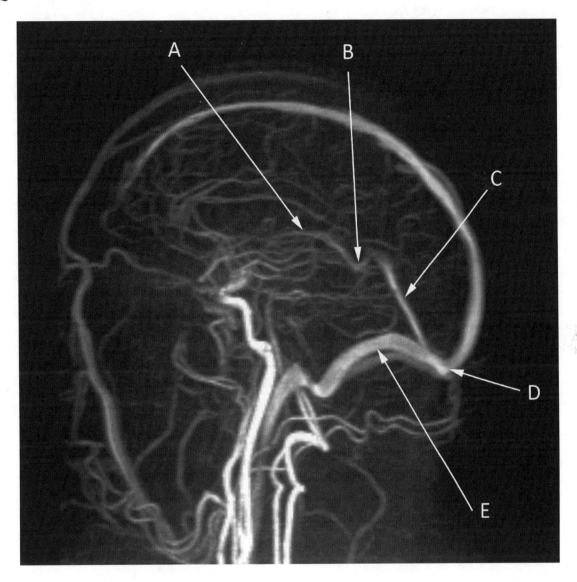

	QUESTION 20	WRITE YOUR ANSWER HERE
A	Name the structure labelled A	
B	Name the structure labelled B	
C	Name the structure labelled C	
D	Name the structure labelled D	
E	Name the structure labelled E	

Paper 10

Answers

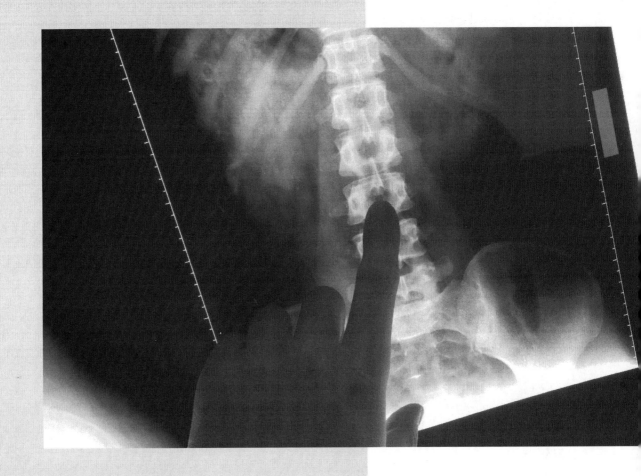

Question 1

A. Middle lobe medial segment
B. Ascending aorta
C. Descending aorta
D. Left hemi-diaphragm
E. Pericardium

Question 2

A. Growth centre for left coracoid process
B. Distal left clavicle
C. Left acromion
D. Growth centre for left humeral head
E. Anterior rib

Question 3

A. Right renal artery
B. Right renal pelvis
C. Right renal vein
D. Loops of small bowel
E. Portal vein

Question 4

A. Right sternocleidomastoid muscle
B. Medial end of right clavicle
C. Anterior costal cartilage of right second rib
D. Trachea
E. Left sterno-clavicular joint

Question 5

A. Brachiocephalic artery
B. Ascending aorta
C. Right atrium
D. Left ventricle
E. Left and right coronary arteries

Question 6

A. Medial tubercle of talus
B. Distal tibia
C. Distal tibiofibular joint
D. Lateral malleolus of the fibula
E. Fourth metatarsal

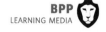

Question 7

A. Right obturator externus muscle
B. Left pectineus muscle
C. Left obturator internus muscle
D. Right gluteus maximus muscle
E. Right ischial tuberosity

Question 8

A. Anterior pituitary gland
B. Pituitary stalk
C. Mammillary body
D. Thalamus
E. Pre-pontine cistern

Question 9

A. Ascending colon
B. Caecal pole
C. Appendix
D. Right acetabular roof
E. Terminal ileum

Question 10

A. Superior vena cava
B. Azygous vein
C. Left superior intercostal vein
D. Left brachiocephalic vein, accessory hemi-azygous vein
E. Right main bronchus

Question 11

A. Right thyroid cartilage lamina
B. Left infrahyoid strap muscle
C. Right sternocleidomastoid muscle
D. Right transverse foramen
E. Left lamina of cervical vertebra

Question 12

A. Left subtalar joint
B. Left talo-navicular joint
C. Left cuboid bone
D. Base of left fifth metatarsal
E. Sesamoid bone in flexor hallucis brevis

Question 13

A. Right mastoid air cells
B. Corpus callosum
C. Outer table
D. Superior sagittal sinus
E. Left superior colliculus

Question 14

A. Right mandibular ramus
B. Right mandibular condylar neck
C. Right mandibular condylar head
D. C2 vertebral body
E. Inferior alveolar canal

Question 15

A. Right temporal lobe (grey matter)
B. Fourth ventricle
C. Ethmoidal air cell (left)
D. Cerebellopontine cistern
E. Left cerebellar hemisphere

Question 16

A. Left peri-renal space / fat
B. Left renal vein
C. Superior mesenteric artery
D. Inferior vena cava
E. Spinal canal

Question 17

A. Vastus intermedius muscle
B. Long saphenous vein
C. Semitendinosus muscle
D. Popliteal artery
E. Biceps femoris muscle

Question 18

A. Right upper lobe
B. Descending aorta
C. Right lower lobe
D. Left hemi diaphragm
E. Middle lobe

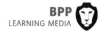

Question 19

A. Growth centre for medial epicondyle
B. Olecranon fossa
C. Growth centre for lateral epicondyle
D. Growth centre for capitellum
E. Growth centre for radial head

Question 20

A. Internal cerebral vein
B. Great cerebral vein of Galen
C. Straight sinus
D. Torcular Herophili
E. Transverse sinus (right)

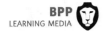

Paper 11

Question Bank

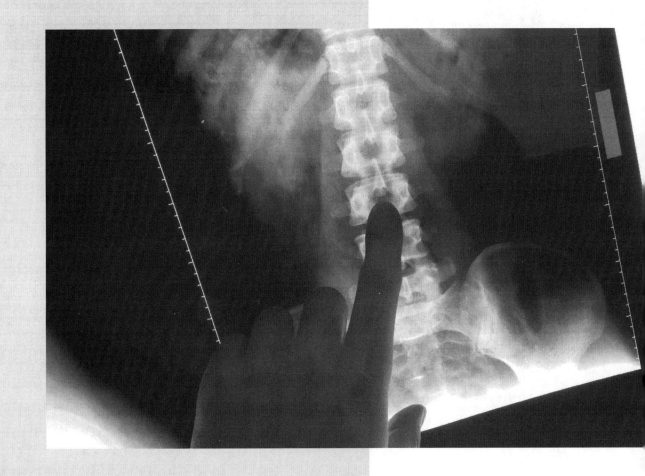

Question 1

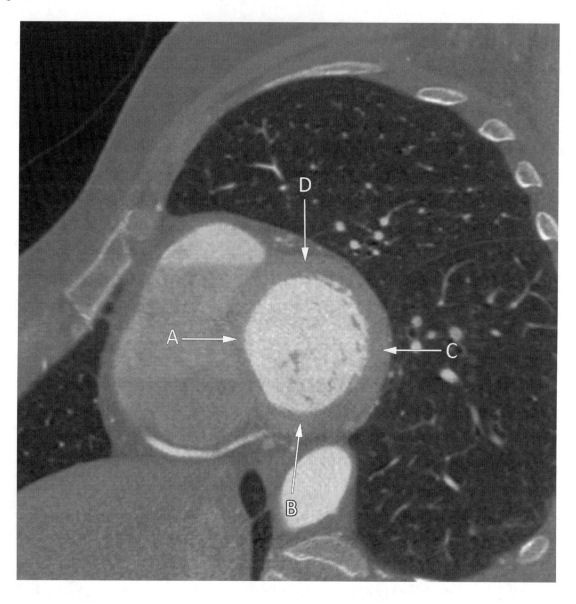

	QUESTION 1	WRITE YOUR ANSWER HERE
A	Name the wall labelled A	
B	Name the wall labelled B	
C	Name the wall labelled C	
D	Name the wall labelled D	
E	What segments are represented?	

Question 2

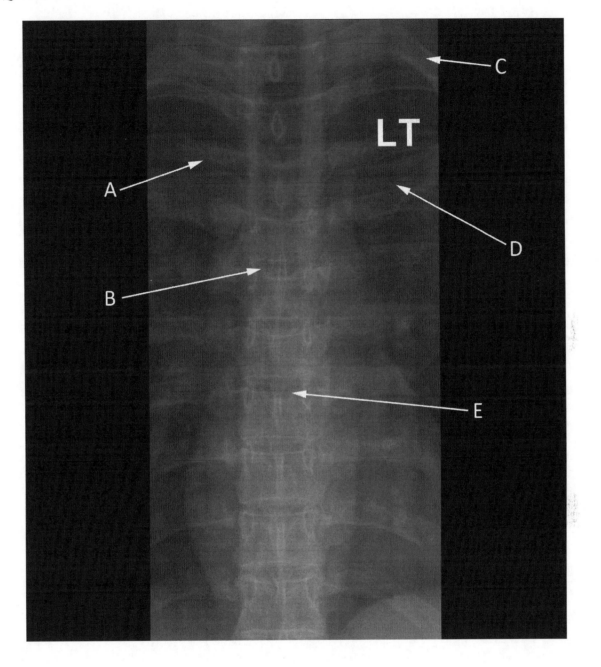

	QUESTION 2	WRITE YOUR ANSWER HERE
A	Name the structure labelled A	
B	Name the structure labelled B	
C	Name the structure labelled C	
D	Name the structure labelled D	
E	Name the structure labelled E	

Question 3

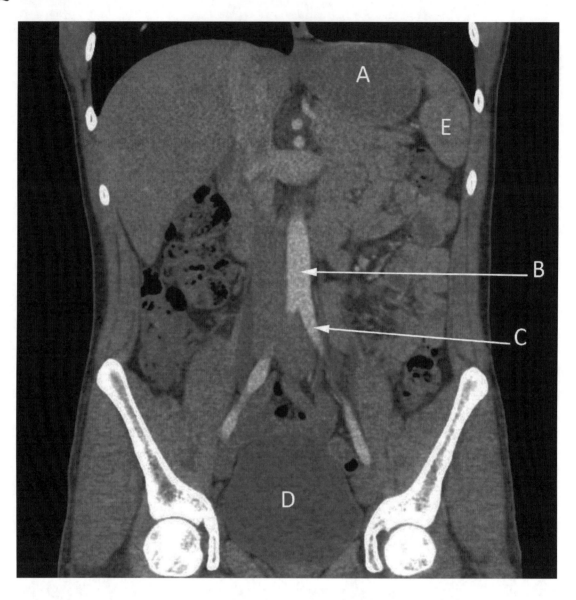

	QUESTION 3	WRITE YOUR ANSWER HERE
A	Name the structure labelled A	
B	Name the structure labelled B	
C	Name the structure labelled C	
D	Name the structure labelled D	
E	Name the structure labelled E	

Question 4

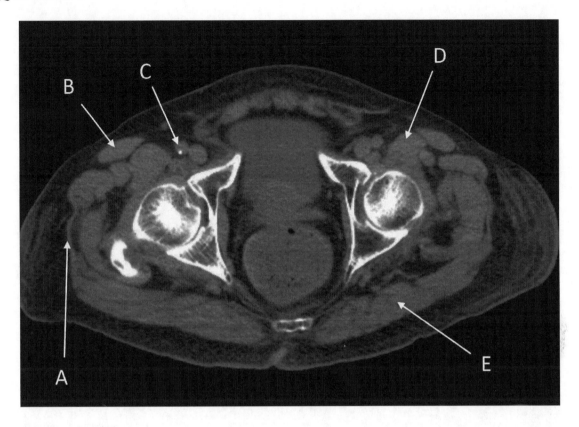

	QUESTION 4	WRITE YOUR ANSWER HERE
A	Name the structure labelled A	
B	Name the structure labelled B	
C	Name the structure labelled C	
D	Name the structure labelled D	
E	Name the structure labelled E	

Question 5

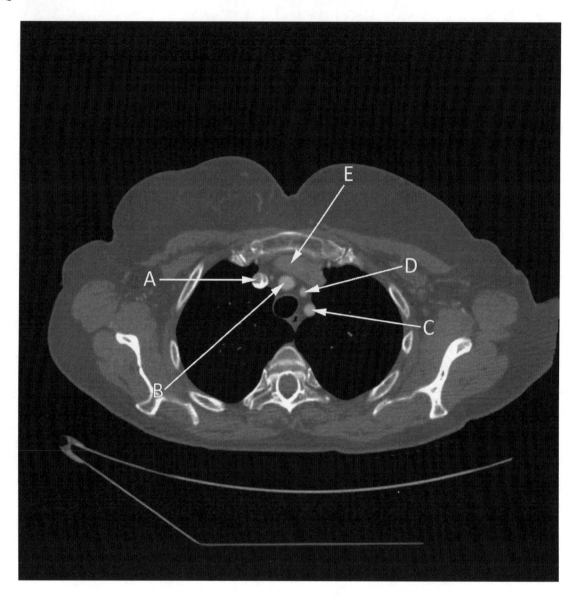

	QUESTION 5	WRITE YOUR ANSWER HERE
A	Name the structure labelled A	
B	Name the structure labelled B	
C	Name the structure labelled C	
D	Name the structure labelled D	
E	Name the structure labelled E	

Question 6

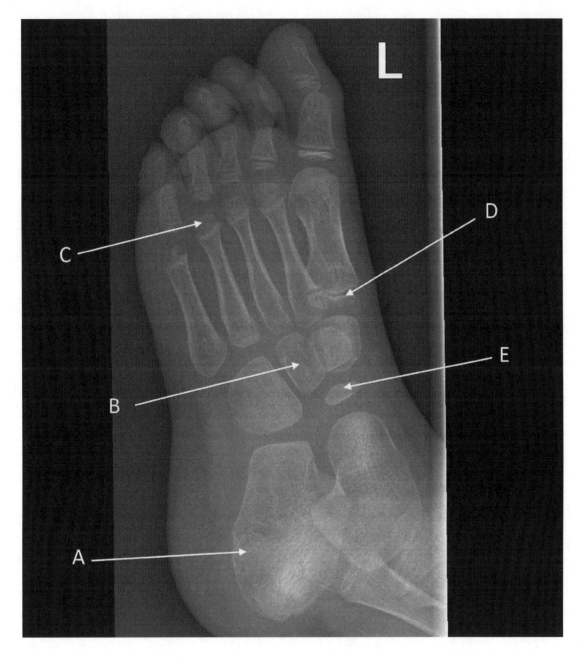

	QUESTION 6	WRITE YOUR ANSWER HERE
A	Name the structure labelled A	
B	Name the structure labelled B	
C	Name the structure labelled C	
D	Name the structure labelled D	
E	Name the structure labelled E	

Question 7

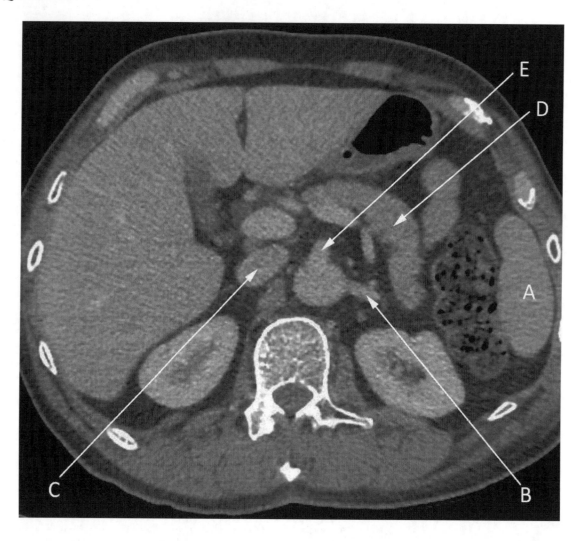

	QUESTION 7	WRITE YOUR ANSWER HERE
A	Name the structure labelled A	
B	Name the structure labelled B	
C	Name the structure labelled C	
D	Name the structure labelled D	
E	Name the structure labelled E	

Question 8

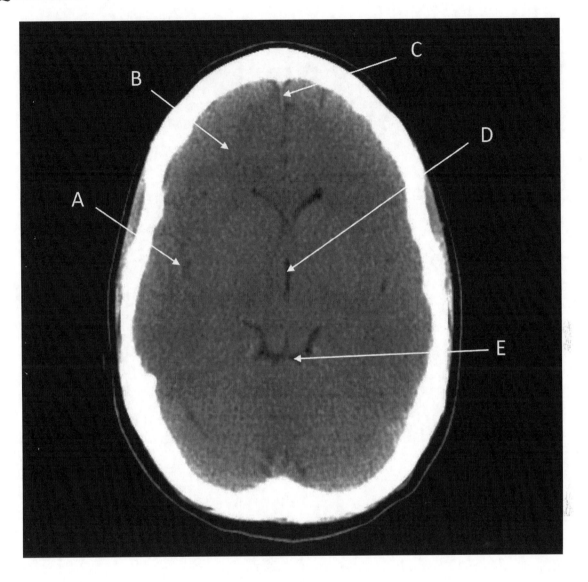

	QUESTION 8	WRITE YOUR ANSWER HERE
A	Name the structure labelled A	
B	Name the structure labelled B	
C	Name the structure labelled C	
D	Name the structure labelled D	
E	Name the structure labelled E	

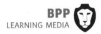

Question 9

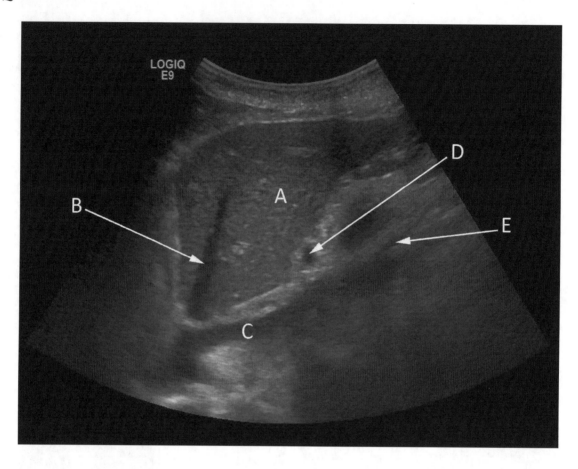

	QUESTION 9	WRITE YOUR ANSWER HERE
A	Name the structure labelled A	
B	Name the structure labelled B	
C	Name the structure labelled C	
D	Name the structure labelled D	
E	Name the structure labelled E	

Question 10

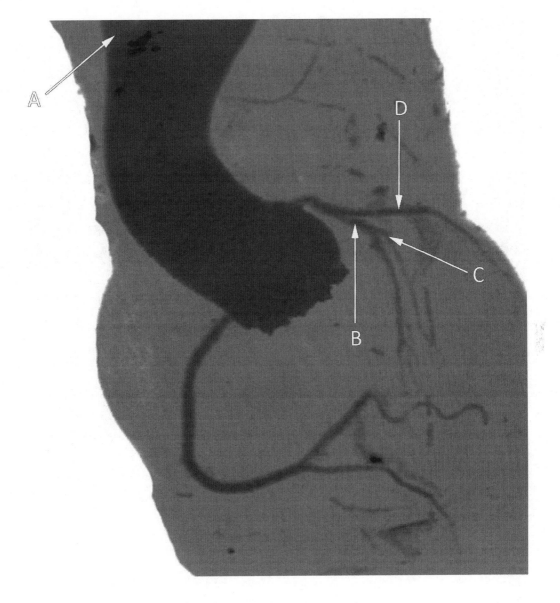

	QUESTION 10	WRITE YOUR ANSWER HERE
A	Name the structure labelled A	
B	Name the structure labelled B	
C	Name the structure labelled C	
D	Name the structure labelled D	
E	Which branches from D supply the left ventricular anterior wall?	

Question 11

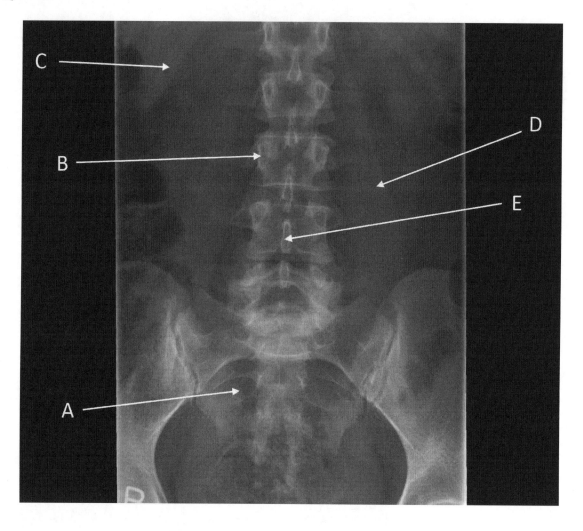

	QUESTION 11	WRITE YOUR ANSWER HERE
A	Name the structure labelled A	
B	Name the structure labelled B	
C	Name the structure labelled C	
D	Name the structure labelled D	
E	Name the structure labelled E	

Question 12

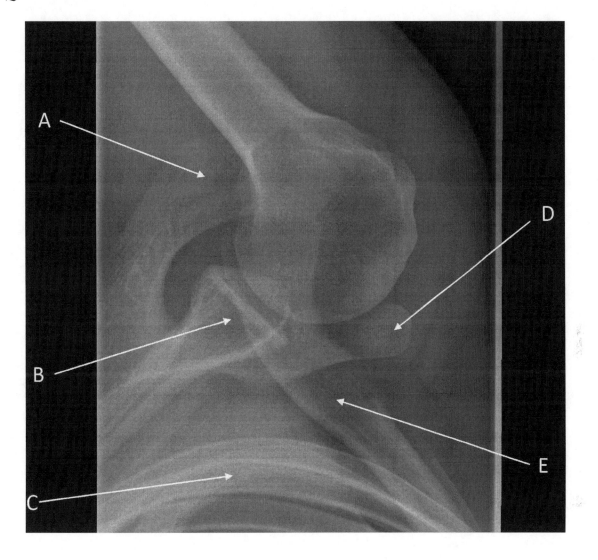

	QUESTION 12	WRITE YOUR ANSWER HERE
A	Name the structure labelled A	
B	Name the structure labelled B	
C	Name the structure labelled C	
D	Name the structure labelled D	
E	Name the structure labelled E	

Question 13

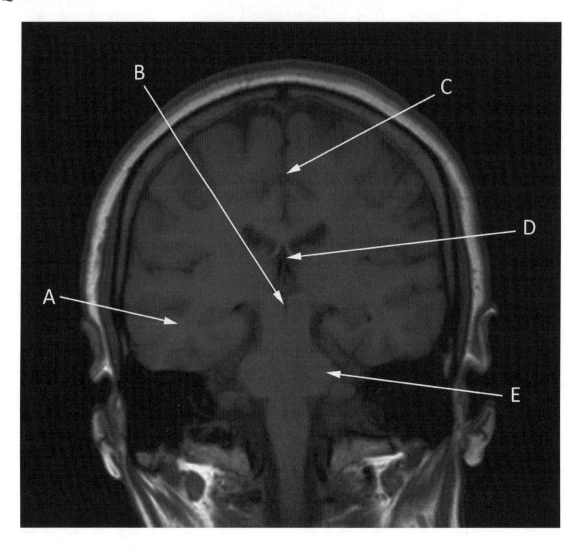

	QUESTION 13	WRITE YOUR ANSWER HERE
A	Name the structure labelled A	
B	Name the structure labelled B	
C	Name the structure labelled C	
D	Name the structure labelled D	
E	Name the structure labelled E	

Question 14

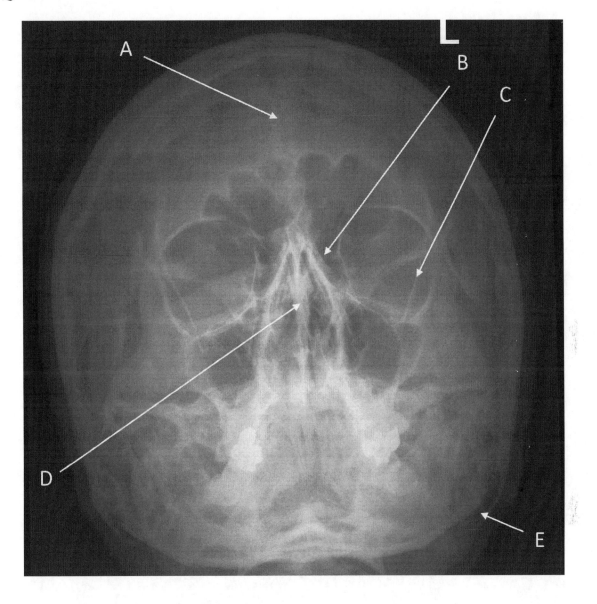

	QUESTION 14	WRITE YOUR ANSWER HERE
A	Name the structure labelled A	
B	Name the structure labelled B	
C	Name the structure labelled C	
D	Name the structure labelled D	
E	Name the structure labelled E	

Question 15

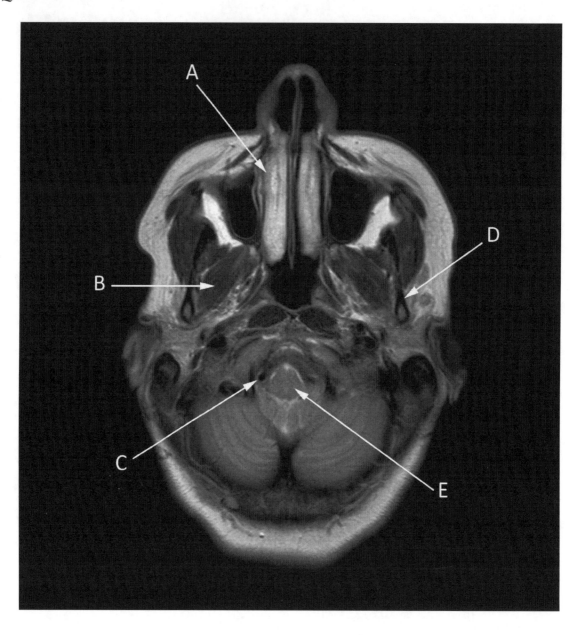

	QUESTION 15	WRITE YOUR ANSWER HERE
A	Name the structure labelled A	
B	Name the structure labelled B	
C	Name the structure labelled C	
D	Name the structure labelled D	
E	Name the structure labelled E	

Question 16

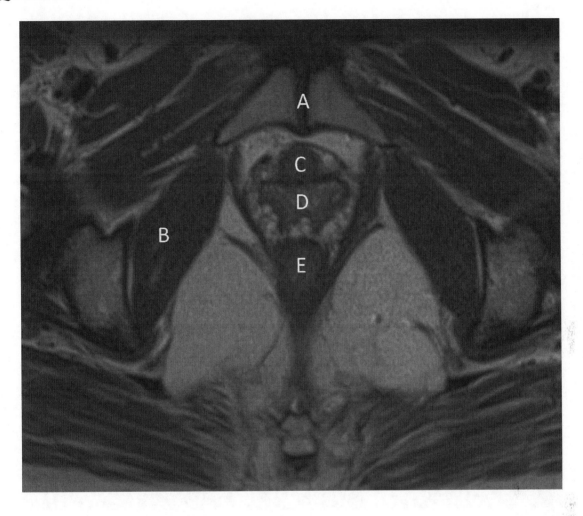

	QUESTION 16	WRITE YOUR ANSWER HERE
A	Name the structure labelled A	
B	Name the structure labelled B	
C	Name the structure labelled C	
D	Name the structure labelled D	
E	Name the structure labelled E	

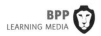

Question 17

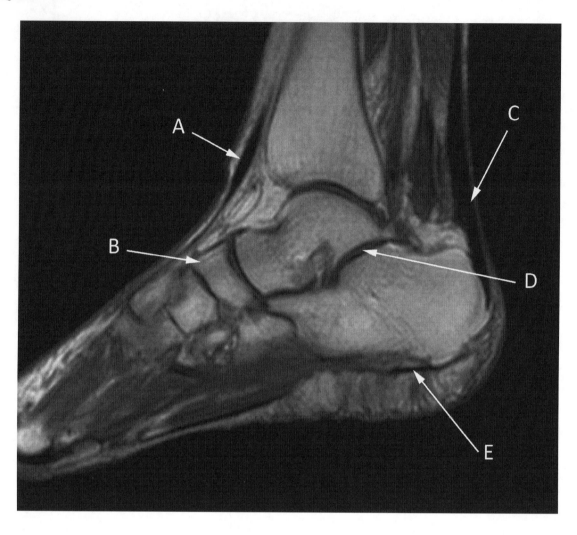

	QUESTION 17	WRITE YOUR ANSWER HERE
A	Name the structure labelled A	
B	Name the structure labelled B	
C	Name the structure labelled C	
D	Name the structure labelled D	
E	Name the structure labelled E	

Question 18

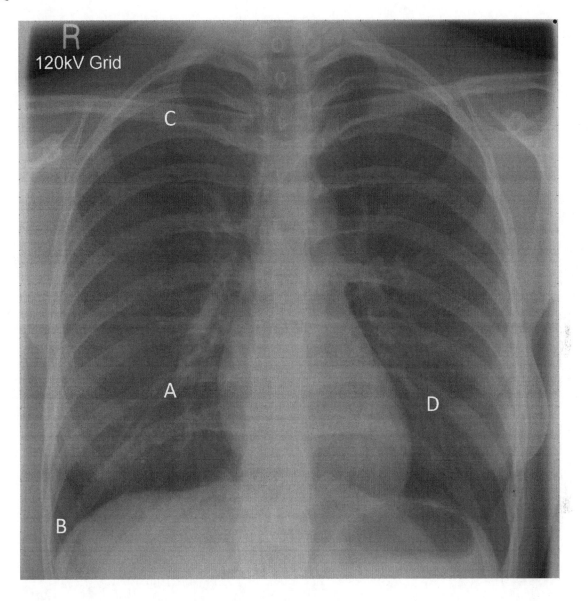

	QUESTION 18	WRITE YOUR ANSWER HERE
A	Name the lobe labelled A	
B	Name the lobe labelled B	
C	Name the lobe labelled C	
D	Name the lobe labelled D	
E	Name the superior anatomical boundary of A	

Question 19

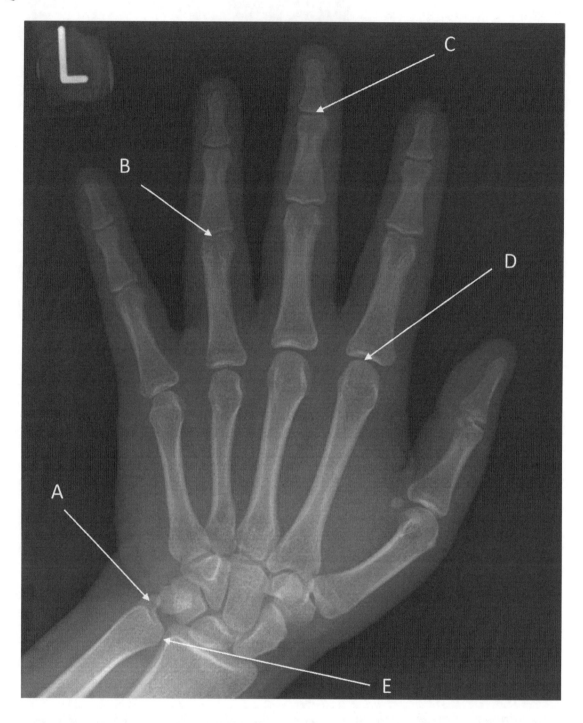

	QUESTION 19	WRITE YOUR ANSWER HERE
A	Name the structure labelled A	
B	Name the structure labelled B	
C	Name the structure labelled C	
D	Name the structure labelled D	
E	Name the structure labelled E	

Question 20

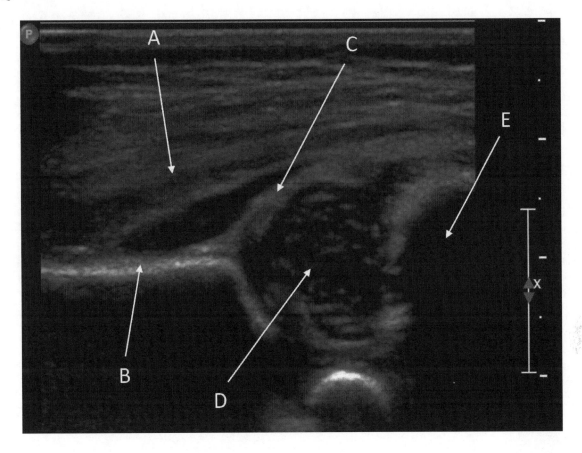

	QUESTION 20	WRITE YOUR ANSWER HERE
A	Name the structure labelled A	
B	Name the structure labelled B	
C	Name the structure labelled C	
D	Name the structure labelled D	
E	Name the structure labelled E	

Paper 11

Answers

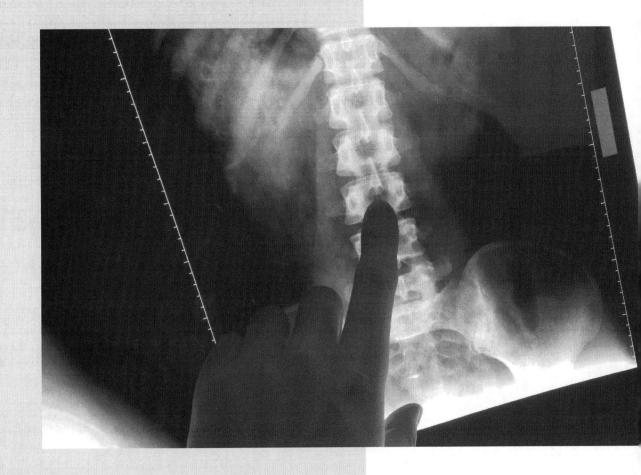

Question 1

A. Left ventricle, septal wall
B. Left ventricle, inferior wall
C. Left ventricle, lateral wall
D. Left ventricle, anterior wall
E. Basal (as opposed to mid or apical)

Question 2

A. Right T3 costovertebral joint
B. T4/T5 intervertebral disc space
C. Left first rib
D. Left clavicle
E. Superior endplate of T7 vertebra

Question 3

A. Stomach
B. Aorta
C. Left common iliac artery
D. Bladder
E. Spleen

Question 4

A. Right iliotibial tract
B. Right sartorius muscle
C. Right external iliac artery
D. Left iliopsoas muscle
E. Left gluteus maximus muscle

Question 5

A. Right brachiocephalic vein
B. Brachiocephalic artery
C. Left subclavian artery
D. Left common carotid artery
E. Left brachiocephalic vein

Question 6

A. Left calcaneus
B. Left lateral cuneiform
C. Epiphysis of left fourth metatarsal
D. Epiphysis of left first metatarsal
E. Left navicular

Question 7

A. Spleen
B. Left renal artery
C. Inferior vena cava
D. Body of pancreas
E. Superior mesenteric artery

Question 8

A. Right Sylvian fissure
B. Right frontal lobe
C. Falx cerebri
D. Third ventricle
E. Quadrigeminal cistern

Question 9

A. Left lobe of liver
B. Left hepatic vein
C. Abdominal aorta
D. Coealic axis
E. Superior mesenteric artery

Question 10

A. Brachio cephalic trunk
B. Circumflex artery
C. Obtuse marginal artery
D. Left anterior descending
E. Diagonal vessels

Question 11

A. Right sacral foramen
B. Right pedicle of L4 vertebra
C. Right 12th rib
D. Left psoas shadow
E. Spinous process of L4

Question 12

A. Acromion
B. Glenoid
C. Rib
D. Coracoid process
E. Clavicle

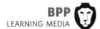

Question 13

A. Right temporal lobe (white matter)
B. Aqueduct of Sylvius
C. Falx cerebri
D. Third ventricle
E. Left middle cerebellar peduncle

Question 14

A. Sagittal suture
B. Left ethmoid air cells
C. Left innominate line
D. Nasal septum
E. Left mastoid process

Question 15

A. Right inferior nasal turbinate
B. Right lateral pterygoid muscle
C. Right vertebral artery
D. Left ramus of mandible
E. Medulla oblongata

Question 16

A. Pubic symphysis
B. Right obturator internus muscle
C. Urethra
D. Vagina
E. Anal canal

Question 17

A. Tendon of tibialis anterior muscle
B. Navicular bone
C. Tendo calcaneus (Achilles' tendon)
D. Posterior subtalar joint
E. Plantar aponeurosis

Question 18

A. Middle (right) lobe
B. Right lower lobe
C. Right upper lobe
D. Left upper lobe (lingula)
E. Horizontal fissure

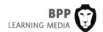

Question 19

A. Left ulnar styloid
B. Proximal interphalangeal joint of the left ring finger
C. Distal interphalangeal joint of the left middle finger
D. Metacarpophalangeal joint of the left index finger
E. Left distal radio-ulnar joint

Question 20

A. Gluteal muscles
B. Ilium
C. Labrum
D. Unossified femoral head
E. Diaphysis of femur

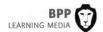

Paper 12

Question Bank

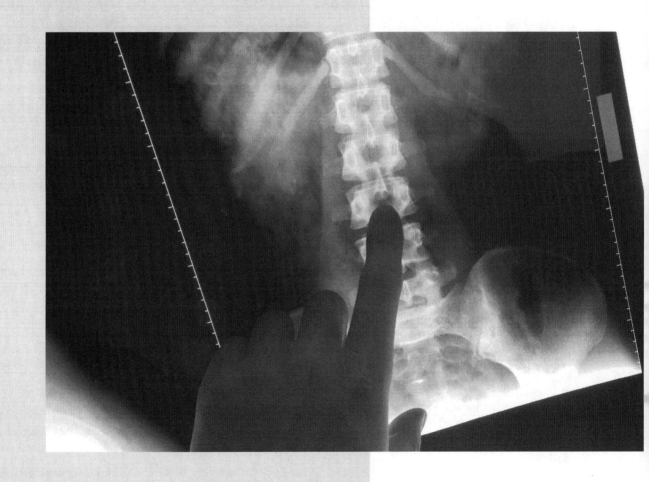

Question 1

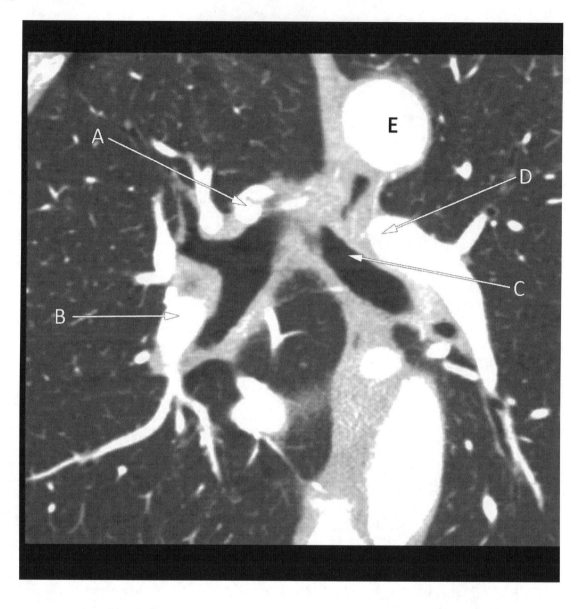

	QUESTION 1	WRITE YOUR ANSWER HERE
A	Name the vessel labelled A	
B	Name the vessel labelled B	
C	Name the structure labelled C	
D	Name the structure labelled D	
E	Name the anatomical region between D and E	

Question 2

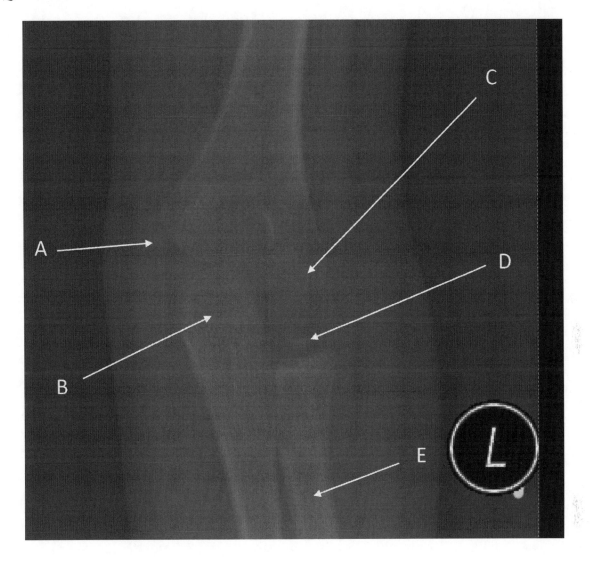

	QUESTION 2	WRITE YOUR ANSWER HERE
A	Name the structure labelled A	
B	Name the structure labelled B	
C	Name the structure labelled C	
D	Name the structure labelled D	
E	Name the structure labelled E	

Question 3

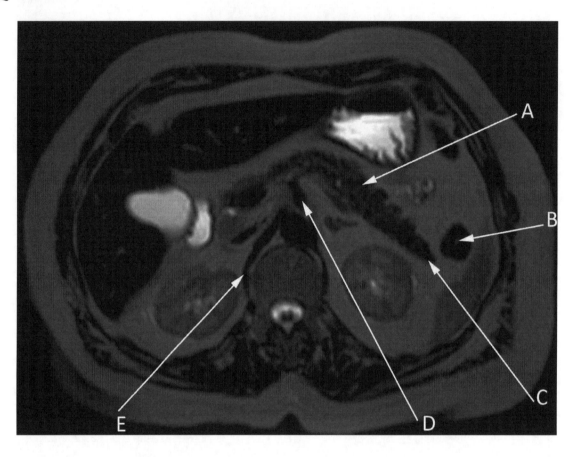

	QUESTION 3	WRITE YOUR ANSWER HERE
A	Name the structure labelled A	
B	Name the structure labelled B	
C	Name the structure labelled C	
D	Name the structure labelled D	
E	Name the structure labelled E	

Question 4

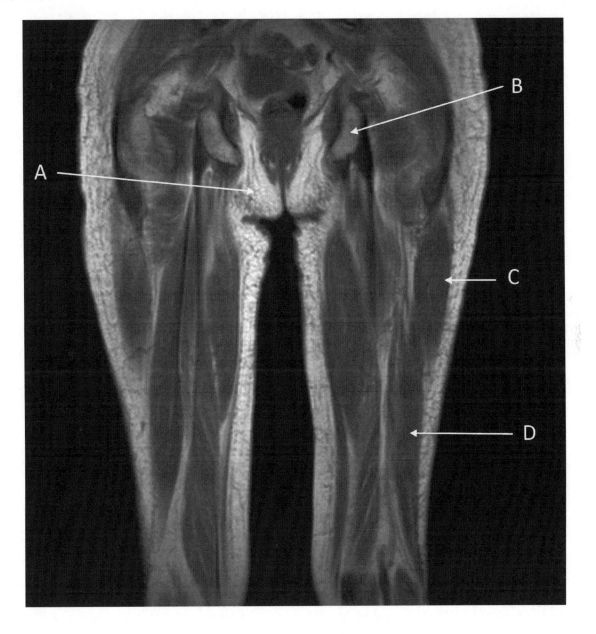

	QUESTION 4	WRITE YOUR ANSWER HERE
A	Name the structure labelled A	
B	Name the structure labelled B	
C	Name the structure labelled C	
D	Name the structure labelled D	
E	What is the distal attachment of D?	

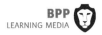

Question 5

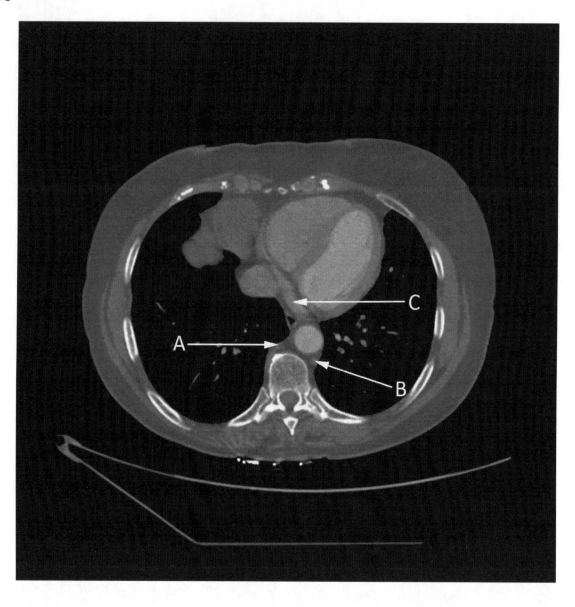

	QUESTION 5	WRITE YOUR ANSWER HERE
A	Name the vessel labelled A	
B	Name the vessel labelled B	
C	Name the vessel labelled C	
D	Where does B drain into?	
E	Where does C drain into?	

Question 6

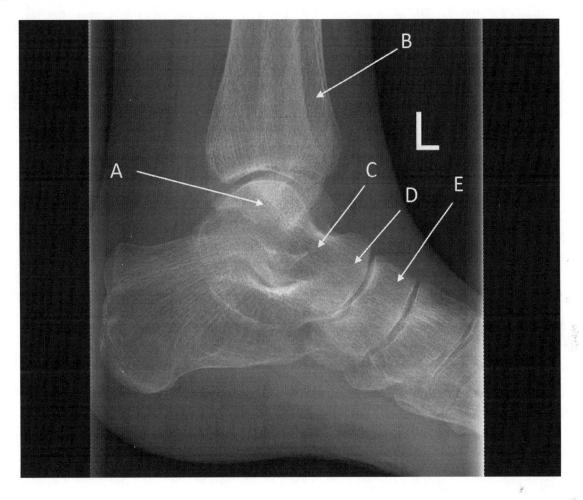

	QUESTION 6	WRITE YOUR ANSWER HERE
A	Name the structure labelled A	
B	Name the structure labelled B	
C	Name the structure labelled C	
D	Name the structure labelled D	
E	Name the structure labelled E	

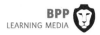

Question 7

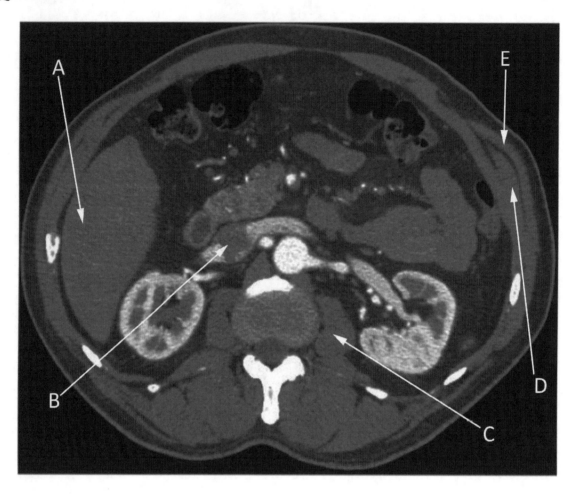

	QUESTION 7	WRITE YOUR ANSWER HERE
A	Name the structure labelled A	
B	Name the structure labelled B	
C	Name the structure labelled C	
D	Name the structure labelled D	
E	Name the structure labelled E	

Question 8

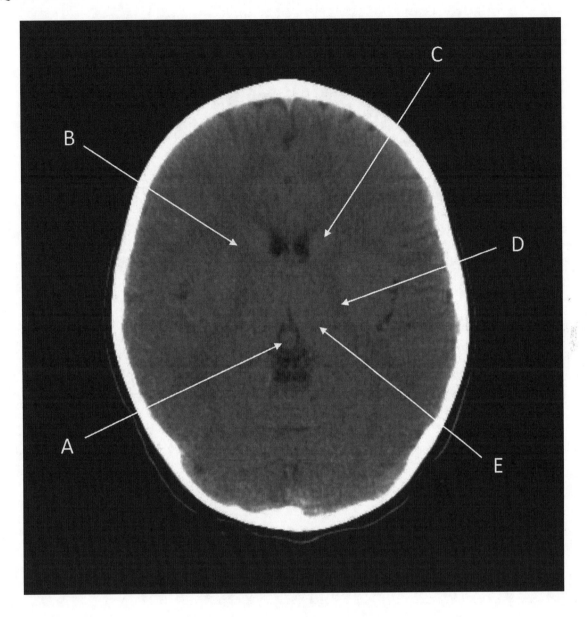

	QUESTION 8	WRITE YOUR ANSWER HERE
A	Name the structure labelled A	
B	Name the structure labelled B	
C	Name the structure labelled C	
D	Name the structure labelled D	
E	Name the structure labelled E	

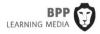

Question 9

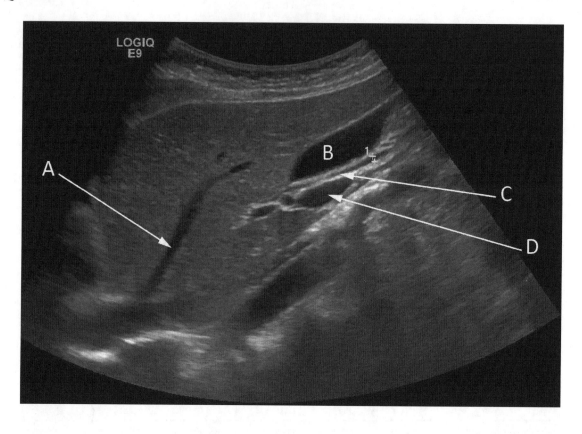

	QUESTION 9	WRITE YOUR ANSWER HERE
A	Name the structure labelled A	
B	Name the structure labelled B	
C	Name the structure labelled C	
D	Name the structure labelled D	
E	What is the normal dimension of the structure labelled C in a 60-year-old patient?	

Question 10

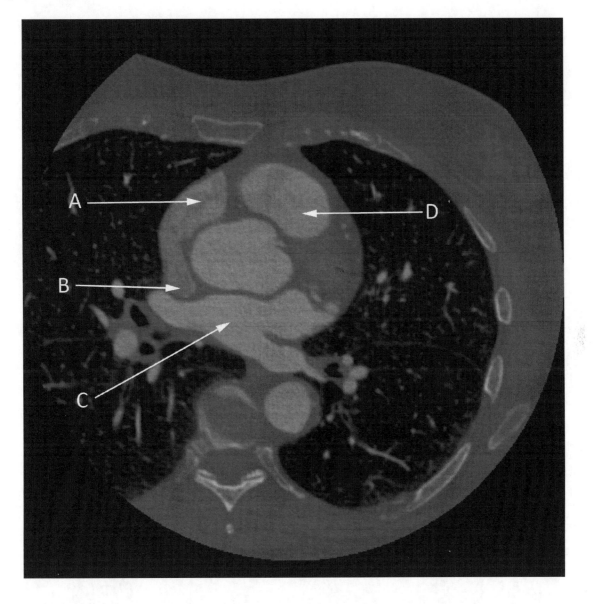

	QUESTION 10	WRITE YOUR ANSWER HERE
A	Name the structure labelled A	
B	Name the structure labelled B	
C	Name the structure labelled C	
D	Name the structure labelled D	
E	Which vessel arises from D?	

Question 11

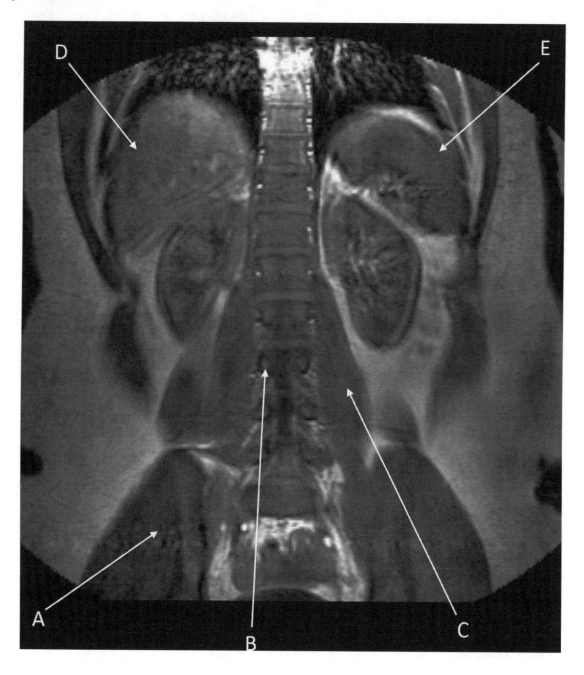

	QUESTION 11	WRITE YOUR ANSWER HERE
A	Name the structure labelled A	
B	Name the structure labelled B	
C	Name the structure labelled C	
D	Name the structure labelled D	
E	Name the structure labelled E	

Question 12

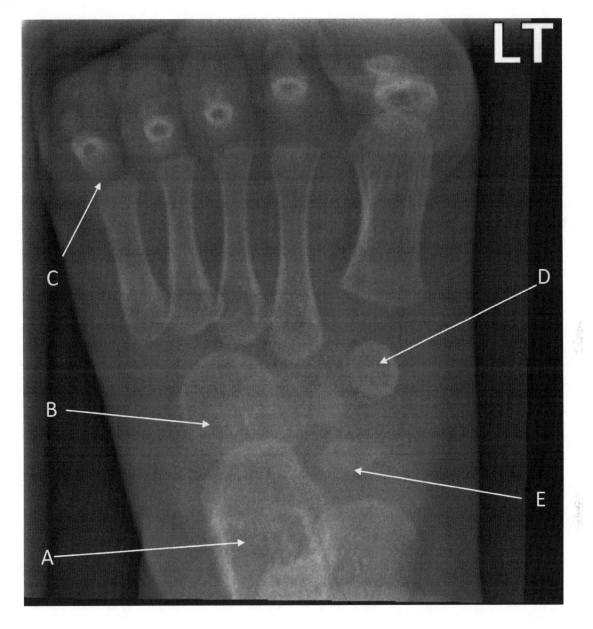

	QUESTION 12	WRITE YOUR ANSWER HERE
A	Name the structure labelled A	
B	Name the structure labelled B	
C	Name the structure labelled C	
D	Name the structure labelled D	
E	Name the structure labelled E	

Question 13

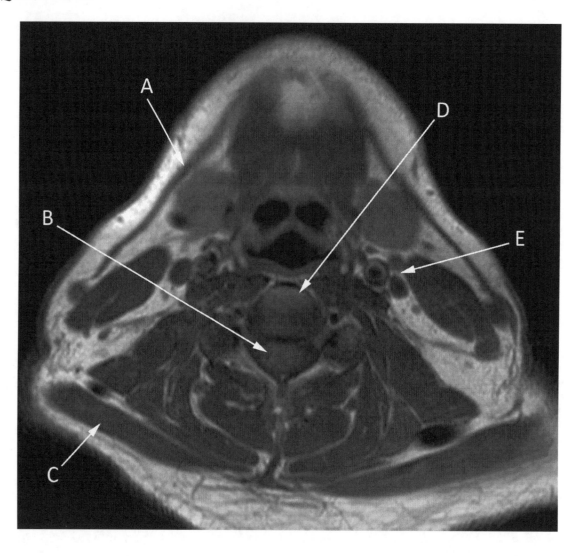

	QUESTION 13	WRITE YOUR ANSWER HERE
A	Name the structure labelled A	
B	Name the structure labelled B	
C	Name the structure labelled C	
D	Name the structure labelled D	
E	Name the space in which the vessels labelled E lie	

Question 14

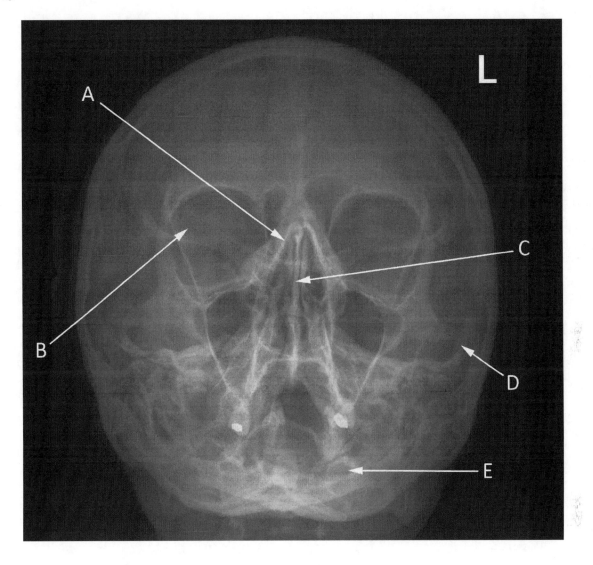

	QUESTION 14	WRITE YOUR ANSWER HERE
A	Name the structure labelled A	
B	Name the structure labelled B	
C	Name the structure labelled C	
D	Name the structure labelled D	
E	Name the structure labelled E	

Question 15

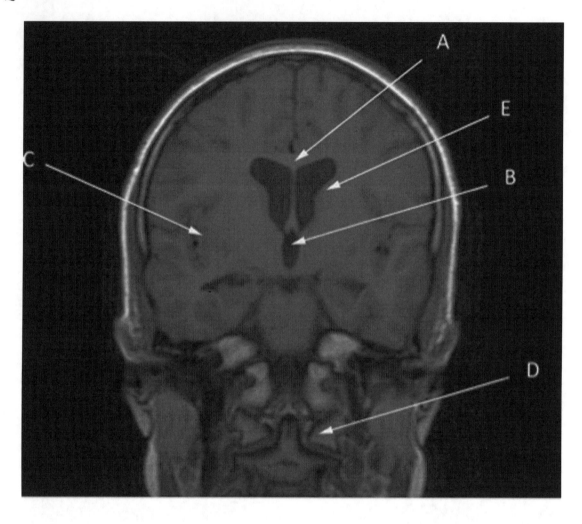

	QUESTION 15	WRITE YOUR ANSWER HERE
A	Name the structure labelled A	
B	Name the structure labelled B	
C	Name the structure labelled C	
D	Name the structure labelled D	
E	Name the structure labelled E	

Question 16

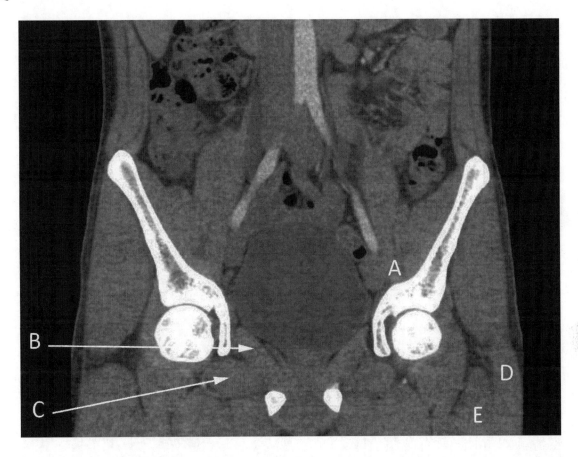

	QUESTION 16	WRITE YOUR ANSWER HERE
A	Name the structure labelled A	
B	Name the structure labelled B	
C	Name the structure labelled C	
D	Name the structure labelled D	
E	Name the structure labelled E	

Question 17

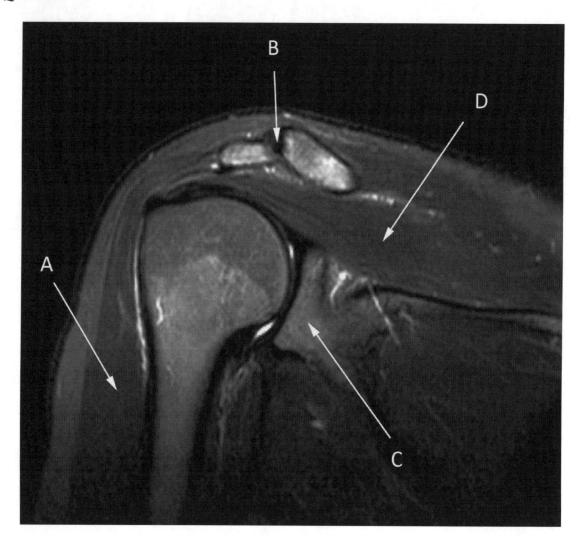

	QUESTION 17	WRITE YOUR ANSWER HERE
A	Name the structure labelled A	
B	Name the structure labelled B	
C	Name the structure labelled C	
D	Name the structure labelled D	
E	What is the distal attachment of D?	

Question 18

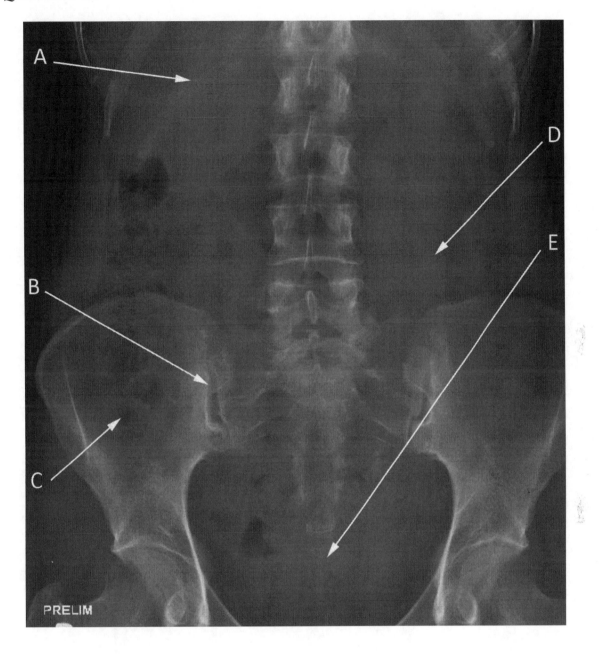

	QUESTION 18	WRITE YOUR ANSWER HERE
A	Name the structure labelled A	
B	Name the structure labelled B	
C	Name the structure labelled C	
D	Name the structure labelled D	
E	Name the structure labelled E	

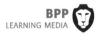

Question 19

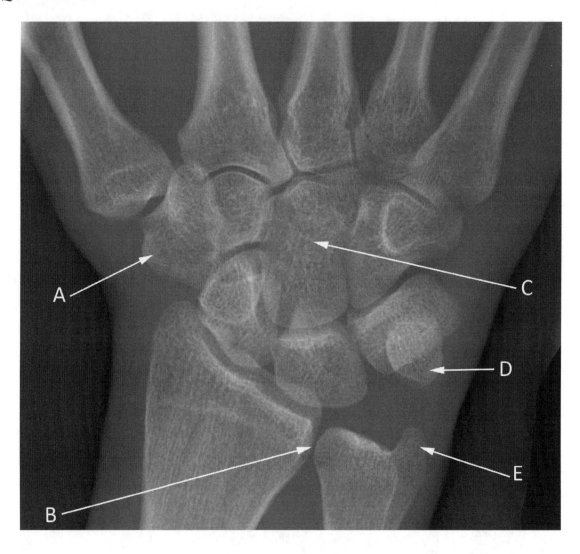

	QUESTION 19	WRITE YOUR ANSWER HERE
A	Name the structure labelled A	
B	Name the structure labelled B	
C	Name the structure labelled C	
D	Name the structure labelled D	
E	Name the structure labelled E	

Question 20

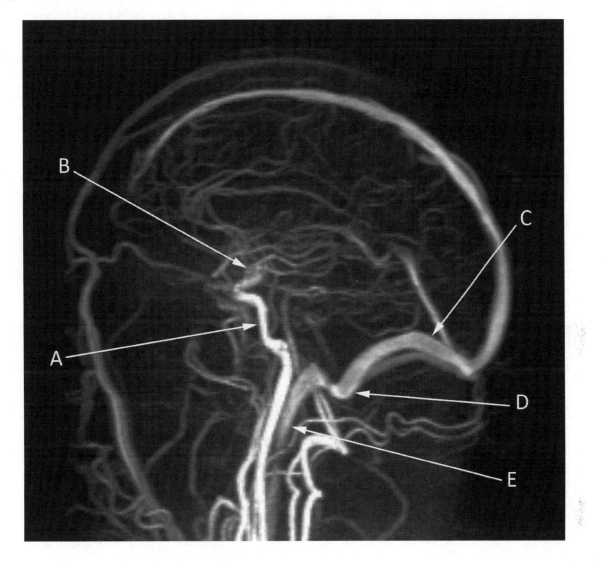

	QUESTION 20	WRITE YOUR ANSWER HERE
A	Name the structure labelled A	
B	Name the structure labelled B	
C	Name the structure labelled C	
D	Name the structure labelled D	
E	Name the structure labelled E	

Paper 12

Answers

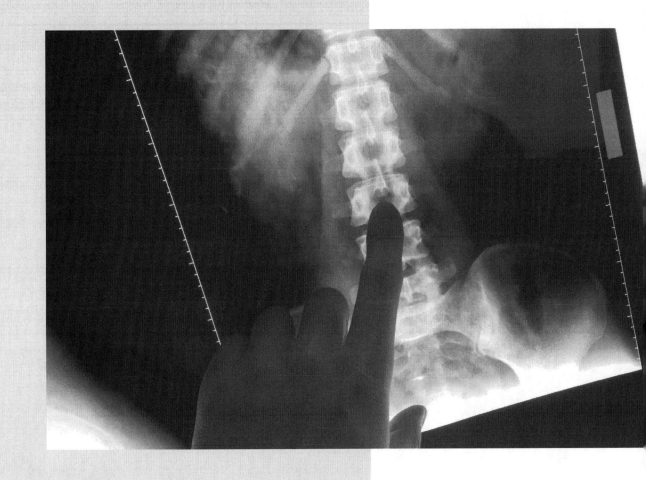

Question 1

A. Azygous vein
B. Interlobar artery
C. Left main bronchus
D. Left main pulmonary artery
E. Aorto-pulmonary window

Question 2

A. Growth centre for left medial epicondyle
B. Left ulna
C. Growth centre for left capitellum
D. Growth centre for left radial head
E. Left radius

Question 3

A. Body of pancreas
B. Descending colon
C. Tail of pancreas
D. Coeliac axis
E. Right crus of diaphragm

Question 4

A. Right ischioanal fossa
B. Left ischium
C. Left vastus lateralis muscle
D. Left biceps femoris muscle
E. Head of left fibula

Question 5

A. Azygous vein
B. Hemi-azygous vein
C. Coronary sinus
D. A (the azygous vein)
E. The right atrium

Question 6

A. Dome of left talus
B. Distal left tibia
C. Neck of left talus
D. Head of left talus
E. Left navicular

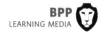

Question 7

A. Right lobe of liver
B. Inferior vena cava
C. Left psoas muscle
D. Left internal oblique muscle
E. Left external oblique muscle

Question 8

A. Pineal gland
B. Anterior limb of right internal capsule
C. Left caudate nucleus
D. Posterior limb of the left internal capsule
E. Left thalamus

Question 9

A. Left hepatic vein
B. Gallbladder
C. Common bile duct
D. Portal vein
E. 6mm

Question 10

A. Right atrial appendage
B. Superior vena cava
C. Left atrium
D. Right ventricular outflow tract
E. Main pulmonary artery

Question 11

A. Right gluteus maximus muscle
B. Right pedicle L3 vertebra
C. Left psoas muscle
D. Liver
E. Spleen

Question 12

A. Left calcaneus
B. Left cuboid
C. Metatarsophalangeal joint of the left fifth toe
D. Left medial cuneiform
E. Left navicular

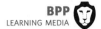

Question 13

A. Right platysma muscle
B. Spinal cord
C. Right trapezius muscle
D. Vertebral body
E. Carotid space

Question 14

A. Nasal bone
B. Body of sphenoid bone (right)
C. Bony nasal septum
D. Left zygomatic arch
E. Left lateral mass of C1

Question 15

A. Corpus callosum
B. Third ventricle
C. Right insula cortex
D. Left lateral mass of C1
E. Left caudate nucleus

Question 16

A. Left iliopsoas muscle
B. Right obturator internus muscle
C. Right obturator externus
D. Left gluteus maximus muscle
E. Left gluteus medius muscle

Question 17

A. Deltoid muscle
B. Acromioclavicular joint
C. Glenoid
D. Supraspinatus
E. Greater tubercle of humerus

Question 18

A. Right 12th rib
B. Right sacro-iliac joint
C. Gas in caecum
D. Left psoas muscle
E. Coccyx

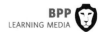

Question 19

A. Trapezium
B. Distal radioulnar joint
C. Capitate
D. Pisiform
E. Styloid process of ulna

Question 20

A. Internal carotid artery (right)
B. Cavernous sinus
C. Transverse sinus
D. Sigmoid sinus (right)
E. Internal jugular vein (right)

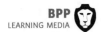

Paper 13

Question Bank

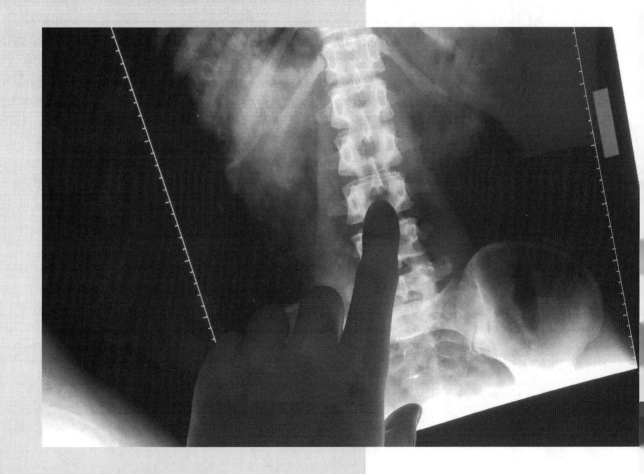

Question 1

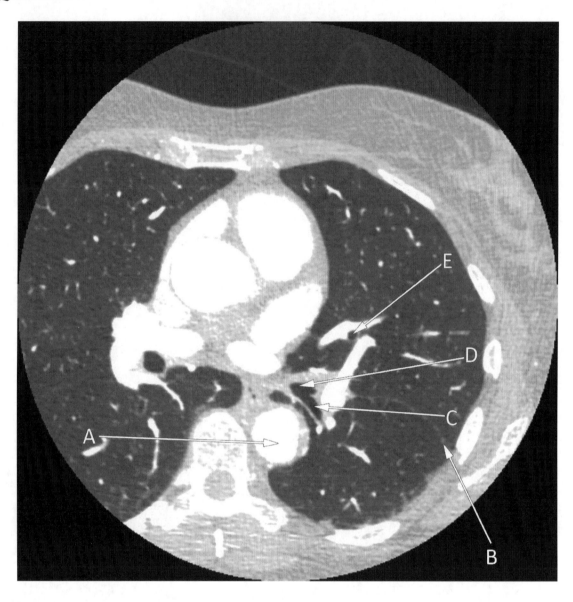

	QUESTION 1	WRITE YOUR ANSWER HERE
A	Name the structure labelled A	
B	Name the structure labelled B	
C	Name the structure labelled C	
D	Name the structure labelled D	
E	Name the structure labelled E	

Question 2

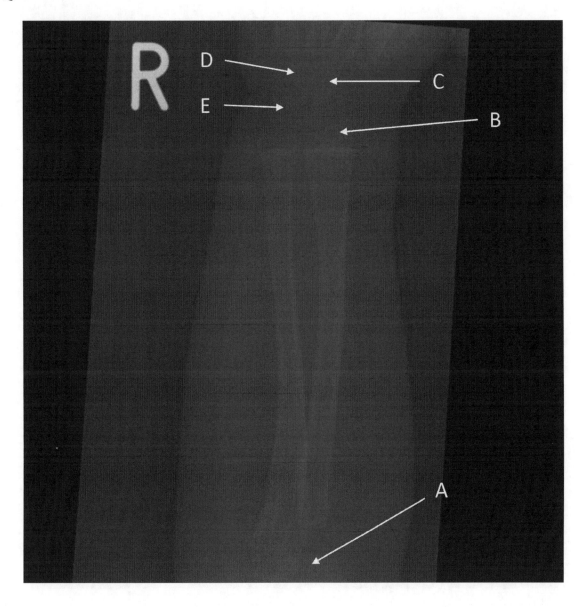

	QUESTION 2	WRITE YOUR ANSWER HERE
A	Name the structure labelled A	
B	Name the structure labelled B	
C	Name the structure labelled C	
D	Name the structure labelled D	
E	Name the structure labelled E	

Question 3

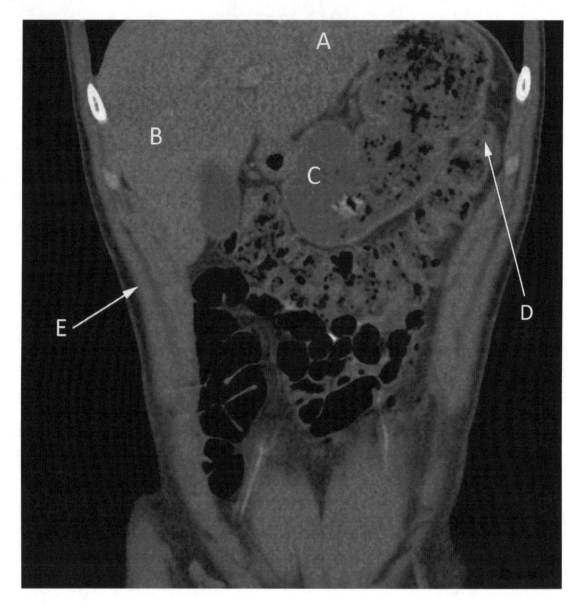

	QUESTION 3	WRITE YOUR ANSWER HERE
A	Name the structure labelled A	
B	Name the structure labelled B	
C	Name the structure labelled C	
D	Name the structure labelled D	
E	Name the structure labelled E	

Question 4

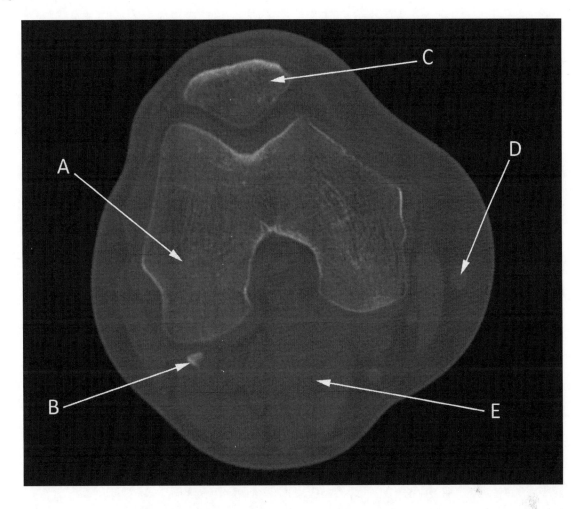

	QUESTION 4	WRITE YOUR ANSWER HERE
A	Name the structure labelled A	
B	Name the structure labelled B	
C	Name the structure labelled C	
D	Name the structure labelled D	
E	Name the structure labelled E	

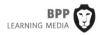

Question 5

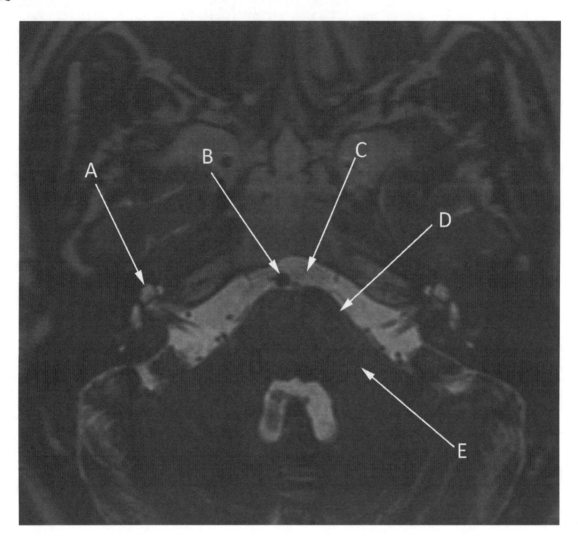

	QUESTION 5	WRITE YOUR ANSWER HERE
A	Name the structure labelled A	
B	Name the structure labelled B	
C	Name the structure labelled C	
D	Name the structure labelled D	
E	Name the structure labelled E	

Question 6

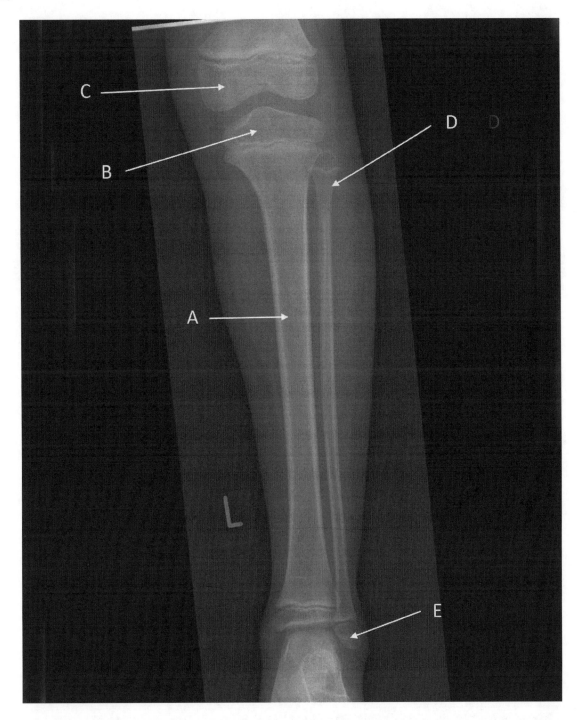

	QUESTION 6	WRITE YOUR ANSWER HERE
A	Name the structure labelled A	
B	Name the structure labelled B	
C	Name the structure labelled C	
D	Name the structure labelled D	
E	Name the structure labelled E	

BPP
LEARNING MEDIA

Question 7

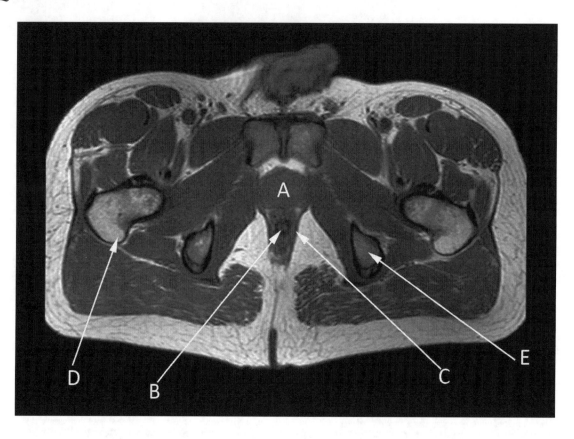

	QUESTION 7	WRITE YOUR ANSWER HERE
A	Name the structure labelled A	
B	Name the structure labelled B	
C	Name the structure labelled C	
D	Name the structure labelled D	
E	Name the structure labelled E	

Question 8

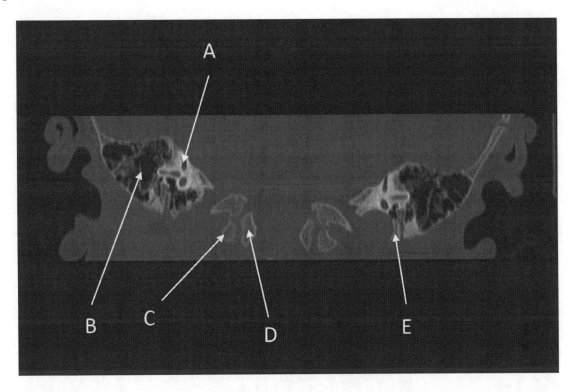

	QUESTION 8	WRITE YOUR ANSWER HERE
A	Name the structure labelled A	
B	Name the structure labelled B	
C	Name the structure labelled C	
D	Name the structure labelled D	
E	Name the structure labelled E	

Question 9

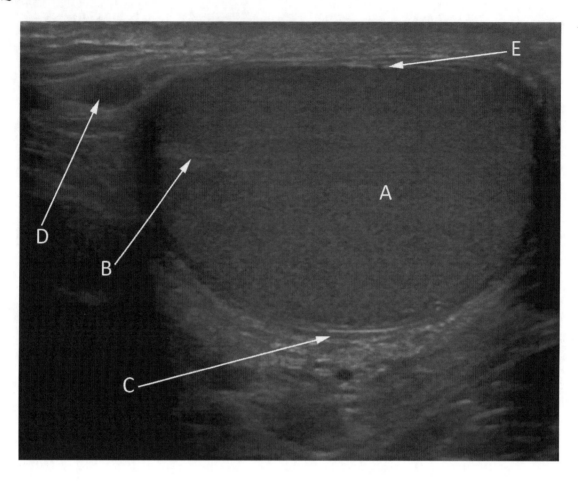

	QUESTION 9	WRITE YOUR ANSWER HERE
A	Name the structure labelled A	
B	Name the structure labelled B	
C	Name the structure labelled C	
D	Name the structure labelled D	
E	Name the structure labelled E	

Question 10

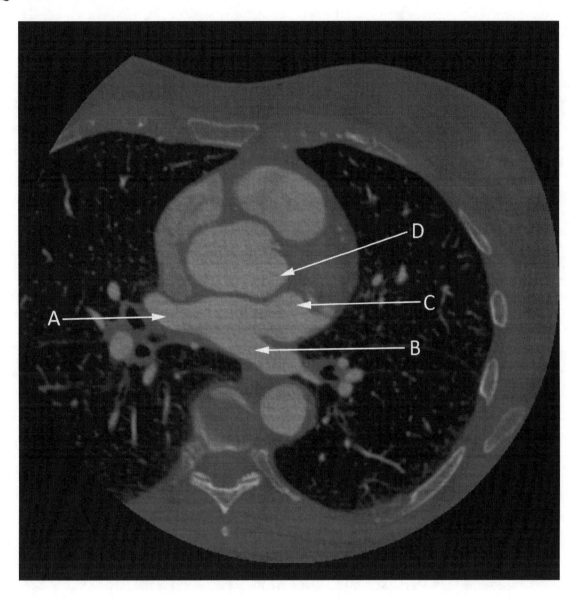

	QUESTION 10	WRITE YOUR ANSWER HERE
A	Name the structure labelled A	
B	Name the structure labelled B	
C	Name the structure labelled C	
D	Name the region of the aortic root labelled D	
E	What vessel arises from D?	

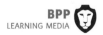

Question 11

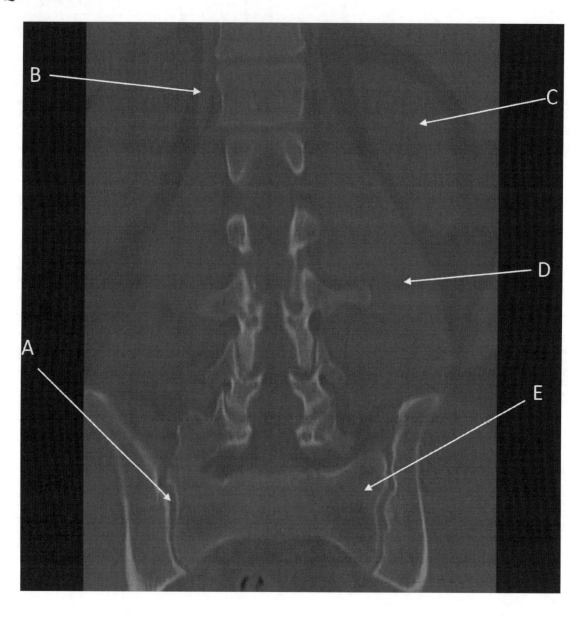

	QUESTION 11	WRITE YOUR ANSWER HERE
A	Name the structure labelled A	
B	Name the structure labelled B	
C	Name the structure labelled C	
D	Name the structure labelled D	
E	Name the structure labelled E	

Question 12

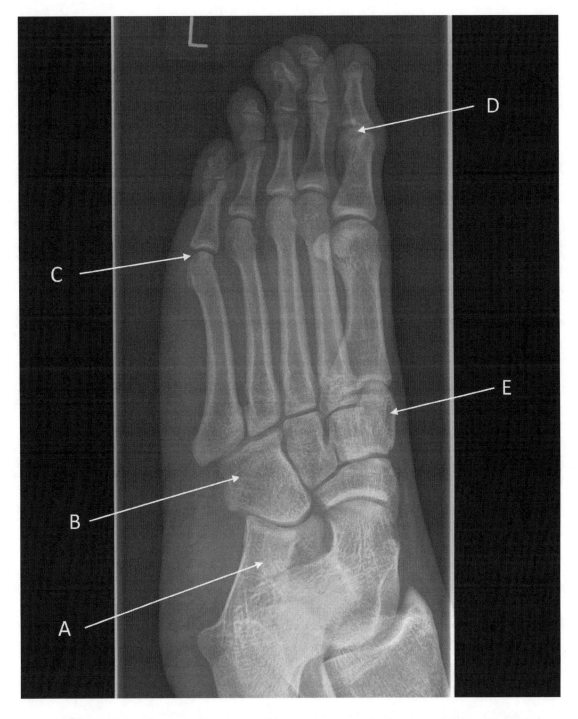

	QUESTION 12	WRITE YOUR ANSWER HERE
A	Name the structure labelled A	
B	Name the structure labelled B	
C	Name the structure labelled C	
D	Name the structure labelled D	
E	Name the structure labelled E	

Question 13

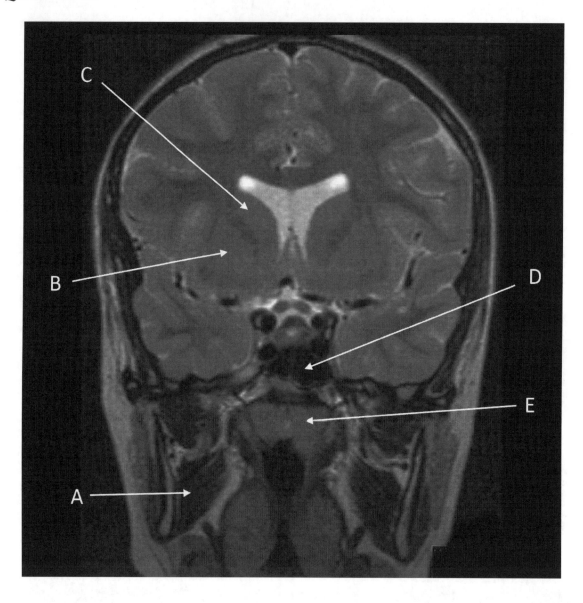

	QUESTION 13	WRITE YOUR ANSWER HERE
A	Name the structure labelled A	
B	Name the structure labelled B	
C	Name the structure labelled C	
D	Name the structure labelled D	
E	Name the structure labelled E	

Question 14

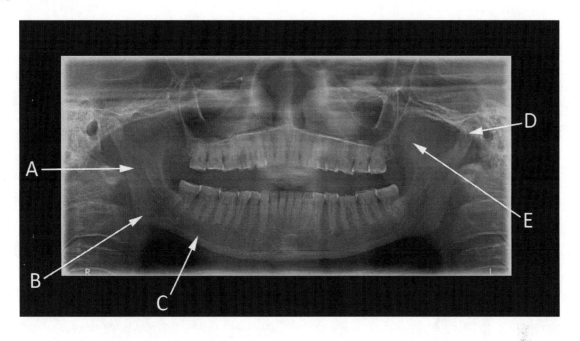

	QUESTION 14	WRITE YOUR ANSWER HERE
A	Name the structure labelled A	
B	Name the structure labelled B	
C	Name the structure labelled C	
D	Name the structure labelled D	
E	Name the structure labelled E	

Question 15

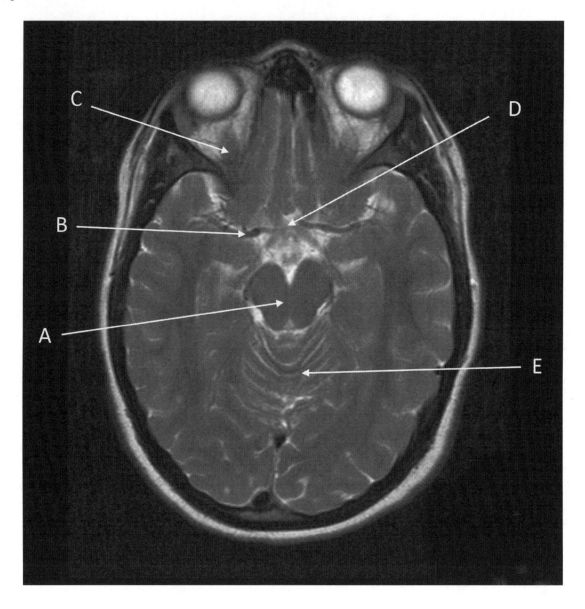

	QUESTION 15	WRITE YOUR ANSWER HERE
A	Name the structure labelled A	
B	Name the structure labelled B	
C	Name the structure labelled C	
D	Name the structure labelled D	
E	Name the structure labelled E	

Question 16

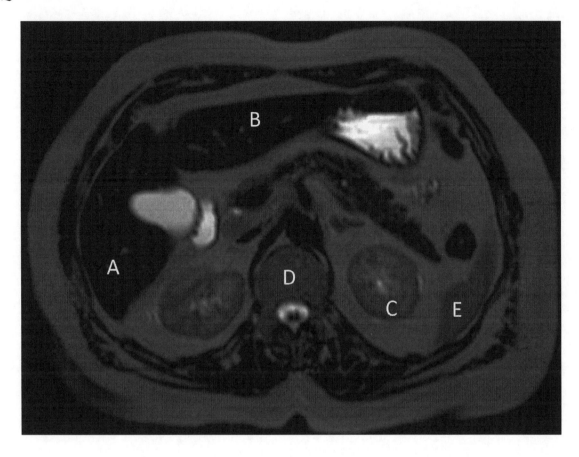

	QUESTION 16	WRITE YOUR ANSWER HERE
A	Name the structure labelled A	
B	Name the structure labelled B	
C	Name the structure labelled C	
D	Name the structure labelled D	
E	Name the structure labelled E	

Question 17

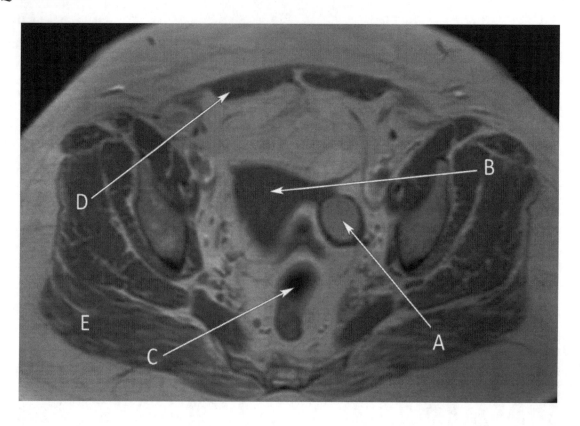

	QUESTION 17	WRITE YOUR ANSWER HERE
A	Name the structure labelled A	
B	Name the structure labelled B	
C	Name the structure labelled C	
D	Name the structure labelled D	
E	Name the structure labelled E	

Question 18

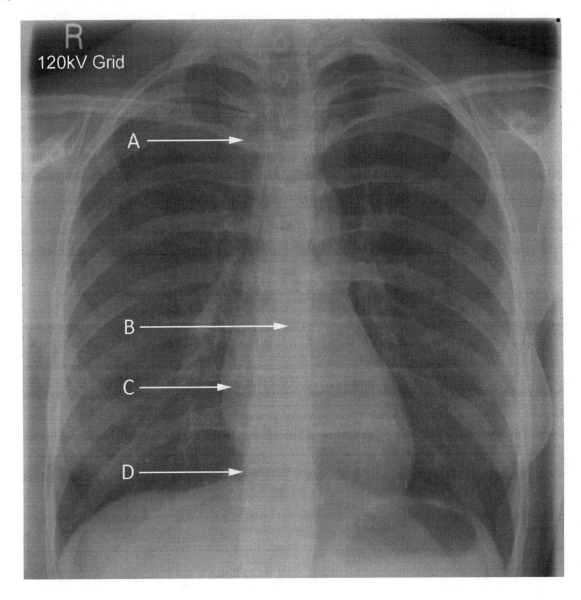

	QUESTION 18	WRITE YOUR ANSWER HERE
A	Name the vessel labelled A	
B	Name the chamber labelled B	
C	Name the chamber labelled C	
D	Name the vessel labelled D	
E	What vessels form structure A?	

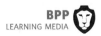

Question 19

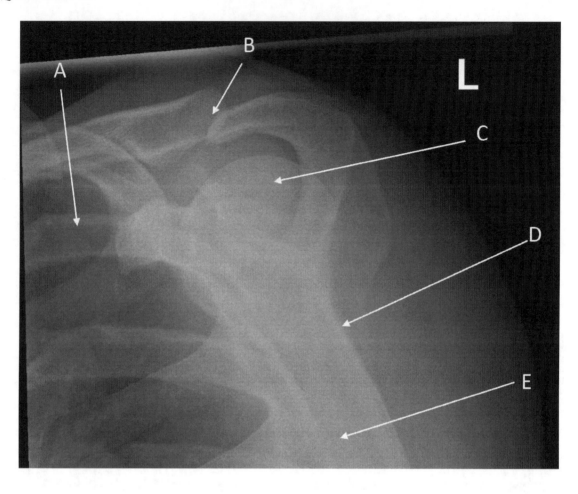

	QUESTION 19	WRITE YOUR ANSWER HERE
A	Name the structure labelled A	
B	Name the structure labelled B	
C	Name the structure labelled C	
D	Name the structure labelled D	
E	Name the structure labelled E	

Question 20

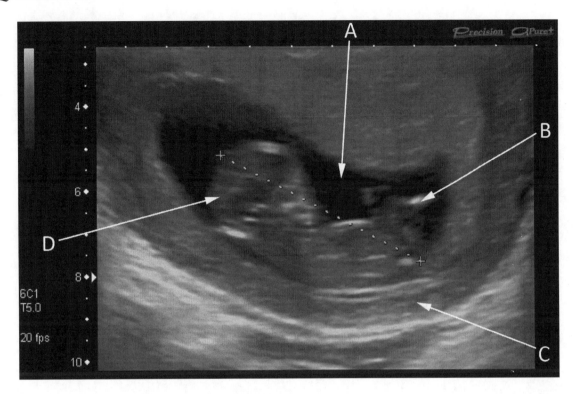

	QUESTION 20	WRITE YOUR ANSWER HERE
A	Name the structure labelled A	
B	Name the structure labelled B	
C	Name the structure labelled C	
D	Name the structure labelled D	
E	Name the measurement (dashed line)	

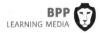

Paper 13

Answers

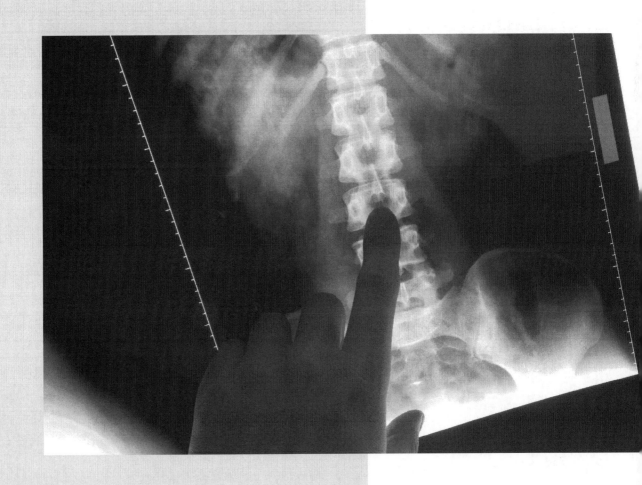

Question 1
A. Descending thoracic aorta
B. Left oblique fissure
C. Left lower lobe apical segmental bronchus
D. Left lower lobe bronchus
E. Lingula bronchus

Question 2
A. Epihpyseal centre of right capitellum
B. Distal epiphysis of right radius
C. Right capitate bone
D. Right hamate bone
E. Right triquetral bone

Question 3
A. Left lobe of liver
B. Right lobe of liver
C. Antrum of stomach
D. Splenic flexure
E. Right external oblique muscle

Question 4
A. Lateral condyle of femur
B. Fabella
C. Patella
D. Long saphenous vein
E. Medial head of gastrocnemius muscle

Question 5
A. Cochlea
B. Basilar artery
C. Pre-pontine cistern
D. Pons
E. Middle cerebellar peduncle

Question 6
A. Left tibial diaphysis
B. Proximal epiphysis of left tibia
C. Distal epiphysis of left femur
D. Left neck of fibula
E. Distal epiphysis of left fibula

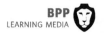

Question 7

A. Prostate
B. Anal canal
C. Levator ani muscle
D. Greater trochanter of right femur
E. Left ischial tuberosity

Question 8

A. Right superior semicircular canal
B. Right mastoid air cells
C. Right transverse process of C1
D. Right lateral mass of C1
E. Left styloid process

Question 9

A. Testis
B. Rete testis
C. Tunica albuginea
D. Head of epididymis
E. Tunica vaginalis

Question 10

A. Right superior pulmonary vein
B. Left superior pulmonary vein
C. Left atrial appendage
D. Left coronary sinus
E. Left coronary artery

Question 11

A. Right sacroiliac joint
B. Right crus of the diaphragm
C. Left kidney
D. Left psoas muscle
E. Left sacral ala

Question 12

A. Left calcaneus
B. Left cuboid
C. Metatarsophalangeal joint of the left fifth toe
D. Interphalangeal joint of the left great toe
E. Left medial cuneiform

Question 13
A. Right medial pterygoid muscle
B. Right putamen
C. Right caudate nucleus
D. Left sphenoid sinus
E. Body of C1 vertebra

Question 14
A. Right ramus of mandible
B. Right angle of mandible
C. Right body of mandible
D. Left condyle of mandible
E. Left coronoid process of mandible

Question 15
A. Midbrain
B. Right middle cerebral artery
C. Right optic nerve
D. Optic chiasm
E. Folia of cerebellum

Question 16
A. Right lobe of liver
B. Left lobe of liver
C. Left kidney
D. Vertebral body
E. Spleen

Question 17
A. Left ovary
B. Uterus
C. Rectum
D. Right rectus abdominis muscle
E. Right gluteus maximus muscle

Question 18
A. Right brachiocephalic vein
B. Left atrium
C. Right atrium
D. Inferior vena cava
E. Right internal jugular vein, right subclavian vein

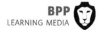

Question 19

A. Left sided rib
B. Left acromioclavicular joint
C. Left humeral head
D. Spine of left scapula
E. Left humerus

Question 20

A. Amniotic fluid
B. Umbilical cord
C. Uterine myometrium
D. Foetal head
E. Crown rump length

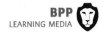

Paper 14

Question Bank

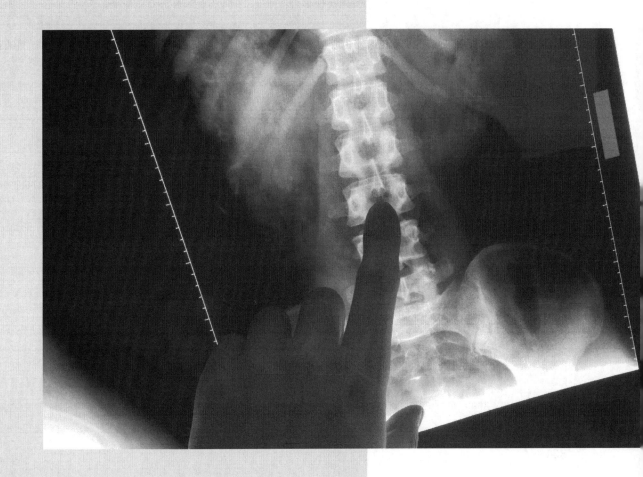

Question 1

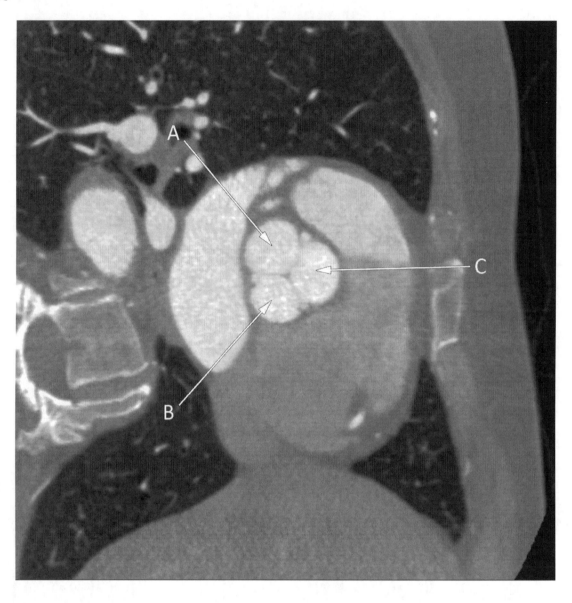

	QUESTION 1	WRITE YOUR ANSWER HERE
A	Name the structure labelled A	
B	Name the structure labelled B	
C	Name the structure labelled C	
D	What valve is represented in the image?	
E	How many leaflets does the valve normally have?	

Question 2

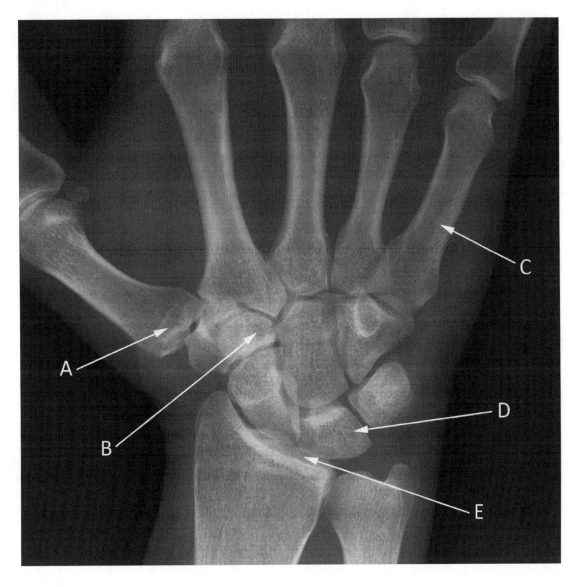

	QUESTION 2	WRITE YOUR ANSWER HERE
A	Name the structure labelled A	
B	Name the structure labelled B	
C	Name the structure labelled C	
D	Name the structure labelled D	
E	Name the structure labelled E	

Question 3

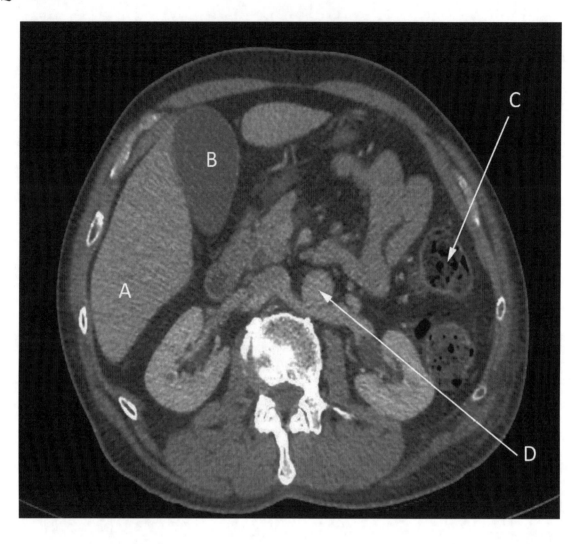

	QUESTION 3	WRITE YOUR ANSWER HERE
A	Name the structure labelled A	
B	Name the structure labelled B	
C	Name the structure labelled C	
D	Name the structure labelled D	
E	Name the anatomical variant depicted on the image	

Question 4

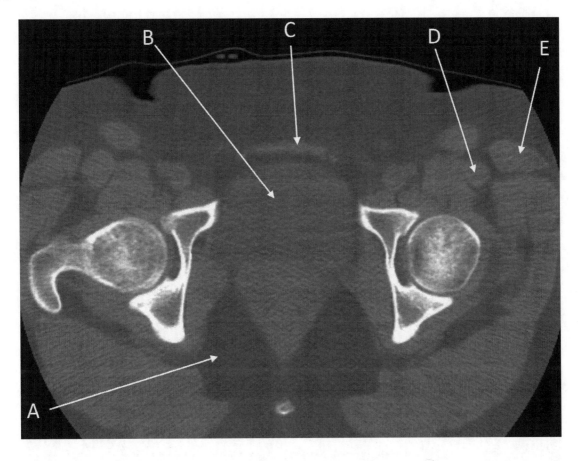

	QUESTION 4	WRITE YOUR ANSWER HERE
A	Name the structure labelled A	
B	Name the structure labelled B	
C	Name the structure labelled C	
D	Name the structure labelled D	
E	Name the structure labelled E	

Question 5

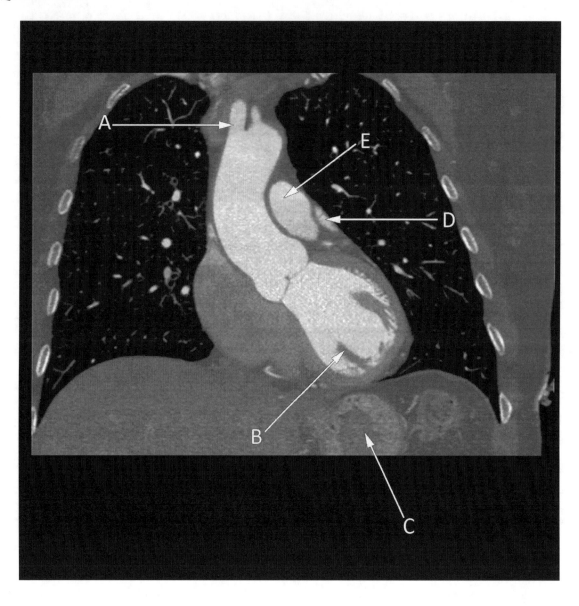

	QUESTION 5	WRITE YOUR ANSWER HERE
A	Name the structure labelled A	
B	Name the structure labelled B	
C	Name the structure labelled C	
D	Name the structure labelled D	
E	Name the structure labelled E	

Question 6

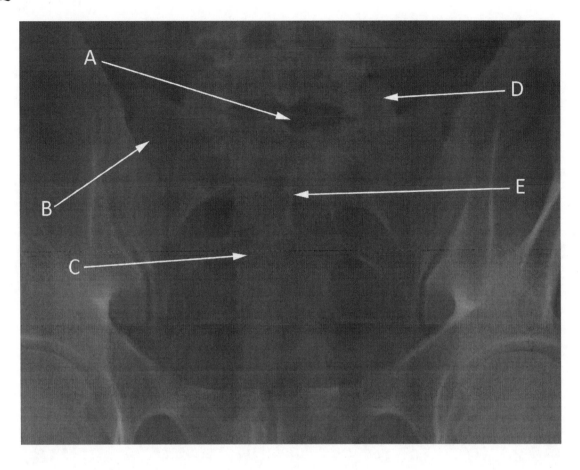

	QUESTION 6	WRITE YOUR ANSWER HERE
A	Name the structure labelled A	
B	Name the structure labelled B	
C	Name the structure labelled C	
D	Name the structure labelled D	
E	Name the structure labelled E	

Question 7

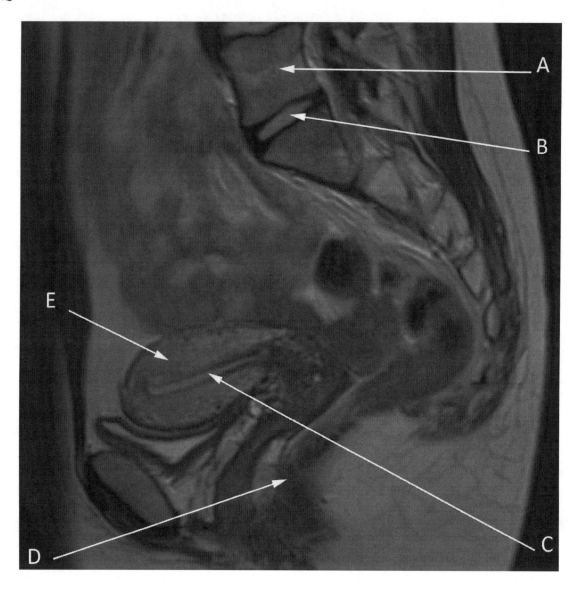

	QUESTION 7	WRITE YOUR ANSWER HERE
A	Name the structure labelled A	
B	Name the structure labelled B	
C	Name the structure labelled C	
D	Name the structure labelled D	
E	Name the structure labelled E	

Question 8

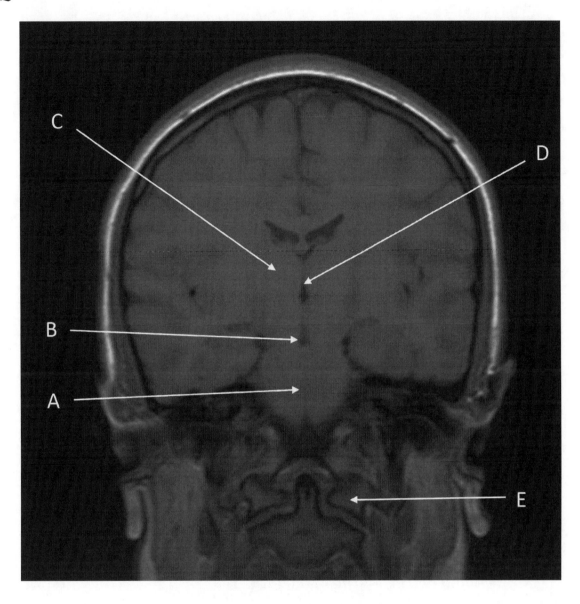

	QUESTION 8	WRITE YOUR ANSWER HERE
A	Name the structure labelled A	
B	Name the structure labelled B	
C	Name the structure labelled C	
D	Name the structure labelled D	
E	Name the structure labelled E	

Question 9

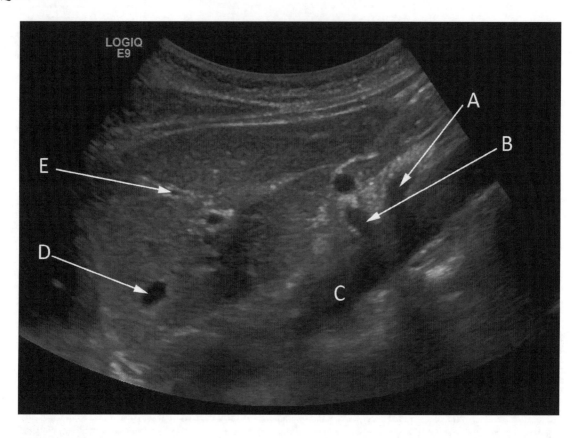

	QUESTION 9	WRITE YOUR ANSWER HERE
A	Name the structure labelled A	
B	Name the structure labelled B	
C	Name the structure labelled C	
D	Name the structure labelled D	
E	Name the structure labelled E	

Question 10

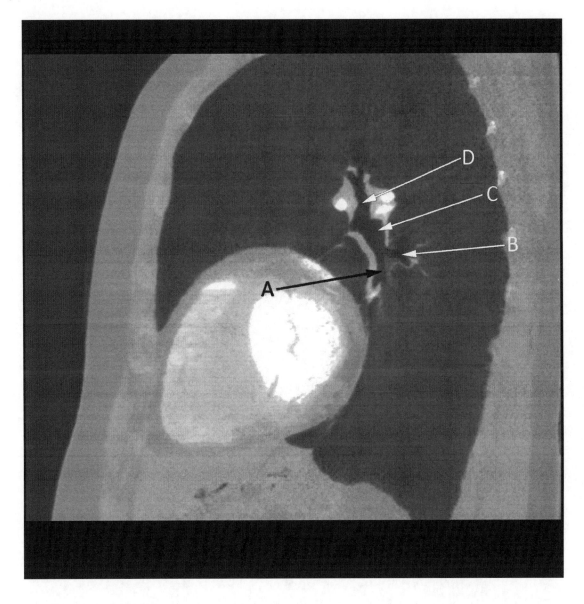

	QUESTION 10	WRITE YOUR ANSWER HERE
A	How many segments will arise from A?	
B	Name the segmental bronchus B	
C	Name the lobar bronchus labelled C	
D	Name the lobar bronchus labelled D	
E	Name the segmental bronchi arising from D	

Question 11

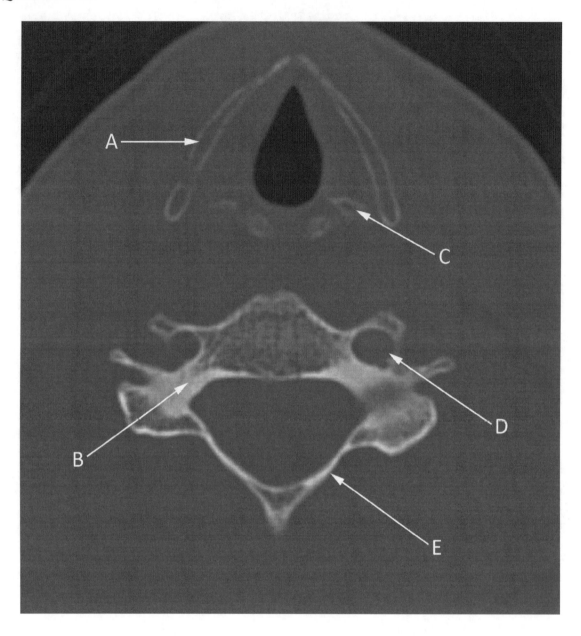

	QUESTION 11	WRITE YOUR ANSWER HERE
A	Name the structure labelled A	
B	Name the structure labelled B	
C	Name the structure labelled C	
D	Name the structure labelled D	
E	Name the structure labelled E	

Question 12

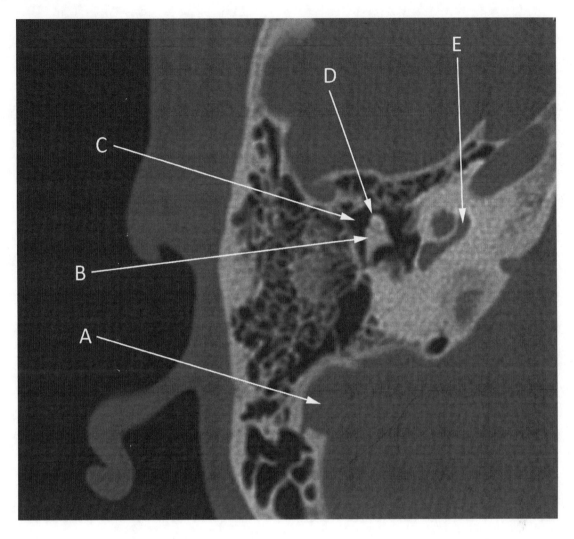

	QUESTION 12	WRITE YOUR ANSWER HERE
A	Name the structure labelled A	
B	Name the structure labelled B	
C	Name the structure labelled C	
D	Name the structure labelled D	
E	Name the structure labelled E	

Question 13

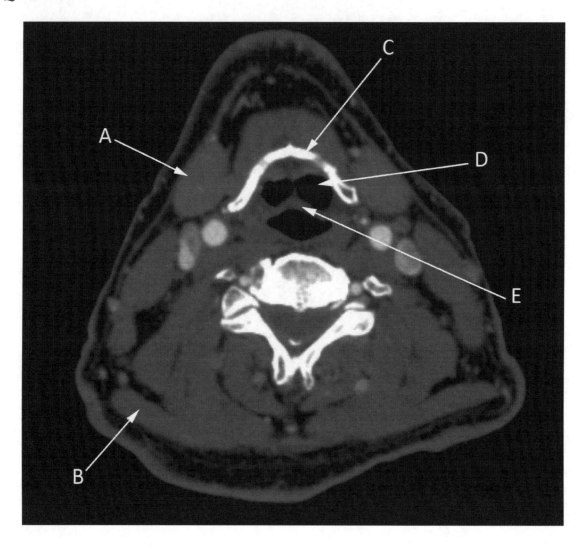

	QUESTION 13	WRITE YOUR ANSWER HERE
A	Name the structure labelled A	
B	Name the structure labelled B	
C	Name the structure labelled C	
D	Name the structure labelled D	
E	Name the structure labelled E	

Question 14

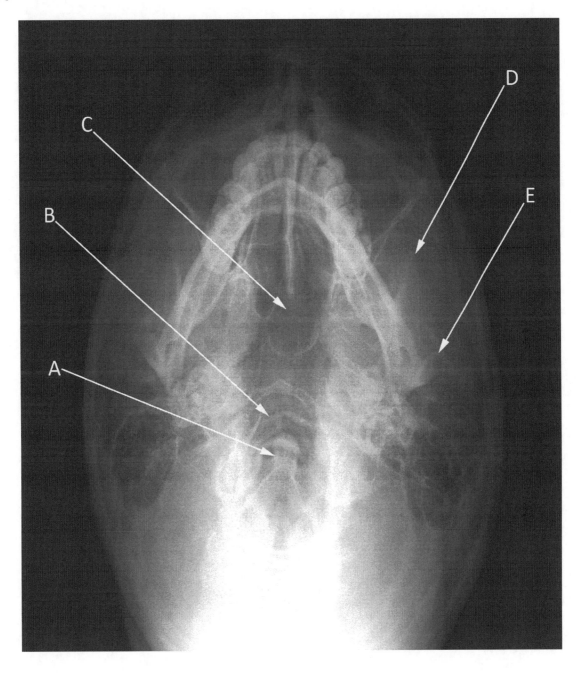

	QUESTION 14	WRITE YOUR ANSWER HERE
A	Name the structure labelled A	
B	Name the structure labelled B	
C	Name the structure labelled C	
D	Name the structure labelled D	
E	Name the structure labelled E	

Question 15

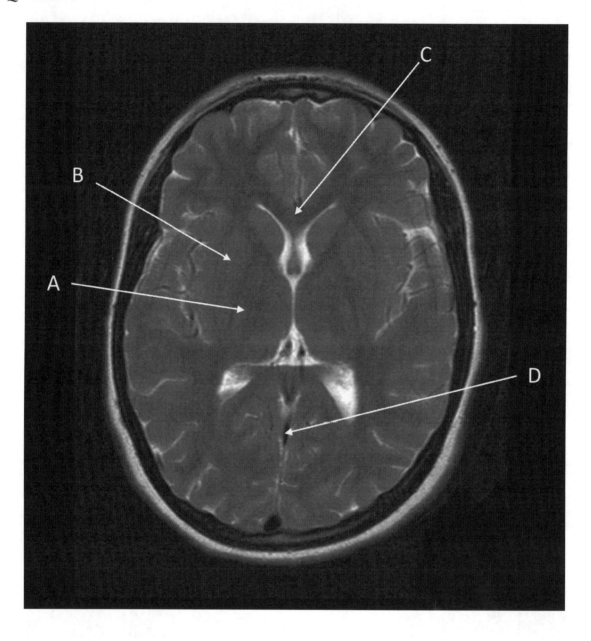

	QUESTION 15	WRITE YOUR ANSWER HERE
A	Name the structure labelled A	
B	Name the structure labelled B	
C	Name the structure labelled C	
D	Name the structure labelled D	
E	What does D drain into?	

Question 16

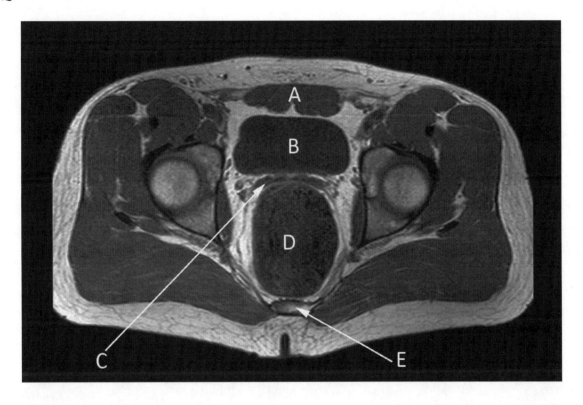

	QUESTION 16	WRITE YOUR ANSWER HERE
A	Name the structure labelled A	
B	Name the structure labelled B	
C	Name the structure labelled C	
D	Name the structure labelled D	
E	Name the structure labelled E	

Question 17

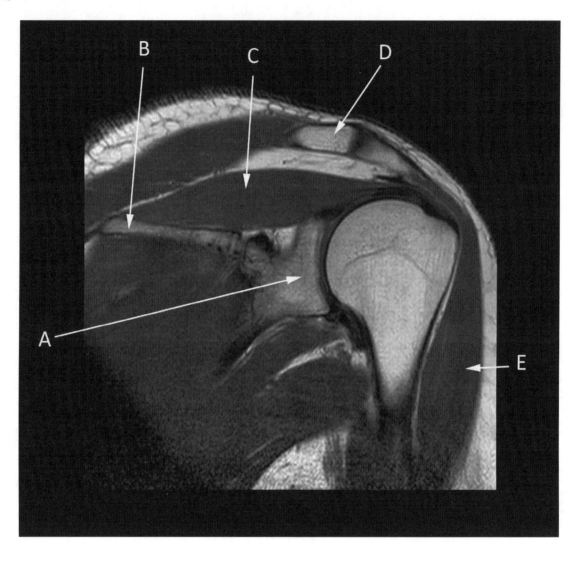

	QUESTION 17	WRITE YOUR ANSWER HERE
A	Name the structure labelled A	
B	Name the structure labelled B	
C	Name the structure labelled C	
D	Name the structure labelled D	
E	Name the structure labelled E	

Question 18

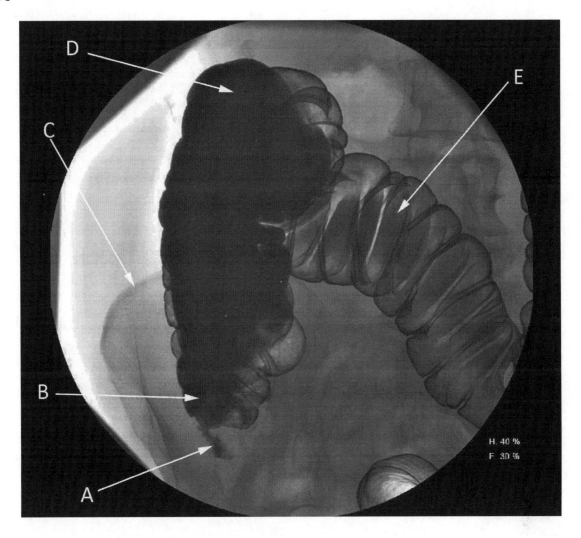

	QUESTION 18	WRITE YOUR ANSWER HERE
A	Name the structure labelled A	
B	Name the structure labelled B	
C	Name the structure labelled C	
D	Name the structure labelled D	
E	Name the structure labelled E	

Question 19

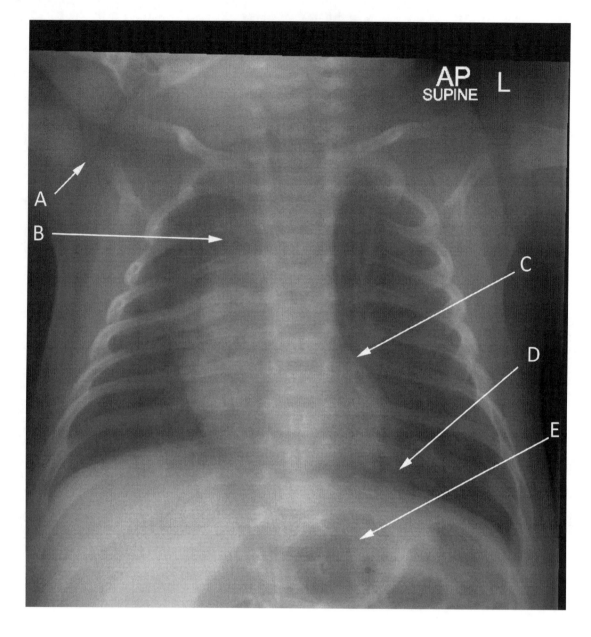

	QUESTION 19	WRITE YOUR ANSWER HERE
A	Name the structure labelled A	
B	Name the structure labelled B	
C	Name the structure labelled C	
D	Name the structure labelled D	
E	Name the structure labelled E	

Question 20

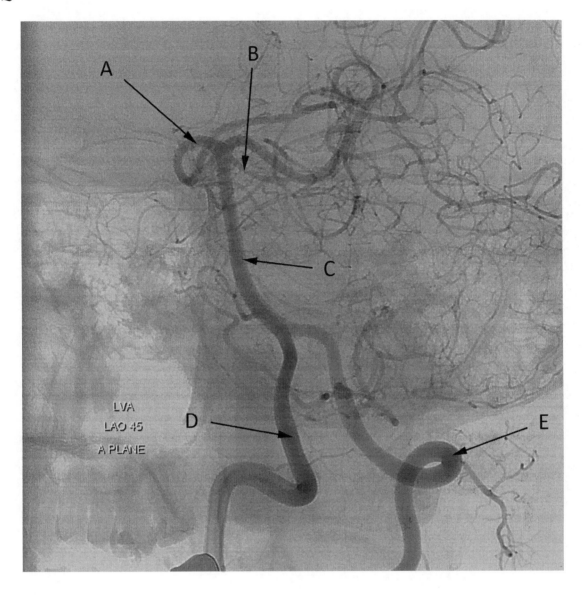

	QUESTION 20	WRITE YOUR ANSWER HERE
A	Name the structure labelled A	
B	Name the structure labelled B	
C	Name the structure labelled C	
D	Name the structure labelled D	
E	What bony structure is E exiting?	

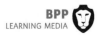

Paper 14

Answers

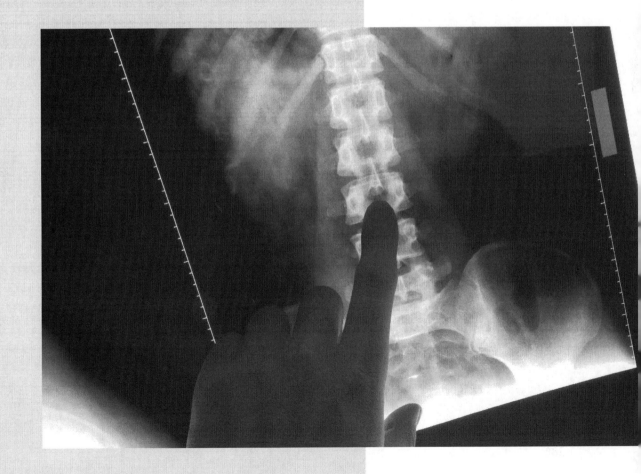

Question 1

A. Left coronary sinus
B. Non coronary Sinus
C. Right coronary Sinus
D. Aortic valve
E. Three

Question 2

A. Base of first metacarpal
B. Trapezoid
C. Shaft of fifth metacarpal
D. Lunate
E. Articular surface of distal radius

Question 3

A. Right lobe of liver
B. Gallbladder
C. Large bowel
D. Aorta
E. Retro-aortic left renal vein

Question 4

A. Right ischioanal fossa
B. Urinary bladder
C. Rectus abdominis muscle
D. Left rectus femoris muscle
E. Left tensor fascia latae muscle

Question 5

A. Brachiocephalic artery
B. Inferior papillary muscle
C. Stomach
D. Left atrial appendage
E. Main pulmonary artery

Question 6

A. L5/S1 intervertebral disc space
B. Right sacral ala
C. Right intermediate sacral crest
D. Left superior articular process
E. Median sacral crest

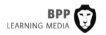

Question 7

A. L5 vertebral body
B. L5/S1 intervertebral disc
C. Endometrium
D. Anal canal
E. Myometrium

Question 8

A. Pons
B. Interpeduncular cistern
C. Right thalamus
D. Third ventricle
E. Left lateral mass of C1

Question 9

A. Superior mesenteric artery
B. Coeliac axis
C. Abdominal aorta
D. Branch of hepatic vein
E. Branch of portal vein

Question 10

A. Four: medial, lateral, posterior and anterior basal segemental bronchi
B. Apical segment of the left lower lobe
C. Left lower lobe bronchus
D. Left upper lobe bronchus
E. Left upper lobe anterior and apico-posterior segmental bronchi

Question 11

A. Thyroid cartilage
B. Pedicle
C. Cricoid cartilage
D. Transverse foramen
E. Lamina

Question 12

A. Sigmoid sinus
B. Incus
C. Prussak's space
D. Head of the malleus
E. Cochlea (basal turn)

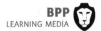

Question 13

A. Right submandibular gland
B. Right trapezius muscle
C. Hyoid bone
D. Left vallecula
E. Epiglottis

Question 14

A. Odontoid peg
B. Anterior arch of atlas
C. Sphenoid sinus
D. Left coronoid process of the mandible
E. Left condyle of the mandible

Question 15

A. Right globus pallidus
B. Right putamen
C. Genu of corpus callosum
D. Straight sinus
E. Transverse sinus

Question 16

A. Rectus abdominis muscle
B. Bladder
C. Seminal vesicle
D. Rectum
E. Coccyx

Question 17

A. Glenoid of scapula
B. Spine of scapula
C. Supraspinatus muscle
D. Clavicle
E. Deltoid muscle

Question 18

A. Appendix
B. Caecum / caecal pole
C. Right iliac crest
D. Hepatic flexure
E. Transverse colon

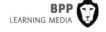

Question 19

A. Growth centre for head of right humerus
B. Thymus
C. Border of left atrial appendage
D. Left cardio-phrenic angle
E. Gastric bubble

Question 20

A. Posterior cerebral artery
B. Superior cerebellar artery
C. Basilar artery
D. Vertebral artery
E. Transverse foramen of atlas

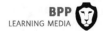

Paper 15

Question Bank

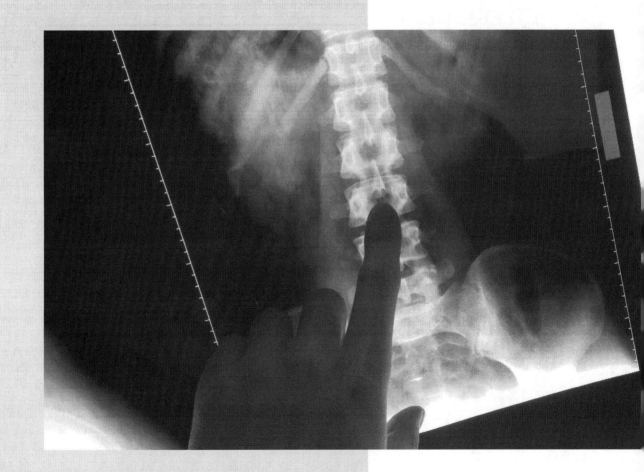

Question 1

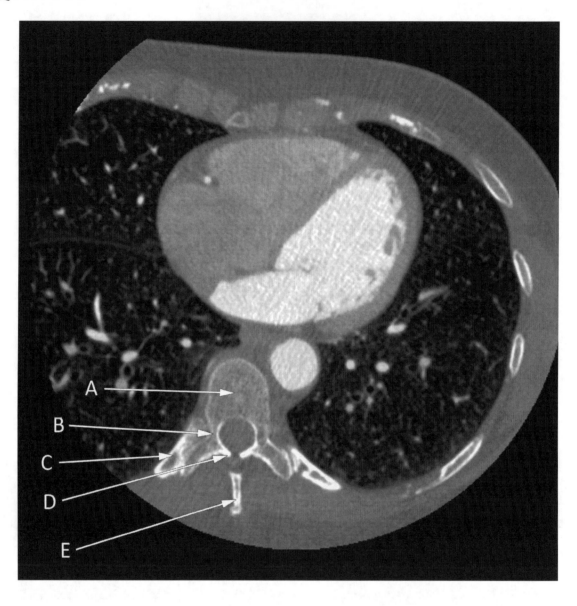

	QUESTION 1	WRITE YOUR ANSWER HERE
A	Name the structure labelled A	
B	Name the structure labelled B	
C	Name the structure labelled C	
D	Name the structure labelled D	
E	Name the structure labelled E	

Question 2

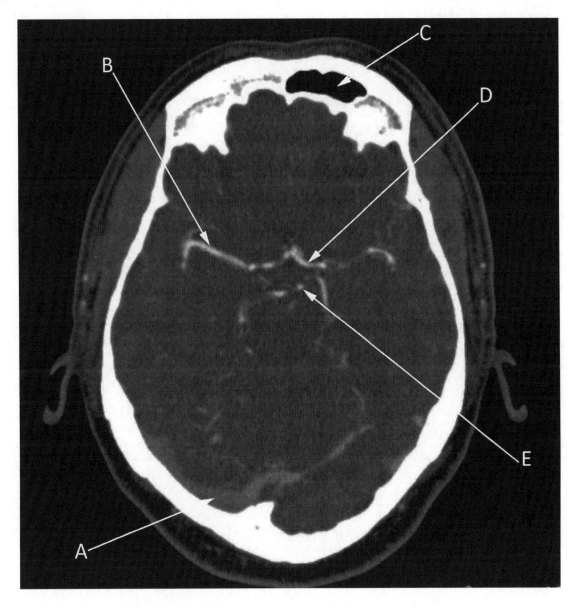

	QUESTION 2	WRITE YOUR ANSWER HERE
A	Name the structure labelled A	
B	Name the structure labelled B	
C	Name the structure labelled C	
D	Name the structure labelled D	
E	Name the structure labelled E	

Question 3

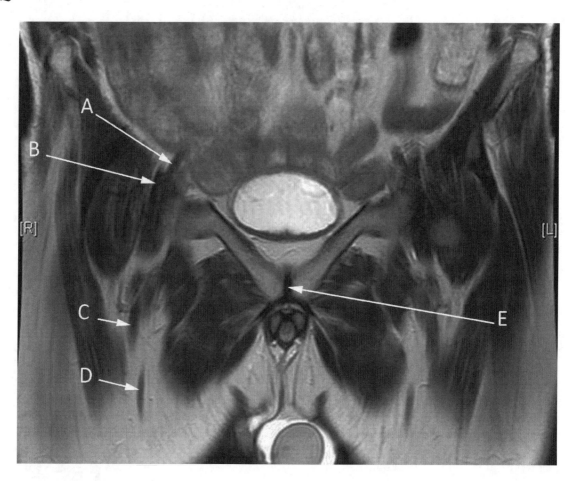

	QUESTION 3	WRITE YOUR ANSWER HERE
A	Name the structure labelled A	
B	Name the structure labelled B	
C	Name the structure labelled C	
D	Name the structure labelled D	
E	Name the structure labelled E	

Question 4

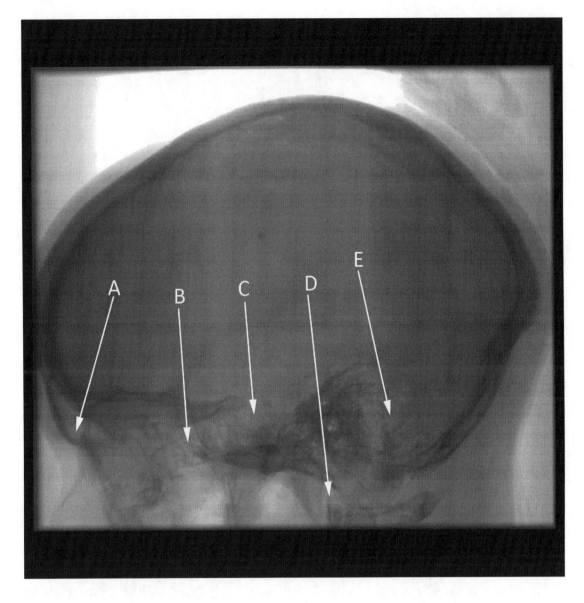

	QUESTION 4	WRITE YOUR ANSWER HERE
A	Name the structure labelled A	
B	Name the structure labelled B	
C	Name the structure labelled C	
D	Name the structure labelled D	
E	Name the structure labelled E	

Question 5

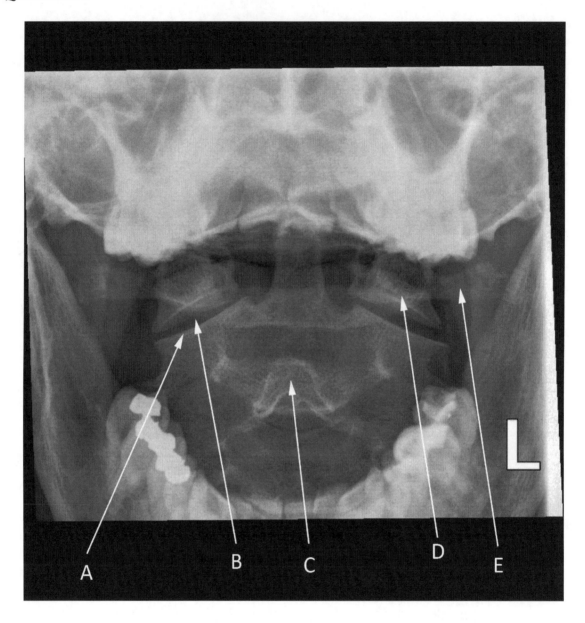

	QUESTION 5	WRITE YOUR ANSWER HERE
A	Name the structure labelled A	
B	Name the structure labelled B	
C	Name the structure labelled C	
D	Name the structure labelled D	
E	Name the structure labelled E	

Question 6

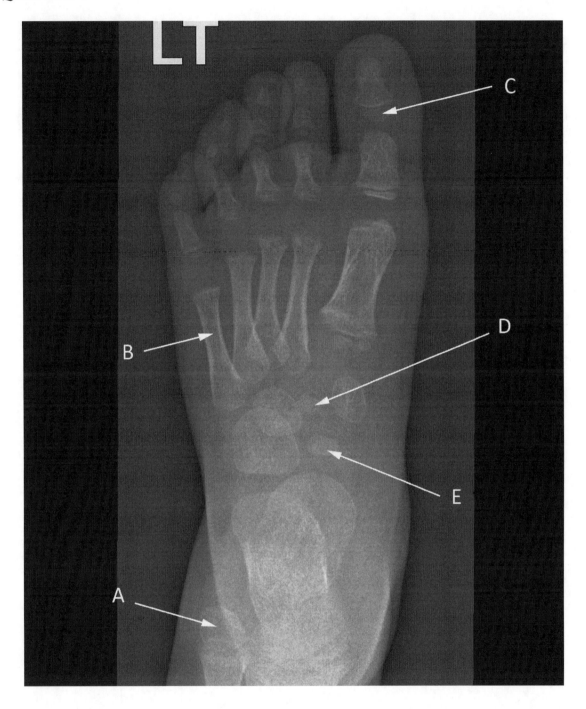

	QUESTION 6	WRITE YOUR ANSWER HERE
A	Name the structure labelled A	
B	Name the structure labelled B	
C	Name the structure labelled C	
D	Name the structure labelled D	
E	Name the structure labelled E	

Question 7

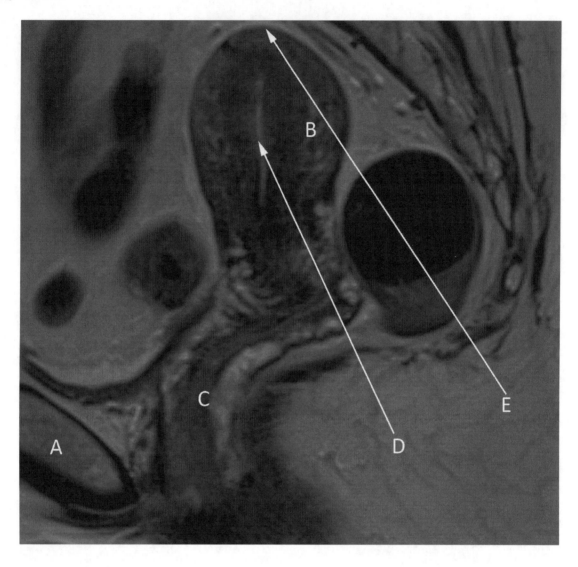

	QUESTION 7	WRITE YOUR ANSWER HERE
A	Name the structure labelled A	
B	Name the structure labelled B	
C	Name the structure labelled C	
D	Name the structure labelled D	
E	Name the structure labelled E	

Question 8

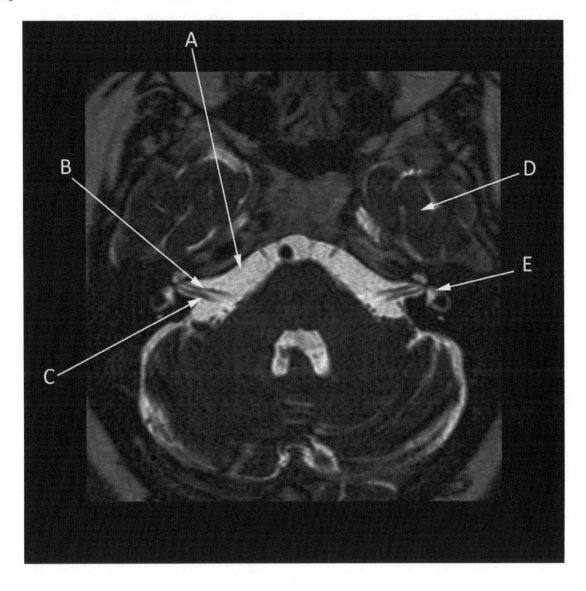

	QUESTION 8	WRITE YOUR ANSWER HERE
A	Name the structure labelled A	
B	Name the structure labelled B	
C	Name the structure labelled C	
D	Name the structure labelled D	
E	Name the structure labelled E	

Question 9

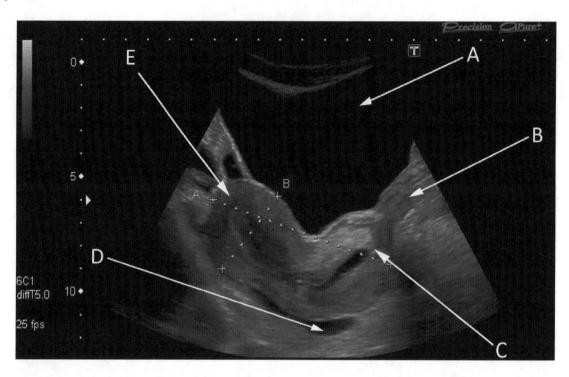

	QUESTION 9	WRITE YOUR ANSWER HERE
A	Name the structure labelled A	
B	Name the structure labelled B	
C	Name the structure labelled C	
D	Name the structure labelled D	
E	Name the structure labelled E	

Question 10

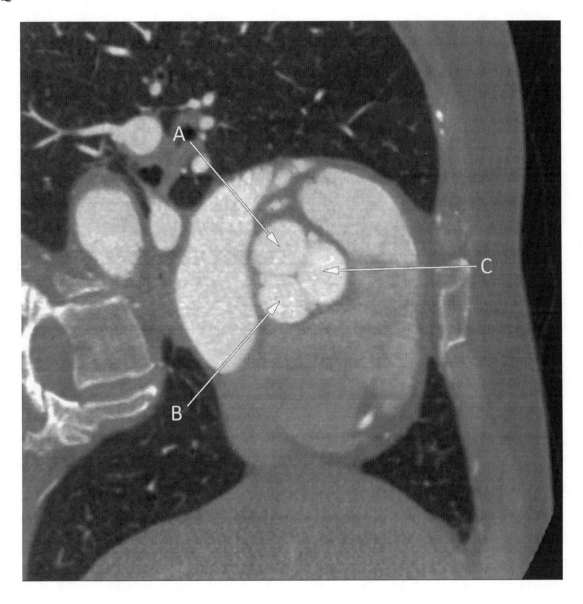

	QUESTION 10	WRITE YOUR ANSWER HERE
A	What coronary artery arises from A?	
B	What coronary artery arises from B?	
C	What coronary artery arises from C?	
D	What do A, B and C form?	
E	Name the anatomical junction just distal to A, B and C	

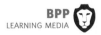

Question 11

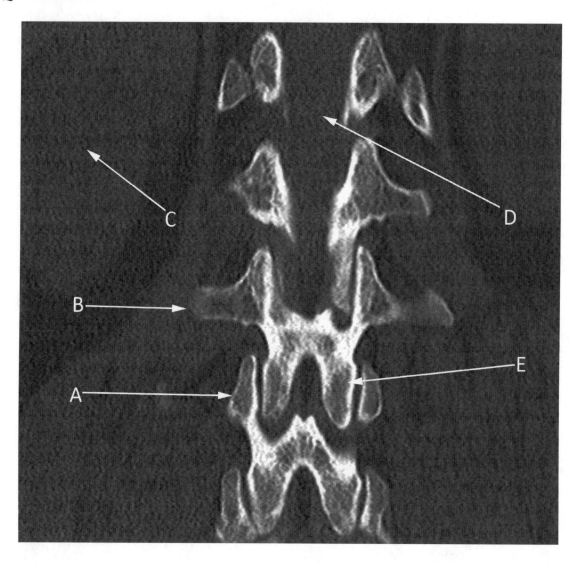

	QUESTION 11	WRITE YOUR ANSWER HERE
A	Name the structure labelled A	
B	Name the structure labelled B	
C	Name the structure labelled C	
D	Name the structure labelled D	
E	Name the structure labelled E	

Question 12

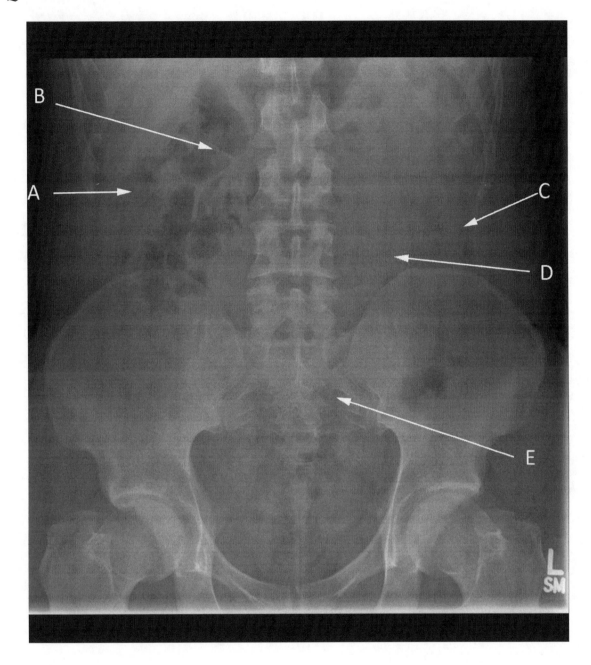

	QUESTION 12	WRITE YOUR ANSWER HERE
A	Name the structure labelled A	
B	Name the structure labelled B	
C	Name the structure labelled C	
D	Name the structure labelled D	
E	Name the structure labelled E	

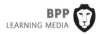

Question 13

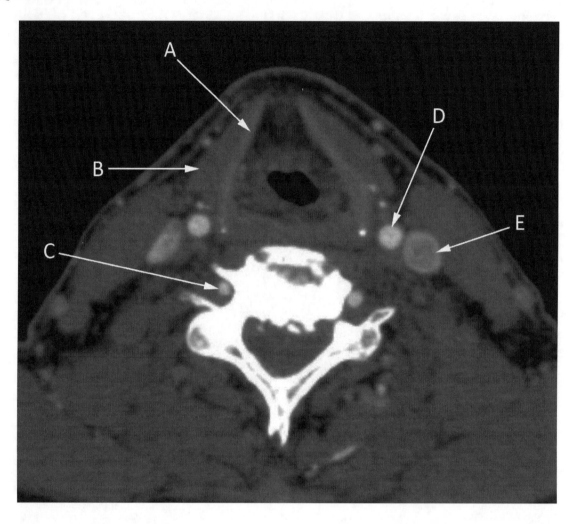

	QUESTION 13	WRITE YOUR ANSWER HERE
A	Name the structure labelled A	
B	Name the structure labelled B	
C	Name the structure labelled C	
D	Name the structure labelled D	
E	Name the structure labelled E	

Question 14

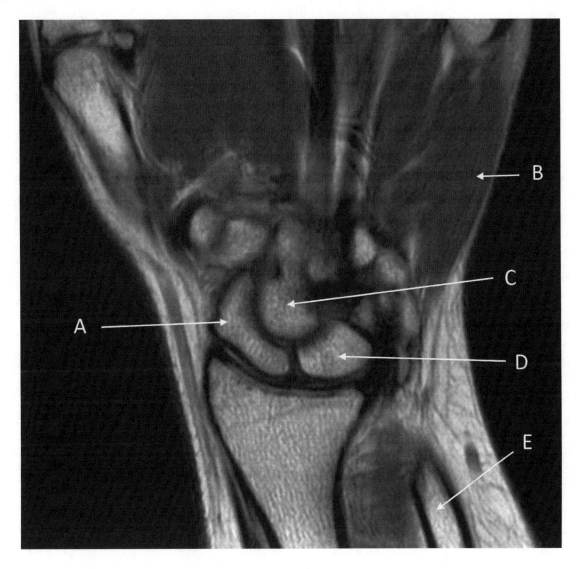

	QUESTION 14	WRITE YOUR ANSWER HERE
A	Name the structure labelled A	
B	Name the structure labelled B	
C	Name the structure labelled C	
D	Name the structure labelled D	
E	Name the structure labelled E	

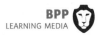

Question 15

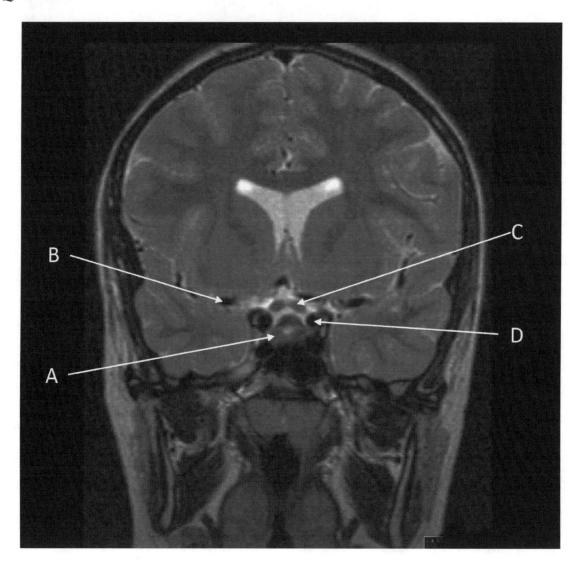

	QUESTION 15	WRITE YOUR ANSWER HERE
A	Name the structure labelled A	
B	Name the structure labelled B	
C	Name the structure labelled C	
D	Name the structure labelled D	
E	Through what bone has D passed through?	

Question 16

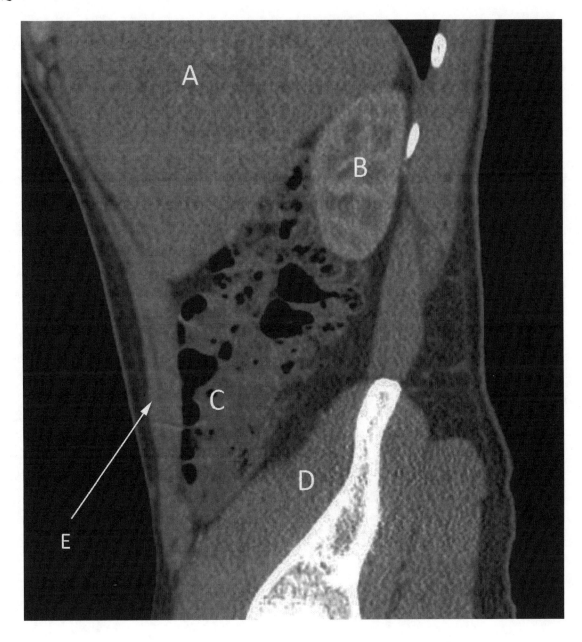

	QUESTION 16	WRITE YOUR ANSWER HERE
A	Name the structure labelled A	
B	Name the structure labelled B	
C	Name the structure labelled C	
D	Name the structure labelled D	
E	Name the structure labelled E	

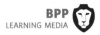

Question 17

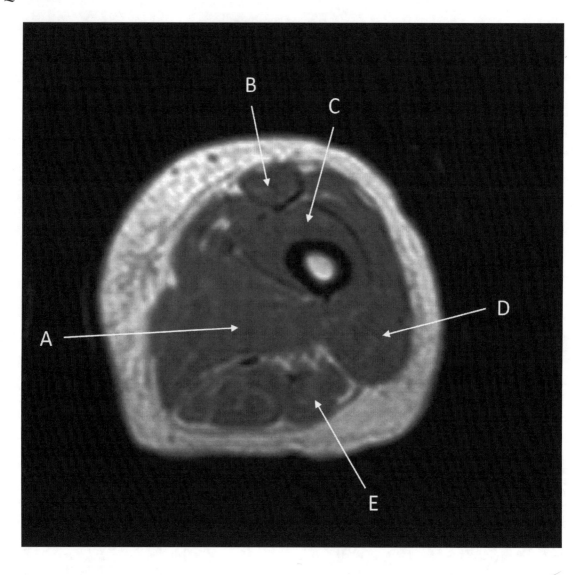

	QUESTION 17	WRITE YOUR ANSWER HERE
A	Name the structure labelled A	
B	Name the structure labelled B	
C	Name the structure labelled C	
D	Name the structure labelled D	
E	Name the structure labelled E	

Question 18

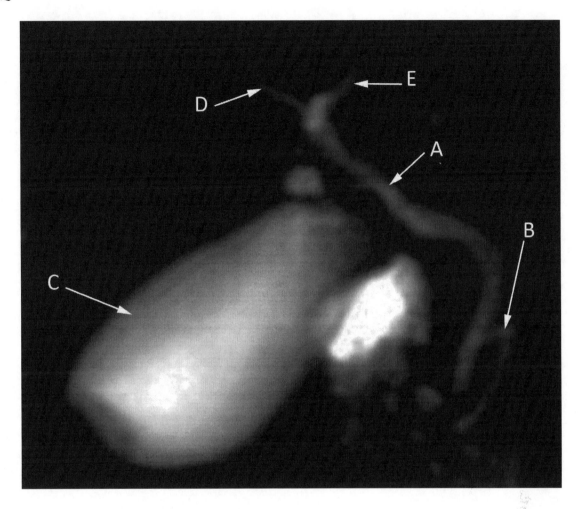

	QUESTION 18	WRITE YOUR ANSWER HERE
A	Name the structure labelled A	
B	Name the structure labelled B	
C	Name the structure labelled C	
D	Name the structure labelled D	
E	Name the structure labelled E	

Question 19

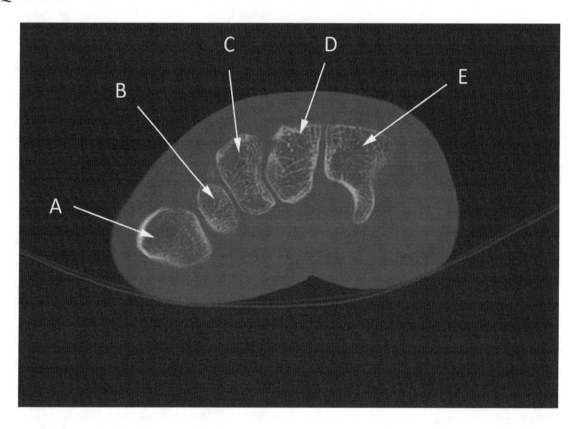

	QUESTION 19	WRITE YOUR ANSWER HERE
A	Name the structure labelled A	
B	Name the structure labelled B	
C	Name the structure labelled C	
D	What carpal bone does D articulate with inferiorly?	
E	Name the structure labelled E	

Question 20

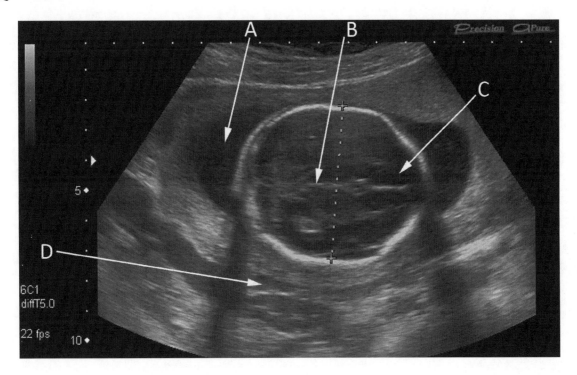

	QUESTION 20	WRITE YOUR ANSWER HERE
A	Name the structure labelled A	
B	Name the structure labelled B	
C	Name the structure labelled C	
D	Name the structure labelled D	
E	Name the measurement (dashed line)	

Paper 15

Answers

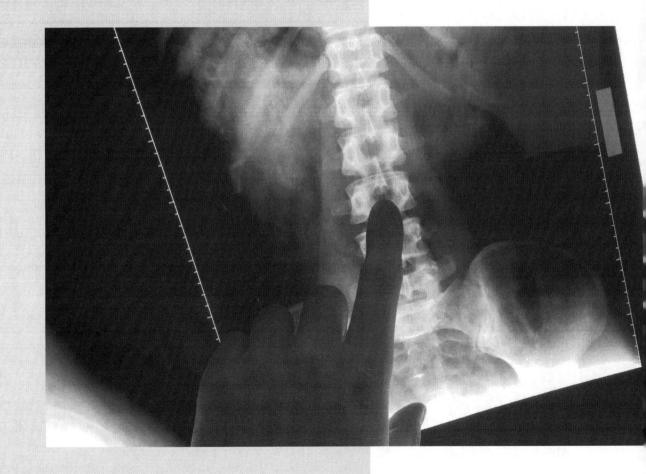

Question 1
A. Vertebral body
B. Right pedicle
C. Right posterior rib
D. Right lamina
E. Spinous process

Question 2
A. Transverse sinus
B. Right middle cerebral artery (M1)
C. Left frontal sinus
D. Left anterior cerebral artery (A1)
E. Left posterior cerebral artery (P1)

Question 3
A. Right external iliac vein
B. Right external iliac artery
C. Right common femoral artery
D. Right common femoral vein
E. Symphysis pubis

Question 4
A. Frontal sinus
B. Ethmoidal sinus
C. Pituitary fossa
D. Anterior arch of atlas
E. Mastoid air cells

Question 5
A. Superior articular process of the second cervical vertebra
B. Atlanto-axial joint
C. Spinous process of the second cervical vertebra
D. Lateral mass of the first cervical vertebra
E. Left transverse process of the first cervical vertebra

Question 6
A. Distal epiphysis of left fibula
B. Diaphysis of left fifth metatarsal
C. Epiphysis of distal phalanx of left big toe
D. Left intermediate cuneiform
E. Left navicular

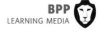

Question 7

A. Pubic bone
B. Myometrium
C. Vagina
D. Endometrium
E. Fundus of uterus

Question 8

A. Right cerebellopontine cistern
B. Right facial nerve
C. Right vestibulocochlear nerve
D. Left temporal lobe
E. Vestibule of left inner ear

Question 9

A. Urinary bladder
B. Vaginal stripe
C. Cervix
D. Free fluid
E. Uterine fundus

Question 10

A. Left coronary artery
B. None
C. Right coronary artery
D. Aortic root
E. Sino-tubular junction

Question 11

A. Superior facet
B. Transverse process
C. Right kidney
D. Spinal cord
E. Inferior facet

Question 12

A. Hepatic flexure
B. Haustra in transverse colon
C. Left properitoneal fat line
D. Left psoas shadow
E. Left first sacral foramen

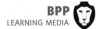

Question 13

A. Thyroid cartilage
B. Right thyrohyoid muscle
C. Right vertebral artery
D. Left common carotid artery
E. Left internal jugular vein

Question 14

A. Scaphoid bone
B. Abductor digiti minimi muscle
C. Capitate bone
D. Lunate bone
E. Ulnar

Question 15

A. Pituitary gland
B. Right middle cerebral artery
C. Optic chiasm
D. Left internal carotid artery
E. Petrous part of the left temporal bone

Question 16

A. Liver
B. Right kidney
C. Ascending colon
D. Right iliacus muscle
E. Rectus abdominis muscle

Question 17

A. Adductor magnus muscle
B. Rectus femoris muscle
C. Vastus intermedius muscle
D. Vastus lateralis muscle
E. Biceps femoris muscle

Question 18

A. Common bile duct
B. Pancreatic bile duct
C. Gallbladder
D. Right hepatic duct
E. Left hepatic duct

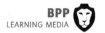

Question 19

A. Base of first metacarpal
B. Trapezium bone
C. Trapezoid bone
D. Lunate bone
E. Hamate bone

Question 20

A. Amniotic fluid
B. Foetal falx cerebri
C. Foetal lateral ventricle
D. Uterine myometrium
E. Biparietal diameter

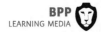

Paper 16

Question Bank

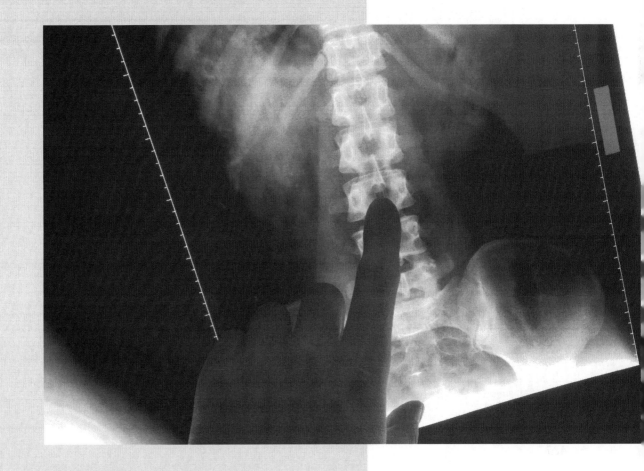

Question 1

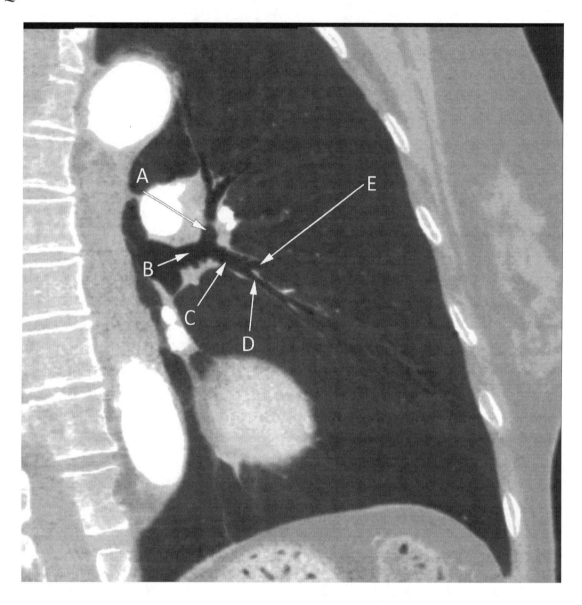

	QUESTION 1	WRITE YOUR ANSWER HERE
A	Name the segmental bronchus A	
B	Name the lobar bronchus B	
C	Name the bronchus labelled C	
D	Name the segmental bronchus D	
E	Name the segmental bronchus E	

Question 2

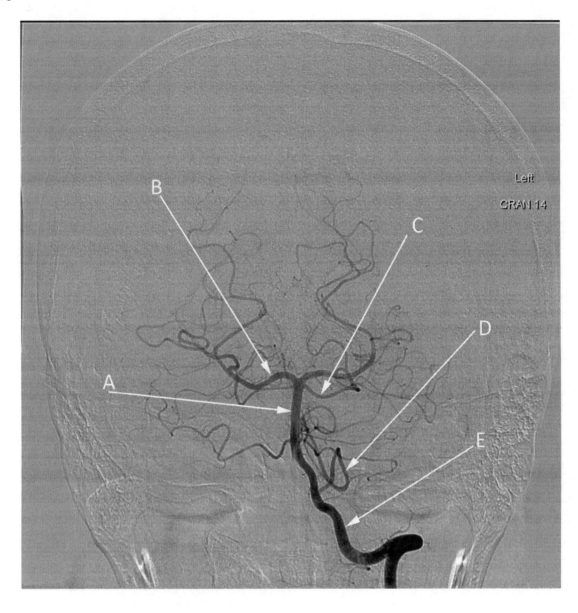

	QUESTION 2	WRITE YOUR ANSWER HERE
A	Name the structure labelled A	
B	Name the structure labelled B	
C	Name the structure labelled C	
D	Name the structure labelled D	
E	Name the structure labelled E	

Question 3

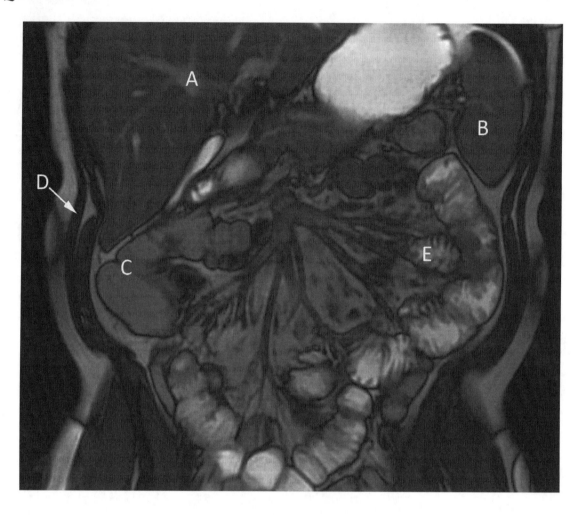

	QUESTION 3	WRITE YOUR ANSWER HERE
A	Name the structure labelled A	
B	Name the structure labelled B	
C	Name the structure labelled C	
D	Name the structure labelled D	
E	Name the structure labelled E	

Question 4

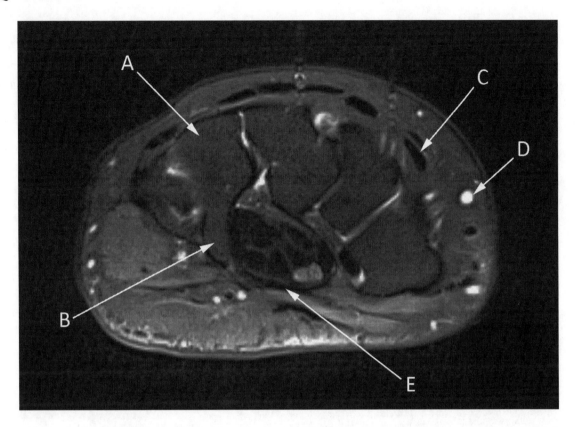

	QUESTION 4	WRITE YOUR ANSWER HERE
A	Name the structure labelled A	
B	Name the structure labelled B	
C	Name the structure labelled C	
D	Name the structure labelled D	
E	Name the structure labelled E	

Question 5

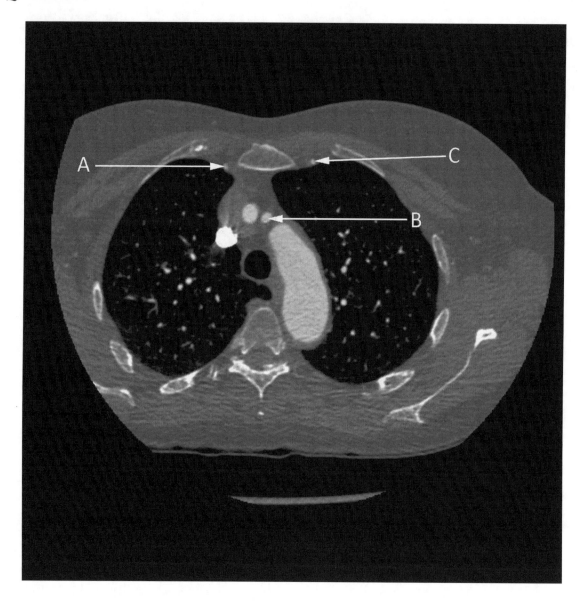

	QUESTION 5	WRITE YOUR ANSWER HERE
A	Name the structure labelled A	
B	Name the structure labelled B	
C	Name the structure labelled C	
D	What vessel does A originate from?	
E	What vessel does C originate from?	

Question 6

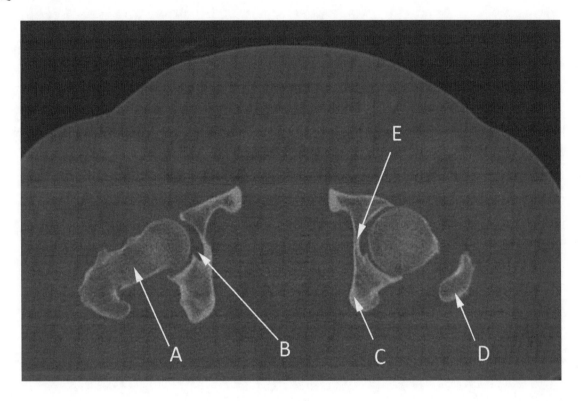

	QUESTION 6	WRITE YOUR ANSWER HERE
A	Name the structure labelled A	
B	What attaches to B?	
C	Name the structure labelled C	
D	Name the structure labelled D	
E	Name the structure labelled E	

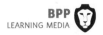

Question 7

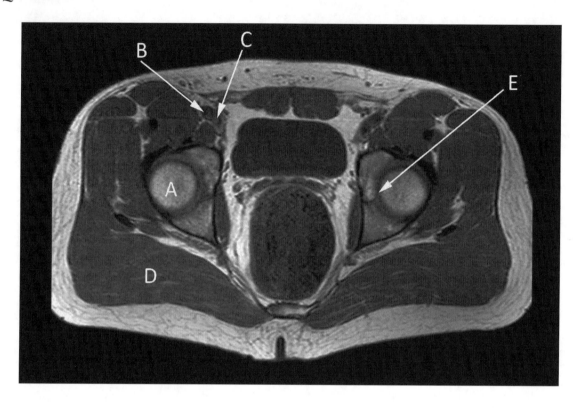

	QUESTION 7	WRITE YOUR ANSWER HERE
A	Name the structure labelled A	
B	Name the structure labelled B	
C	Name the structure labelled C	
D	Name the structure labelled D	
E	Name the structure labelled E	

Question 8

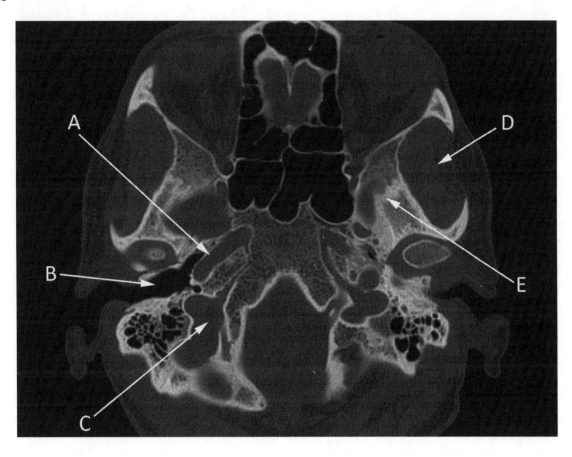

	QUESTION 8	WRITE YOUR ANSWER HERE
A	Name the structure labelled A	
B	Name the structure labelled B	
C	Name the structure labelled C	
D	Name the structure labelled D	
E	Name the structure labelled E	

Question 9

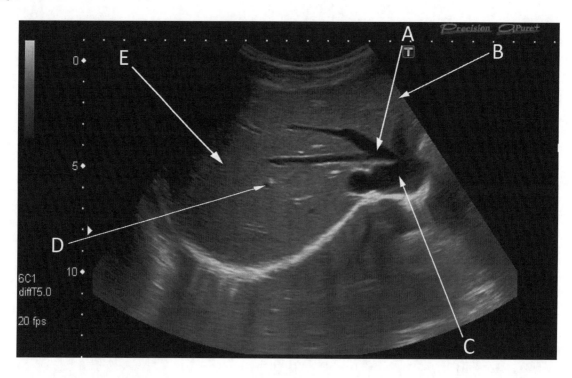

	QUESTION 9	WRITE YOUR ANSWER HERE
A	Name the structure labelled A	
B	Name the structure labelled B	
C	Name the structure labelled C	
D	Name the structure labelled D	
E	Name the structure labelled E	

Question 10

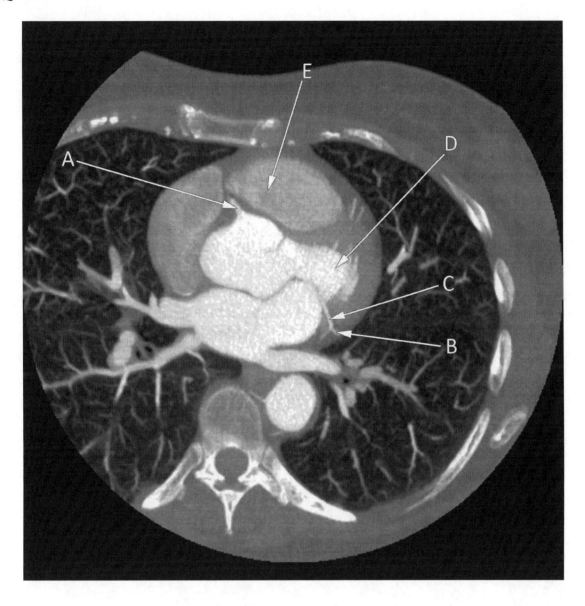

	QUESTION 10	WRITE YOUR ANSWER HERE
A	Name the structure labelled A	
B	Name the structure labelled B	
C	Name the structure labelled C	
D	Name the structure labelled D	
E	Name the structure labelled E	

Question 11

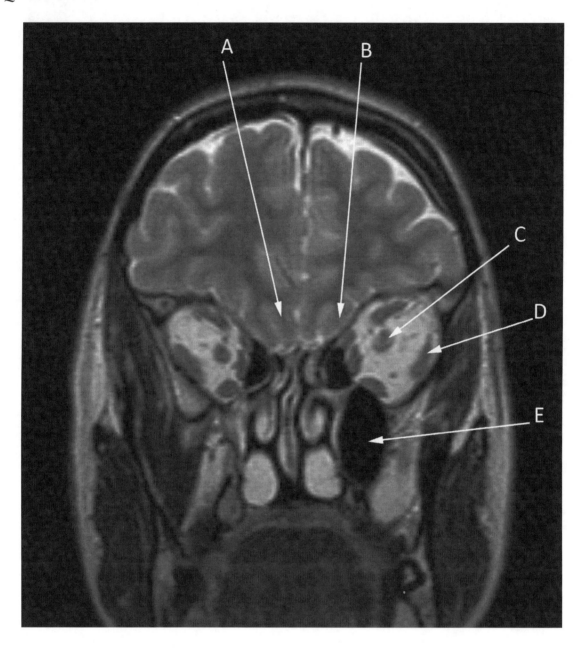

	QUESTION 11	WRITE YOUR ANSWER HERE
A	Name the structure labelled A	
B	Name the structure labelled B	
C	Name the structure labelled C	
D	Name the structure labelled D	
E	Name the structure labelled E	

Question 12

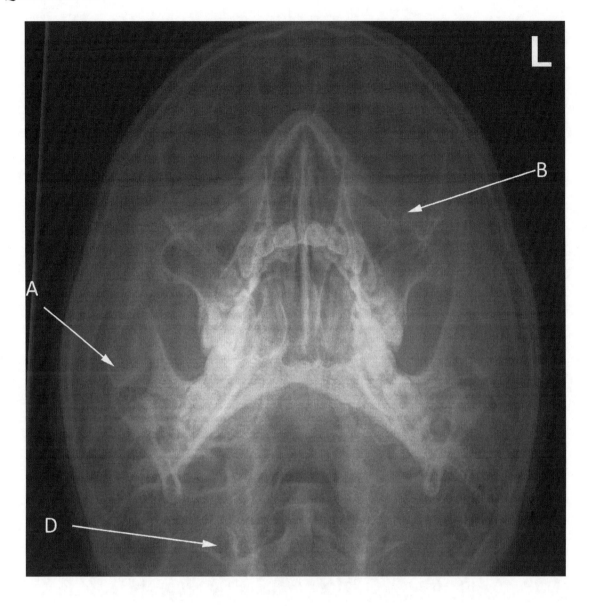

	QUESTION 12	WRITE YOUR ANSWER HERE
A	Name the structure labelled A	
B	Name the structure labelled B	
C	What passes through B?	
D	Name the structure labelled D	
E	What passes through D?	

Question 13

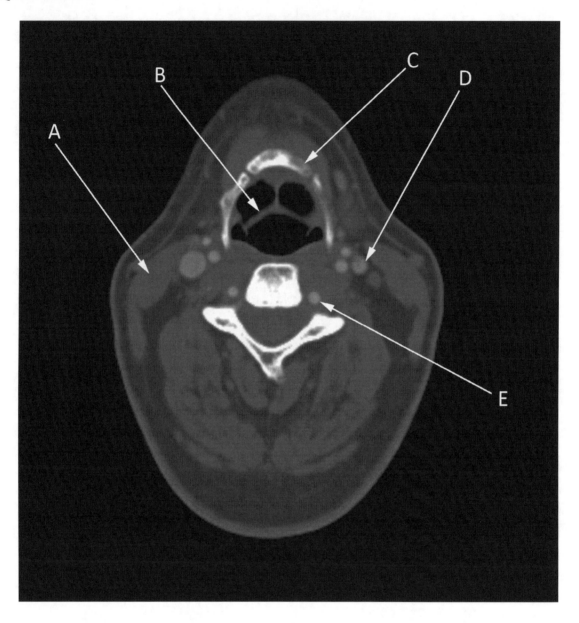

	QUESTION 13	WRITE YOUR ANSWER HERE
A	Name the structure labelled A	
B	Name the structure labelled B	
C	Name the structure labelled C	
D	Name the structure labelled D	
E	Name the structure labelled E	

Question 14

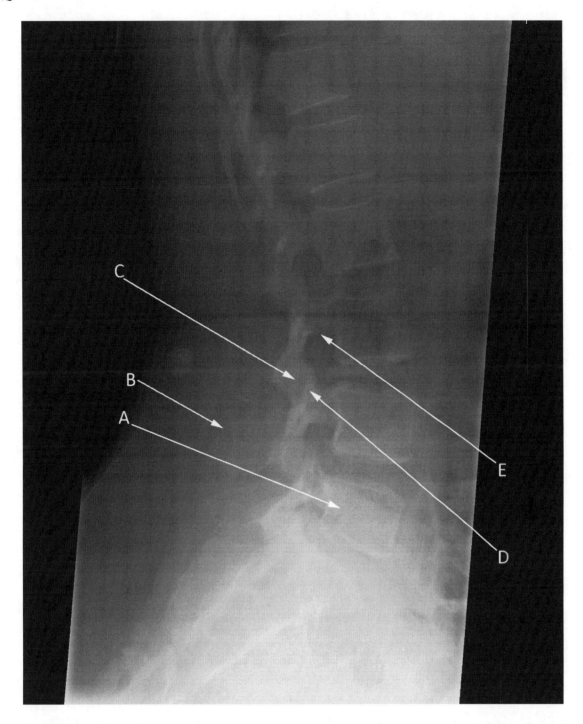

	QUESTION 14	WRITE YOUR ANSWER HERE
A	Name the structure labelled A	
B	Name the structure labelled B	
C	Name the structure labelled C	
D	Name the structure labelled D	
E	Name the structure labelled E	

Question 15

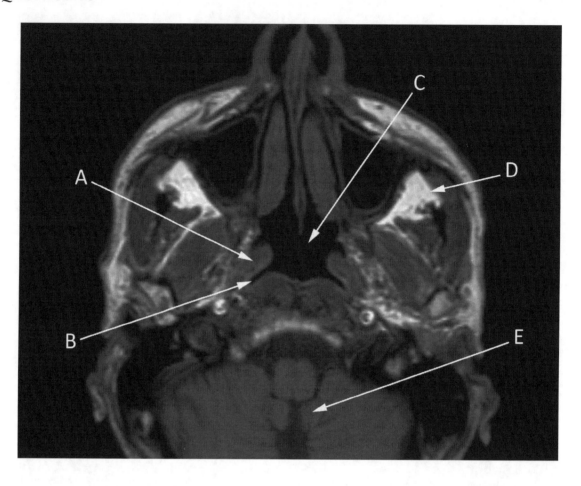

	QUESTION 15	WRITE YOUR ANSWER HERE
A	Name the structure labelled A	
B	Name the structure labelled B	
C	Name the structure labelled C	
D	Name the structure labelled D	
E	Name the structure labelled E	

Question 16

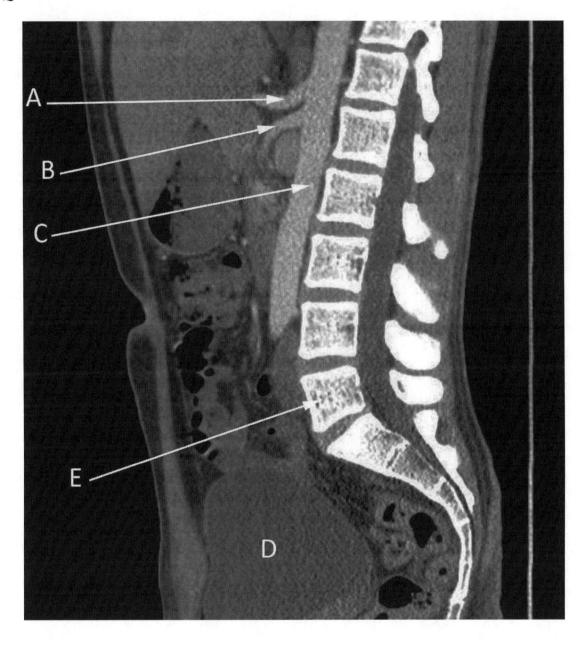

	QUESTION 16	WRITE YOUR ANSWER HERE
A	Name the structure labelled A	
B	Name the structure labelled B	
C	Name the structure labelled C	
D	Name the structure labelled D	
E	Name the structure labelled E	

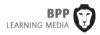

Question 17

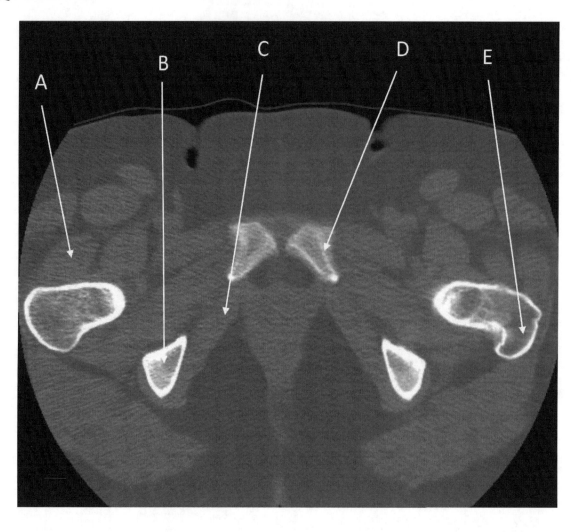

	QUESTION 17	WRITE YOUR ANSWER HERE
A	Name the structure labelled A	
B	Name the structure labelled B	
C	Name the structure labelled C	
D	Name the structure labelled D	
E	Name the structure labelled E	

Question 18

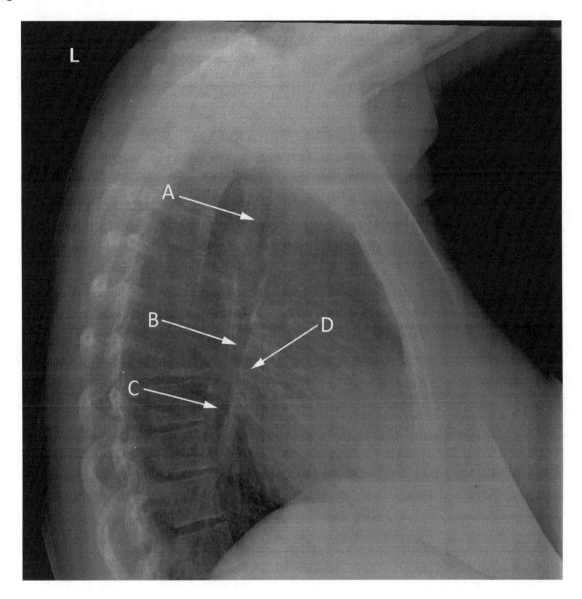

	QUESTION 18	WRITE YOUR ANSWER HERE
A	Name the structure labelled A	
B	Name the structure labelled B	
C	Name the structure labelled C	
D	Name the structure labelled D	
E	Which lower lobe segmental airway arises close to D?	

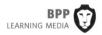

Question 19

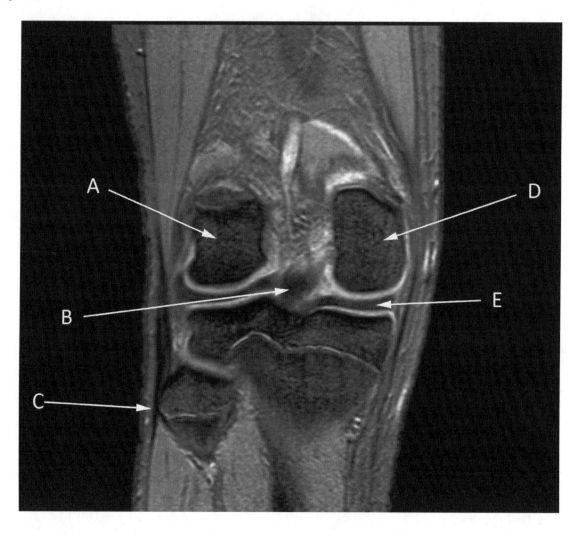

	QUESTION 19	WRITE YOUR ANSWER HERE
A	Name the structure labelled A	
B	Name the structure labelled B	
C	Name the structure labelled C	
D	Name the structure labelled D	
E	Name the structure labelled E	

Question 20

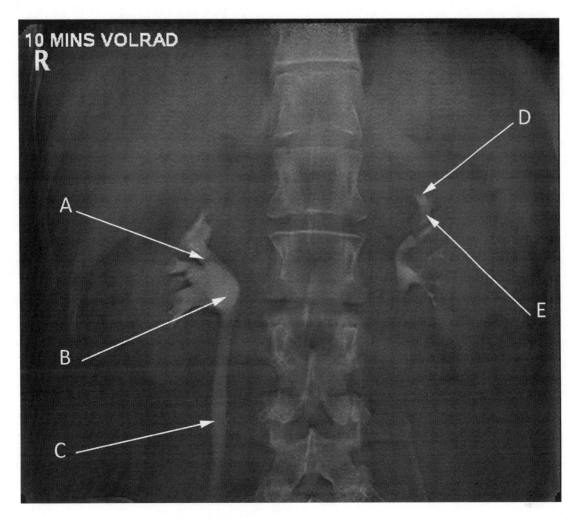

	QUESTION 20	WRITE YOUR ANSWER HERE
A	Name the structure labelled A	
B	Name the structure labelled B	
C	Name the structure labelled C	
D	Name the structure labelled D	
E	Name the structure labelled E	

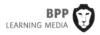

Paper 16

Answers

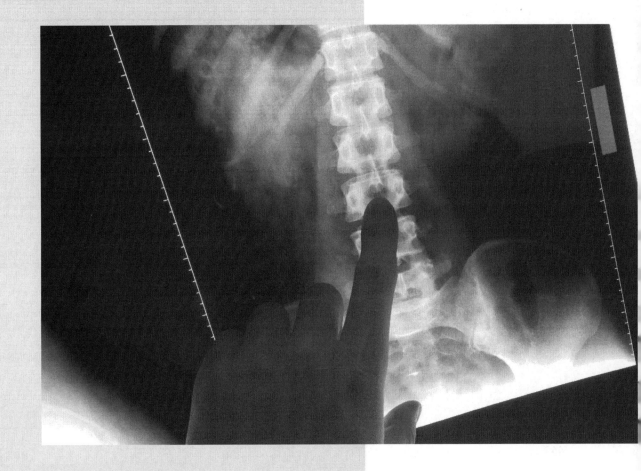

Question 1

A. Left upper lobe apico-posterior segmental bronchus
B. Left upper lobe
C. Lingula bronchus
D. Lingula inferior segmental bronchus
E. Lingula superior segmental bronchus

Question 2

A. Basilar artery
B. Right posterior cerebral artery
C. Left superior cerebellar artery
D. Left posterior inferior cerebellar artery
E. Left vertebral artery

Question 3

A. Portal vein
B. Spleen
C. Hepatic flexure
D. Right external oblique muscle
E. Jejunal loop

Question 4

A. Hamate
B. Hook of hamate
C. Tendon of extensor carpi radialis longus muscle
D. Cephalic vein
E. Flexor retinaculum

Question 5

A. Right internal mammary artery
B. Left common carotid artery
C. Left internal mammary artery
D. Right subclavian artery
E. Left subclavian artery

Question 6

A. Right neck of femur
B. Right ligamentum teres
C. Left ischial spine
D. Left greater trochanter
E. Left acetabulum

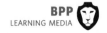

Question 7

A. Right femoral head
B. Right external iliac artery
C. Right external iliac vein
D. Right gluteus maximus muscle
E. Left acetabulum

Question 8

A. Right carotid canal
B. Right external auditory meatus
C. Right jugular foramen
D. Left temporalis muscle
E. Left sphenosquamous suture

Question 9

A. Middle hepatic vein
B. Left lobe of liver
C. Inferior vena cava
D. Branch of portal vein
E. Right lobe of liver

Question 10

A. Right coronary artery
B. Obtuse marginal branch of the circumflex
C. Circumflex artery
D. Left ventricle / left ventricular outflow tract
E. Right ventricle / right ventricular outflow tract

Question 11

A. Gyrus rectus
B. Medial orbital gyrus
C. Optic nerve
D. Lateral rectus muscle
E. Maxillary sinus

Question 12

A. Temporal process of right zygomatic bone
B. Left infra-orbital foramen
C. Infraorbital nerve, artery and vein
D. Right transverse foramen
E. Right vertebral artery

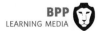

Question 13

A. Right sternocleidomastoid muscle
B. Epiglottis (free margin)
C. Hyoid bone
D. Left internal jugular vein
E. Left verterbral artery

Question 14

A. Body of L5 vertebra
B. Posterior spinous process L4
C. Inferior facet of L3 vertebra
D. Superior facet of L4 vertebra
E. Inferior vertebral notch of L3

Question 15

A. Tensor veli palatini muscle
B. Lateral pharyngeal recess
C. Nasopharynx
D. Fat in infratemporal fossa
E. Left cerebellar tonsil

Question 16

A. Coeliac axis
B. Superior mesenteric artery
C. Aorta
D. Urinary bladder
E. L5 vertebral body

Question 17

A. Right vastus lateralis muscle
B. Right ischium
C. Right obturator internus muscle
D. Left inferior pubic ramus
E. Greater trochanter of left femur

Question 18

A. Trachea
B. Bronchus intermedius
C. Right lower lobe bronchus
D. Middle lobe bronchus
E. Right lower lobe apical segmental bronchus

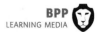

Question 19

A. Lateral femoral condyle
B. Posterior cruciate ligament
C. Iliotibial tract
D. Medial femoral condyle
E. Posterior horn of the medial meniscus

Question 20

A. Major calyx (right kidney upper pole)
B. Right renal pelvis
C. Right ureter
D. Renal papilla (left kidney upper pole)
E. Minor calyx (left kidney upper pole)

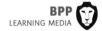

Paper 17

Question Bank

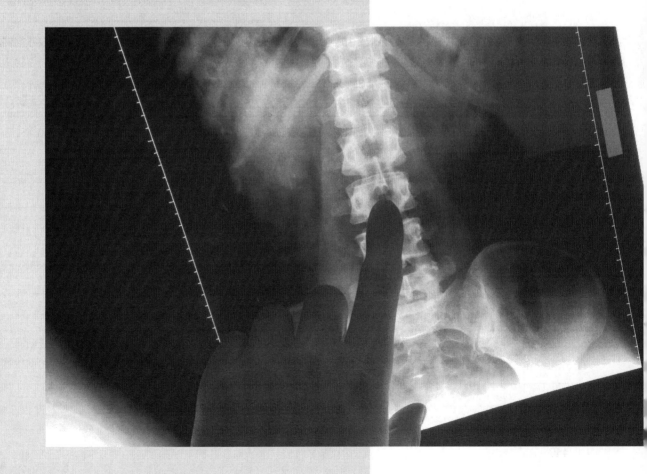

Question 1

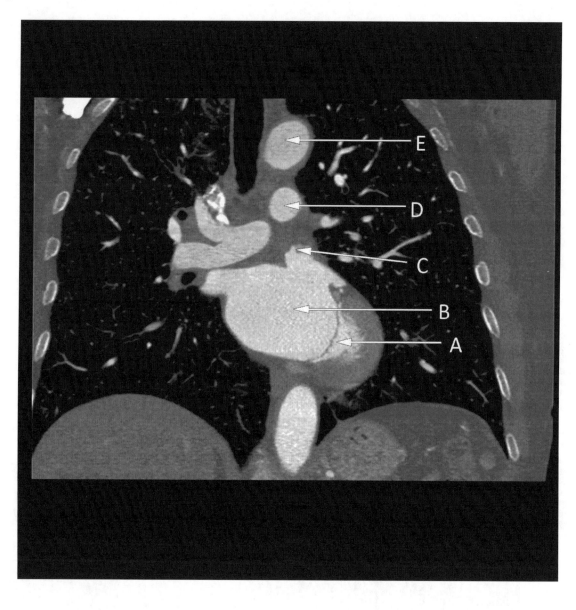

	QUESTION 1	WRITE YOUR ANSWER HERE
A	Name the structure labelled A	
B	Name the structure labelled B	
C	Name the structure labelled C	
D	Name the structure labelled D	
E	Name the structure labelled E	

Question 2

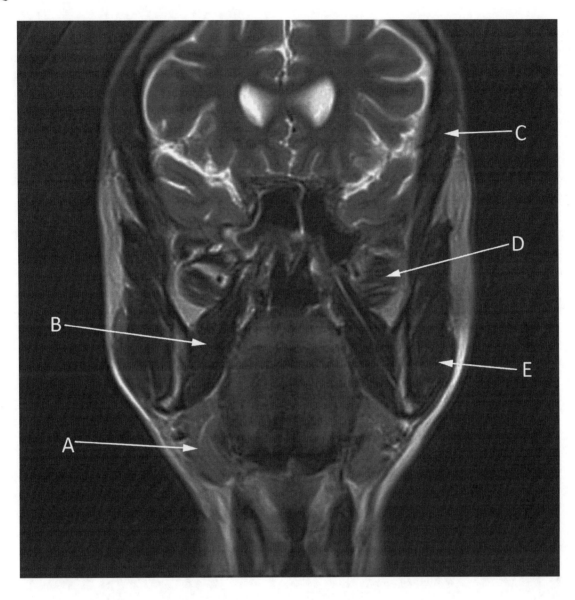

	QUESTION 2	WRITE YOUR ANSWER HERE
A	Name the structure labelled A	
B	Name the structure labelled B	
C	Name the structure labelled C	
D	Name the structure labelled D	
E	Name the structure labelled E	

Question 3

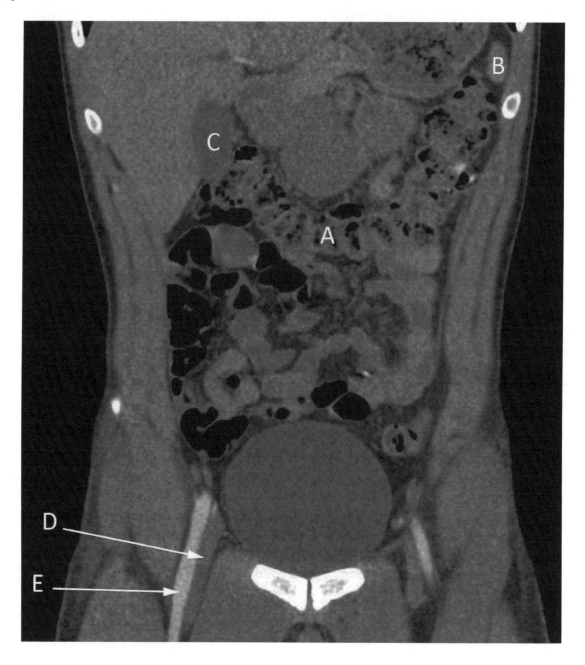

	QUESTION 3	WRITE YOUR ANSWER HERE
A	Name the structure labelled A	
B	Name the structure labelled B	
C	Name the structure labelled C	
D	Name the structure labelled D	
E	Name the structure labelled E	

Question 4

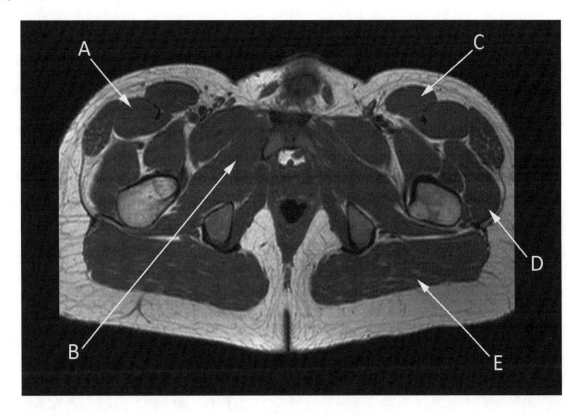

	QUESTION 4	WRITE YOUR ANSWER HERE
A	Name the structure labelled A	
B	Name the structure labelled B	
C	Name the structure labelled C	
D	Name the structure labelled D	
E	Name the structure labelled E	

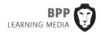

Question 5

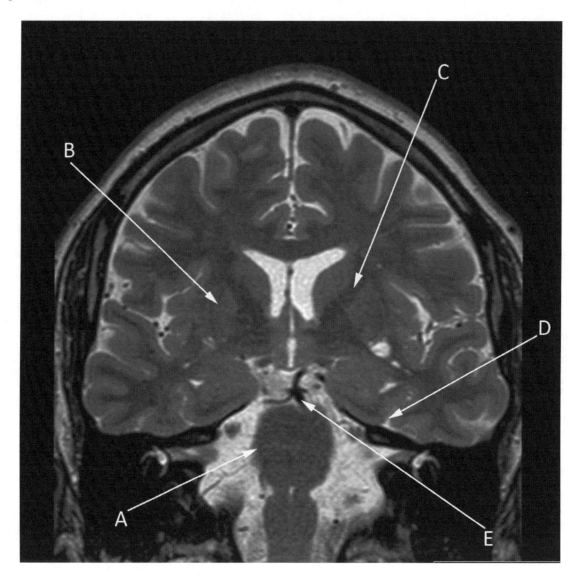

	QUESTION 5	WRITE YOUR ANSWER HERE
A	Name the structure labelled A	
B	Name the structure labelled B	
C	Name the structure labelled C	
D	Name the structure labelled D	
E	Name the structure labelled E	

Question 6

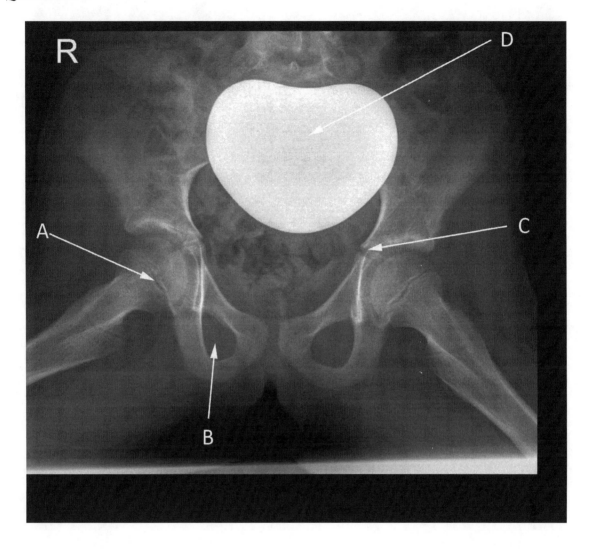

	QUESTION 6	WRITE YOUR ANSWER HERE
A	Name the structure labelled A	
B	Name the structure labelled B	
C	Name the structure labelled C	
D	Name the structure labelled D	
E	What projection is this film?	

Question 7

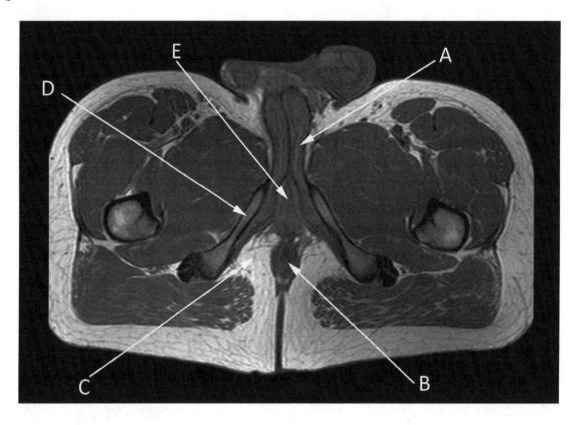

	QUESTION 7	WRITE YOUR ANSWER HERE
A	Name the structure labelled A	
B	Name the structure labelled B	
C	Name the structure labelled C	
D	Name the structure labelled D	
E	Name the structure labelled E	

Question 8

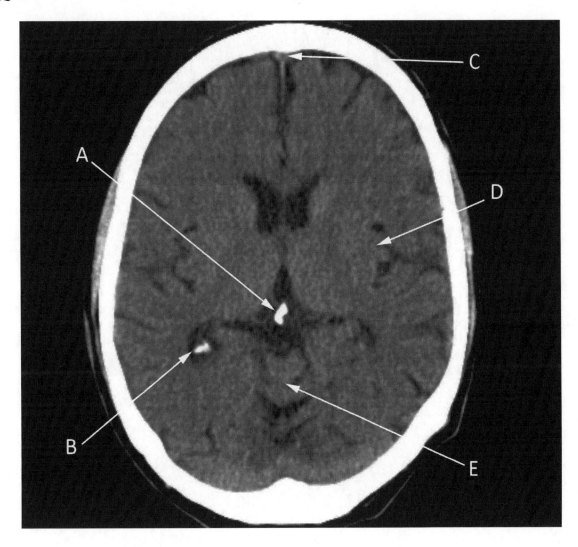

	QUESTION 8	WRITE YOUR ANSWER HERE
A	Name the structure labelled A	
B	Name the structure labelled B	
C	Name the structure labelled C	
D	Name the structure labelled D	
E	Name the structure labelled E	

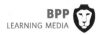

Question 9

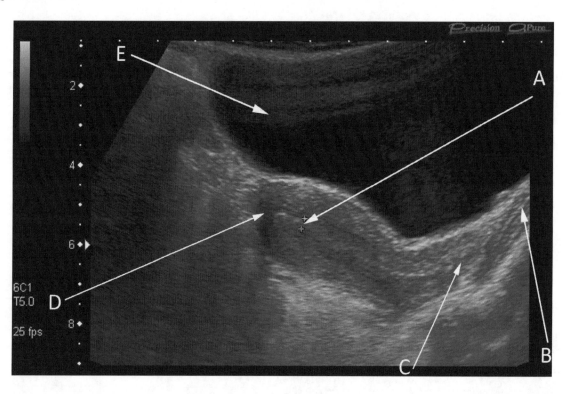

	QUESTION 9	WRITE YOUR ANSWER HERE
A	Name the measurement labelled A	
B	Name the structure labelled B	
C	Name the structure labelled C	
D	Name the structure labelled D	
E	Name the structure labelled E	

Question 10

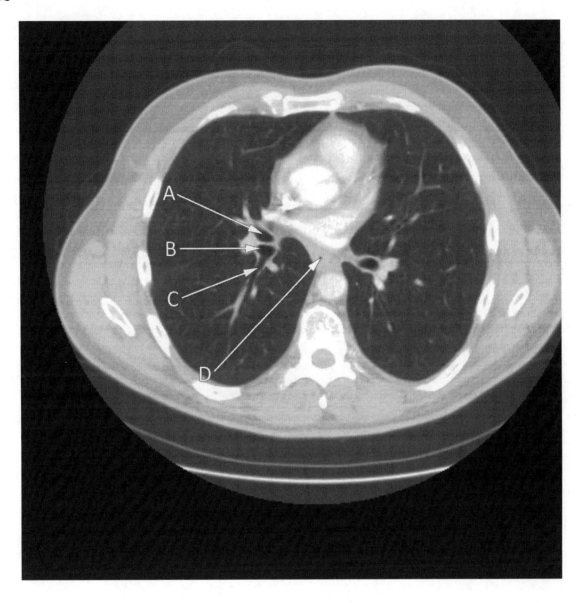

	QUESTION 10	WRITE YOUR ANSWER HERE
A	Name the lobar bronchus labelled A	
B	Name the lobar bronchus labelled B	
C	Name the structure labelled C	
D	Name the structure labelled D	
E	'A' runs inferior to which lung fissure?	

Question 11

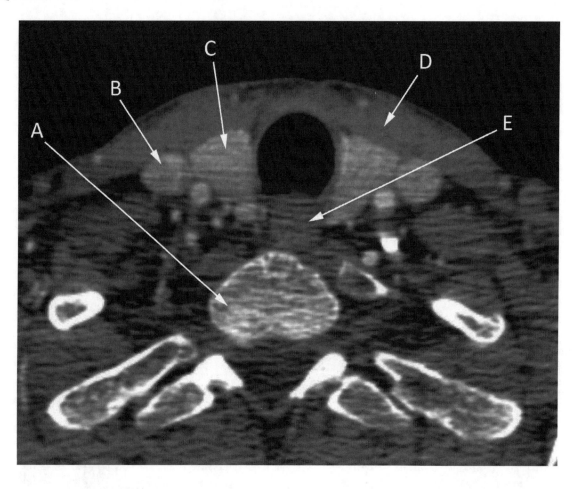

	QUESTION 11	WRITE YOUR ANSWER HERE
A	Name the structure labelled A	
B	Name the structure labelled B	
C	Name the structure labelled C	
D	Name the structure labelled D	
E	Name the structure labelled E	

Question 12

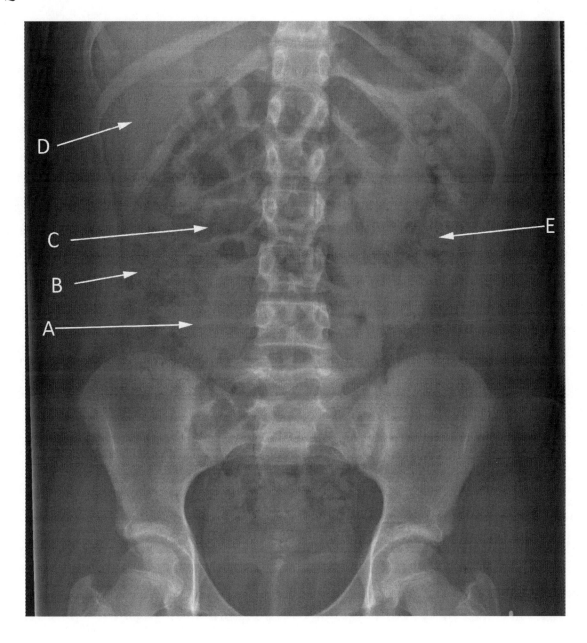

	QUESTION 12	WRITE YOUR ANSWER HERE
A	Name the structure labelled A	
B	Name the structure labelled B	
C	Name the structure labelled C	
D	Name the structure labelled D	
E	Name the structure labelled E	

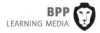

Question 13

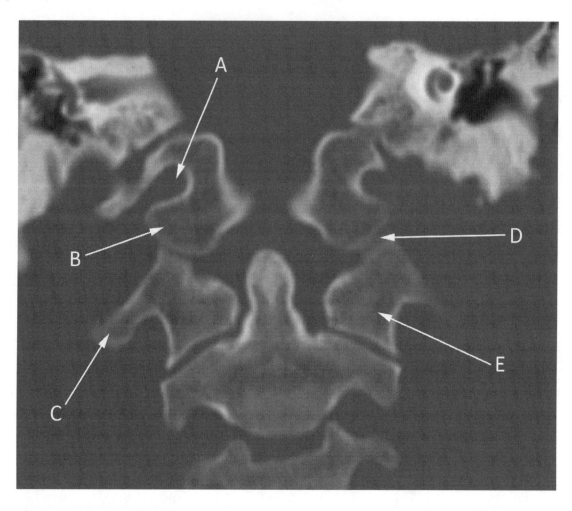

	QUESTION 13	WRITE YOUR ANSWER HERE
A	Name the structure labelled A	
B	Name the structure labelled B	
C	Name the structure labelled C	
D	Name the structure labelled D	
E	Name the structure labelled E	

Question 14

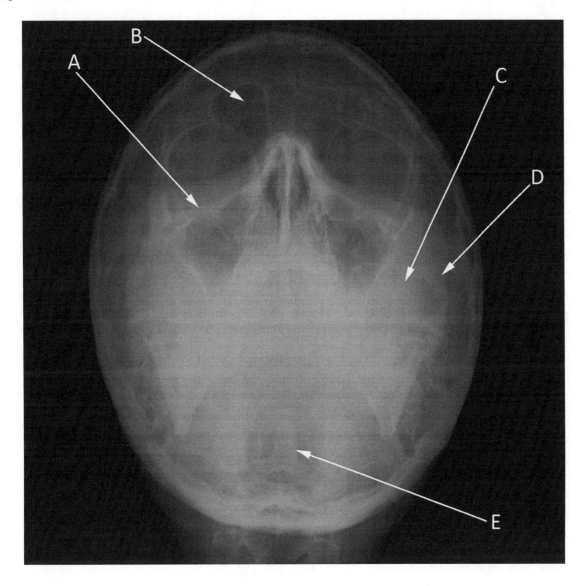

	QUESTION 14	WRITE YOUR ANSWER HERE
A	Name the structure labelled A	
B	Name the structure labelled B	
C	Name the structure labelled C	
D	Name the structure labelled D	
E	Name the structure labelled E	

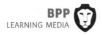

Question 15

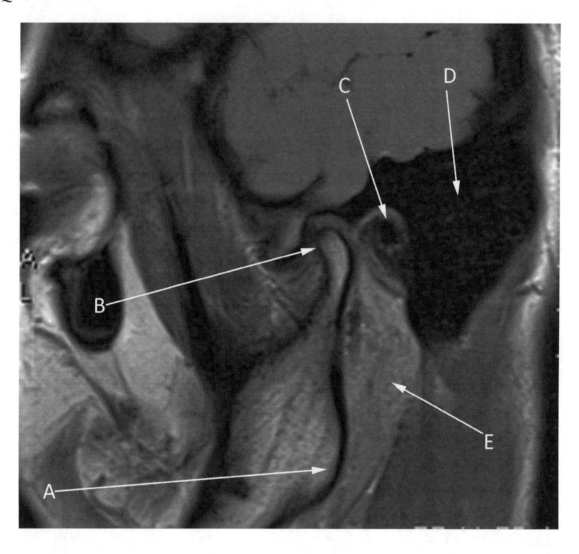

	QUESTION 15	WRITE YOUR ANSWER HERE
A	Name the structure labelled A	
B	Name the structure labelled B	
C	Name the structure labelled C	
D	Name the structure labelled D	
E	Name the structure labelled E	

Question 16

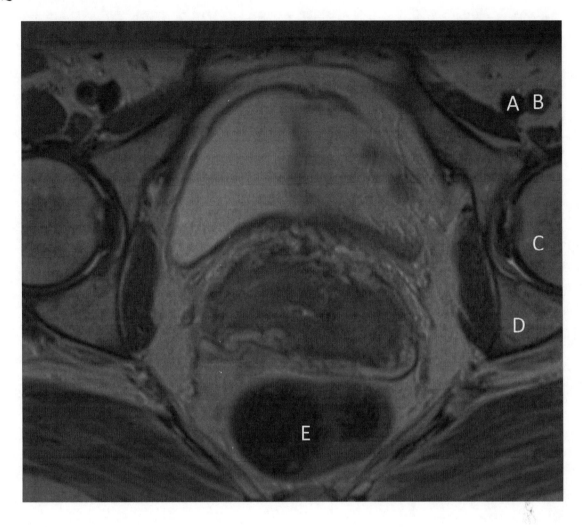

	QUESTION 16	WRITE YOUR ANSWER HERE
A	Name the structure labelled A	
B	Name the structure labelled B	
C	Name the structure labelled C	
D	Name the structure labelled D	
E	Name the structure labelled E	

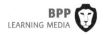

Question 17

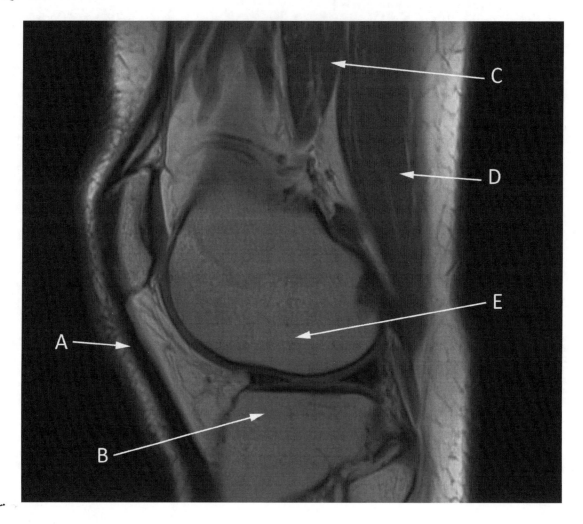

	QUESTION 17	WRITE YOUR ANSWER HERE
A	Name the structure labelled A	
B	Name the structure labelled B	
C	Name the structure labelled C	
D	Name the structure labelled D	
E	Name the structure labelled E	

Question 18

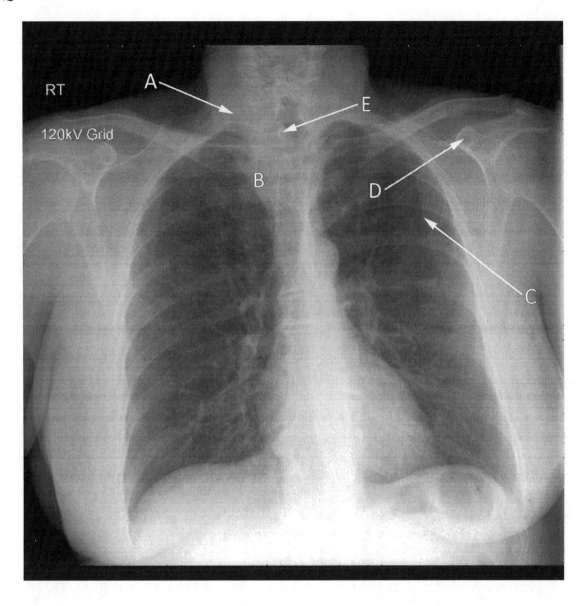

	QUESTION 18	WRITE YOUR ANSWER HERE
A	Name the bony structure labelled A	
B	Which vessels converge to form B?	
C	Which structure forms line C?	
D	Name the structure labelled D	
E	Name the bony structure labelled E	

Question 19

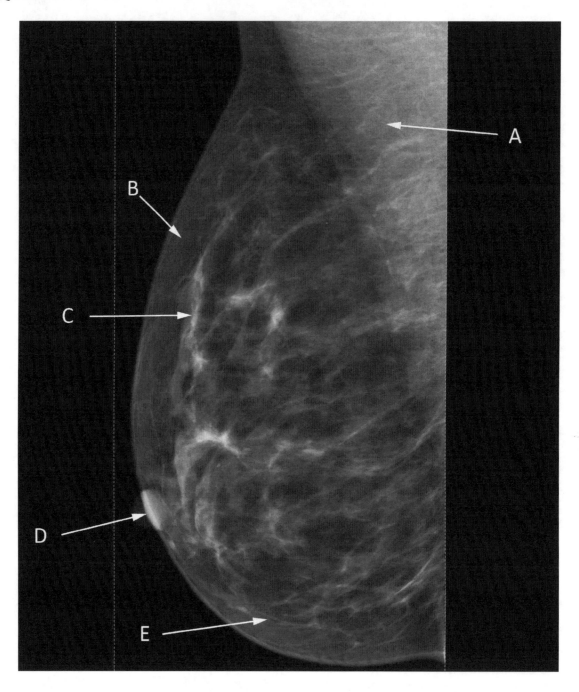

	QUESTION 19	WRITE YOUR ANSWER HERE
A	Name the structure labelled A	
B	Name the structure labelled B	
C	Name the structure labelled C	
D	Name the structure labelled D	
E	What projection is this film?	

Question 20

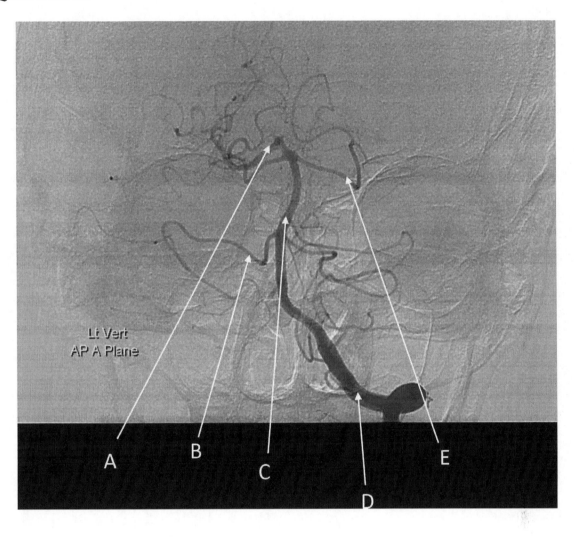

	QUESTION 20	WRITE YOUR ANSWER HERE
A	Name the structure labelled A	
B	Name the structure labelled B	
C	Name the structure labelled C	
D	Name the structure labelled D	
E	Name the structure labelled E	

Paper 17

Answers

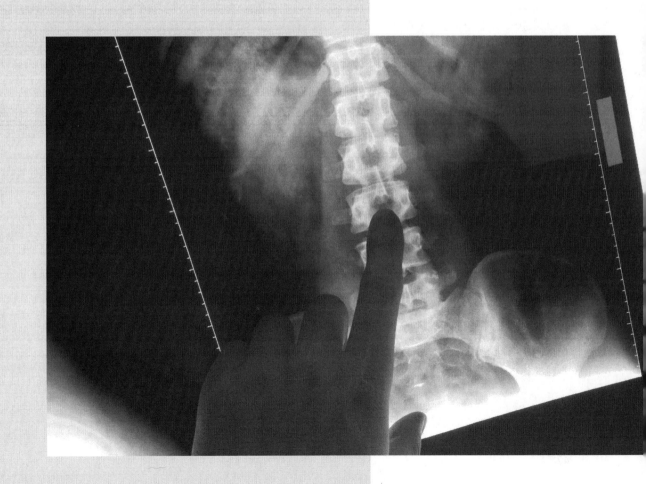

Question 1

A. Left ventricle
B. Left atrium
C. Left atrial appendage
D. Left main pulmonary artery
E. Aortic arch

Question 2

A. Right submandibular gland
B. Right medial pterygoid muscle
C. Left temporalis muscle
D. Left lateral pterygoid muscle
E. Left masseter muscle

Question 3

A. Transverse colon
B. Spleen
C. Gallbladder
D. Right common femoral vein
E. Right common femoral artery

Question 4

A. Right rectus femoris muscle
B. Right adductor longus muscle
C. Left sartorius muscle
D. Left vastus medialis muscle
E. Left gluteus maximus muscle

Question 5

A. Pons
B. Right putamen
C. Left internal capsule (anterior limb)
D. Collateral sulcus
E. Basilar artery

Question 6

A. Epiphyseal line
B. Right obturator foramen
C. Left tri-radiate cartilage
D. Gonadal shield
E. Frog leg

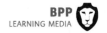

Question 7

A. Corpus cavernosum
B. Anal canal
C. Ischio-anal fossa
D. Right inferior pubic ramus
E. Urethra

Question 8

A. Calcification in pineal gland
B. Calcification in choroid plexus
C. Superior sagittal sinus
D. Left insular cortex
E. Superior cerebellar vermis

Question 9

A. Endometrial thickness
B. Vagina
C. Cervix
D. Uterine myometrium of fundus
E. Urinary bladder

Question 10

A. Middle (right) lobe bronchus
B. Right lower lobe bronchus
C. Right lower lobe apical segmental bronchus
D. Oesophagus
E. Horizontal fissure

Question 11

A. Vertebral body
B. Right internal jugular vein
C. Right lobe of thyroid gland
D. Left sternocleidomastoid muscle
E. Oesophagus

Question 12

A. Right psoas margin
B. Ascending colon
C. Loops of jejunum
D. Liver
E. Descending colon

Question 13

A. Right hypoglossal canal
B. Right occipital condyle
C. Right transverse process of atlas
D. Left atlanto-occipital joint
E. Left lateral mass of atlas

Question 14

A. Inferior margin of the right orbit
B. Right frontal sinus
C. Left coronoid process of the mandible
D. Left zygomatic arch
E. Odontoid peg

Question 15

A. Angle of the mandible
B. Condyle of the mandible
C. External auditory canal
D. Mastoid air cells
E. Parotid gland

Question 16

A. Left external iliac vein
B. Left external iliac artery
C. Left femoral head
D. Left ischium
E. Rectum

Question 17

A. Patellar tendon
B. Lateral condyle of tibia
C. Vastus lateralis muscle
D. Short head of biceps femoris muscle
E. Lateral condyle of femur

Question 18

A. Right transverse process T1/ right 1st rib
B. Right internal jugular vein, right subclavian vein
C. Left scapula
D. Left coracoid process
E. Spinous process

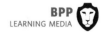

Question 19

A. Pectoralis major muscle
B. Adipose tissue
C. Fibroglandular tissue
D. Nipple
E. Cooper's ligament

Question 20

A. Right posterior cerebral artery
B. Anterior inferior cerebellar artery
C. Basilar artery
D. Left vertebral artery
E. Left superior cerebellar artery

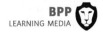

Paper 18

Question Bank

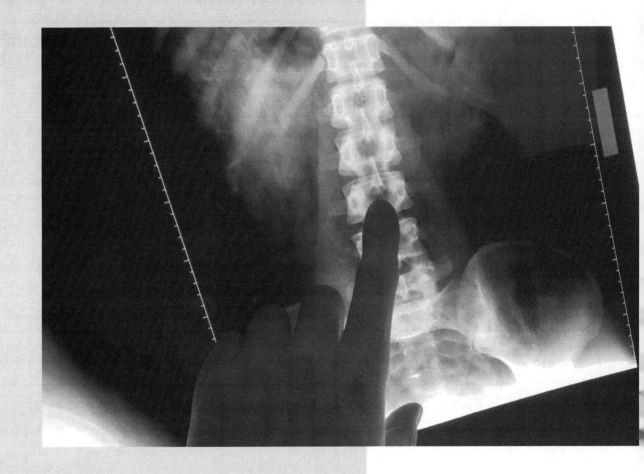

Question 1

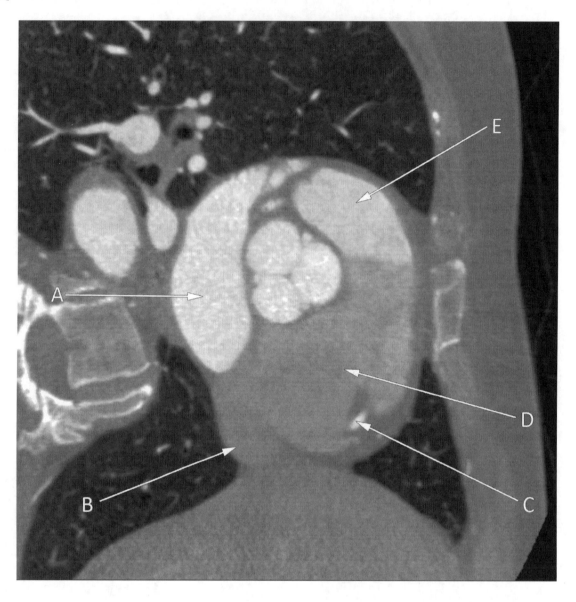

	QUESTION 1	WRITE YOUR ANSWER HERE
A	Name the structure labelled A	
B	Name the structure labelled B	
C	Name the structure labelled C	
D	Name the structure labelled D	
E	Name the structure labelled E	

Question 2

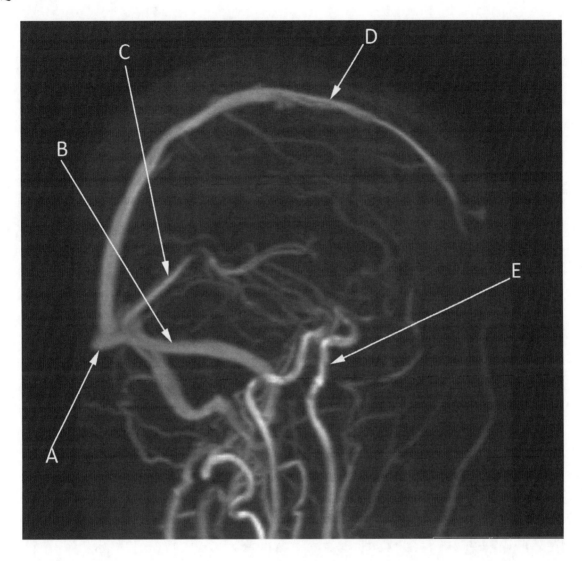

	QUESTION 2	WRITE YOUR ANSWER HERE
A	Name the structure labelled A	
B	Name the structure labelled B	
C	Name the structure labelled C	
D	Name the structure labelled D	
E	Name the structure labelled E	

Question 3

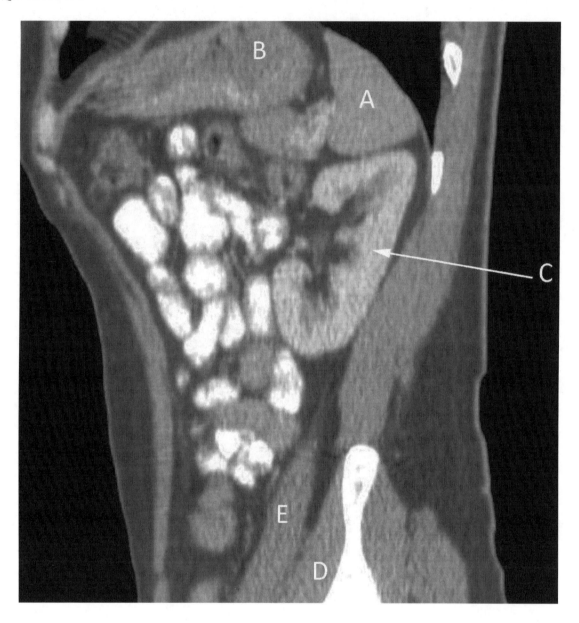

	QUESTION 3	WRITE YOUR ANSWER HERE
A	Name the structure labelled A	
B	Name the structure labelled B	
C	Name the structure labelled C	
D	Name the structure labelled D	
E	Name the structure labelled E	

Question 4

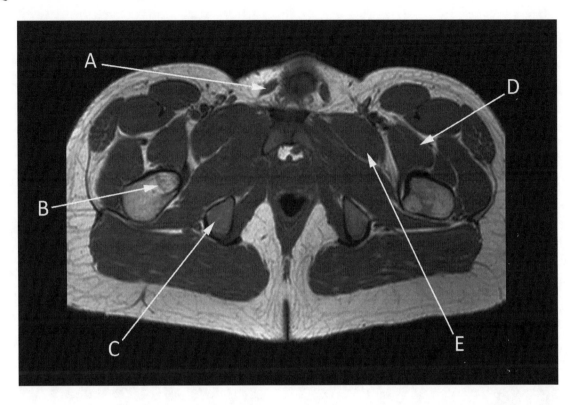

	QUESTION 4	WRITE YOUR ANSWER HERE
A	Name the structure labelled A	
B	Name the structure labelled B	
C	Name the structure labelled C	
D	Name the structure labelled D	
E	Name the insertion of the structure labelled E	

Question 5

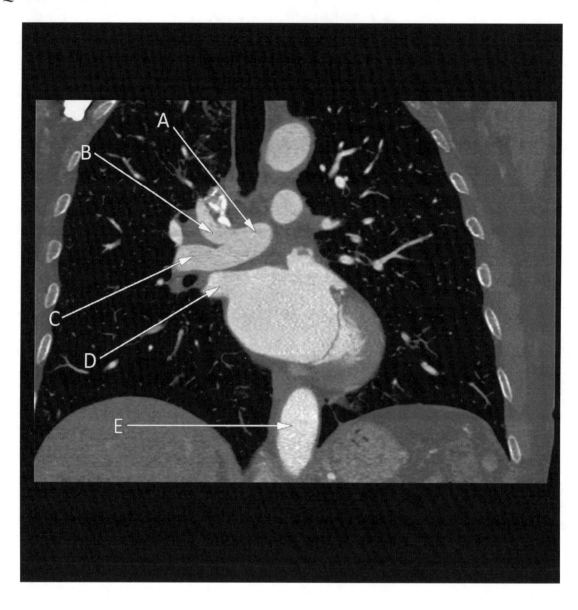

	QUESTION 5	WRITE YOUR ANSWER HERE
A	Name the structure labelled A	
B	Name the structure labelled B	
C	Name the structure labelled C	
D	Name the structure labelled D	
E	Name the structure labelled E	

Question 6

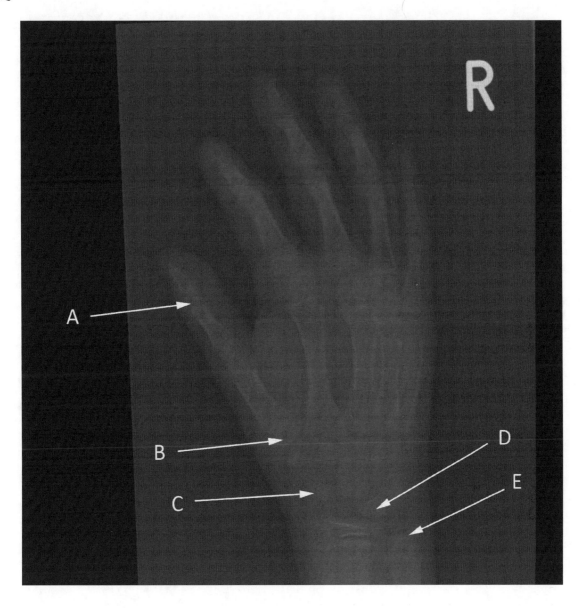

	QUESTION 6	WRITE YOUR ANSWER HERE
A	Name the structure labelled A	
B	Name the structure labelled B	
C	Name the structure labelled C	
D	Name the structure labelled D	
E	Name the structure labelled E	

Question 7

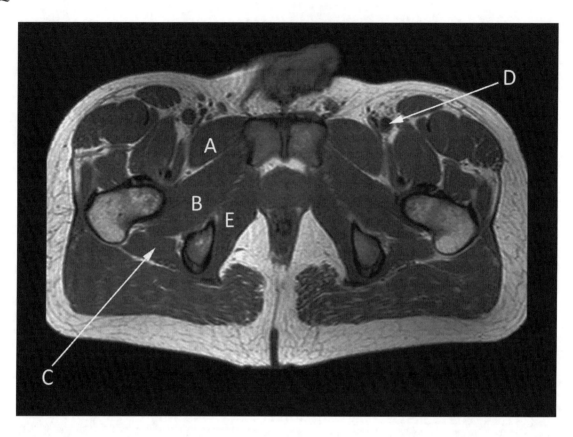

	QUESTION 7	WRITE YOUR ANSWER HERE
A	Name the structure labelled A	
B	Name the structure labelled B	
C	Name the structure labelled C	
D	Name the structure labelled D	
E	Name the structure labelled E	

Question 8

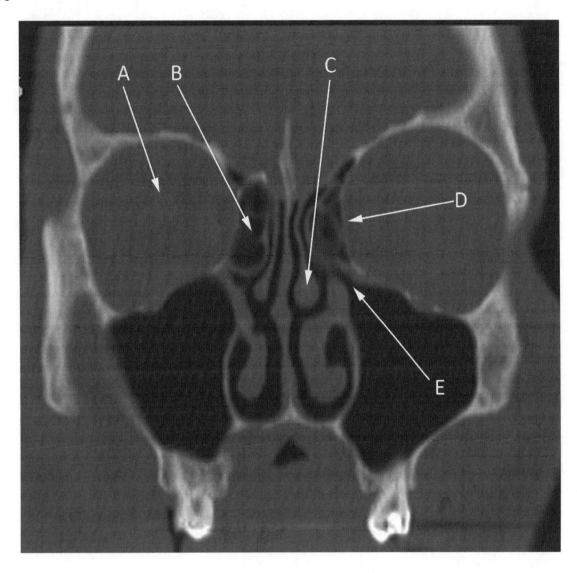

	QUESTION 8	WRITE YOUR ANSWER HERE
A	Name the structure labelled A	
B	Name the structure labelled B	
C	Name the structure labelled C	
D	Name the structure labelled D	
E	Name the structure labelled E	

Question 9

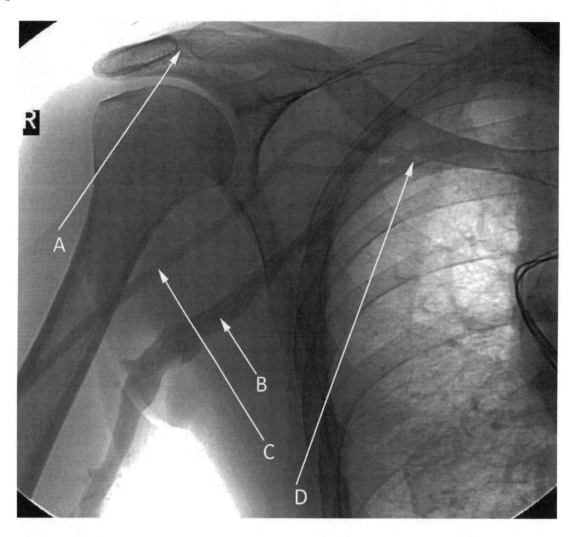

	QUESTION 9	WRITE YOUR ANSWER HERE
A	Name the structure labelled A	
B	Name the structure labelled B	
C	Name the structure labelled C	
D	Name the structure labelled D	
E	Name the investigation shown	

Question 10

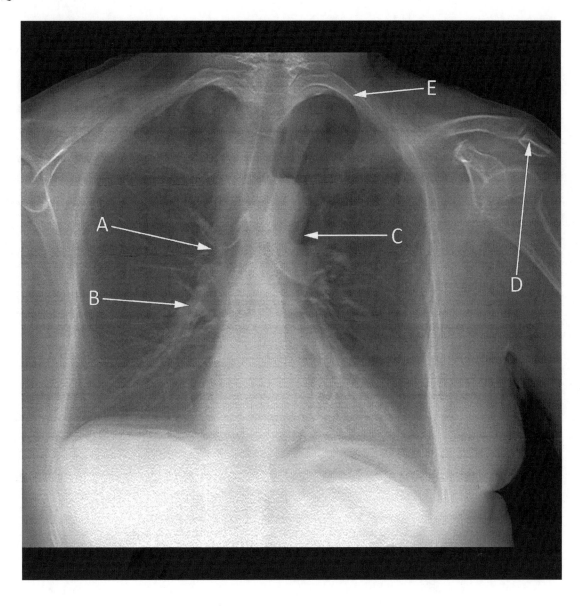

	QUESTION 10	WRITE YOUR ANSWER HERE
A	Name the lobar airway labelled A	
B	Name the vessel labelled B	
C	Name the structure forming border line C	
D	Name the structure labelled D	
E	Name the structure labelled E	

Question 11

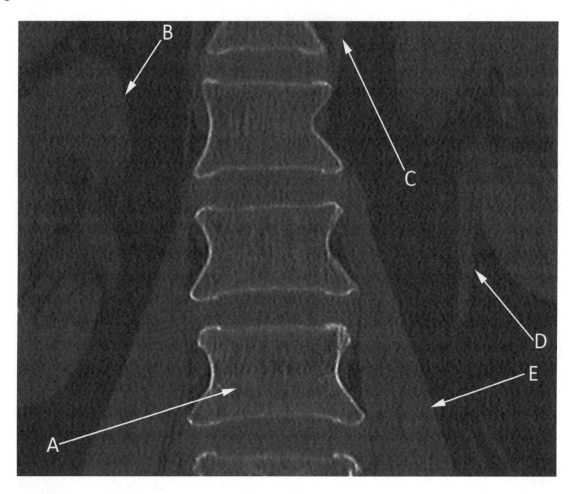

	QUESTION 11	WRITE YOUR ANSWER HERE
A	Name the structure labelled A	
B	Name the structure labelled B	
C	Name the structure labelled C	
D	Name the structure labelled D	
E	Name the structure labelled E	

Question 12

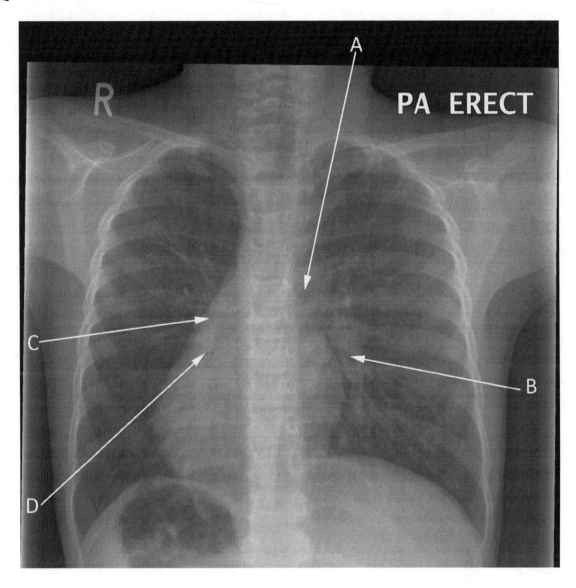

	QUESTION 12	WRITE YOUR ANSWER HERE
A	Name the structure labelled A	
B	Name the structure labelled B	
C	Name the structure labelled C	
D	Name the structure labelled D	
E	What is the normal variant on this film?	

Question 13

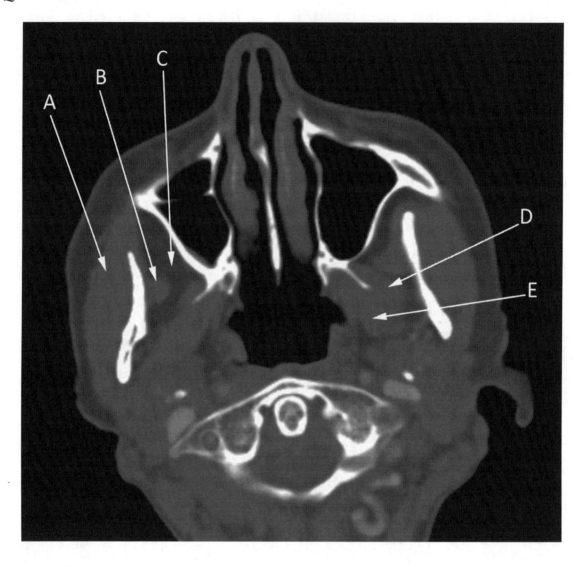

	QUESTION 13	WRITE YOUR ANSWER HERE
A	Name the structure labelled A	
B	Name the structure labelled B	
C	Name the structure labelled C	
D	Name the structure labelled D	
E	Name the structure labelled E	

Question 14

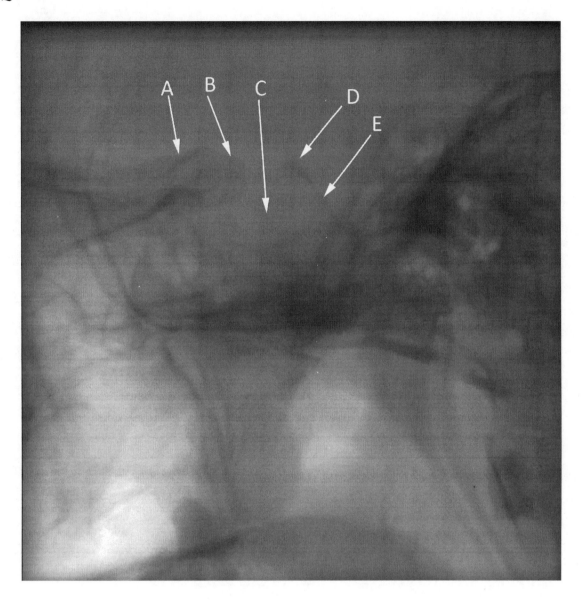

	QUESTION 14	WRITE YOUR ANSWER HERE
A	Name the structure labelled A	
B	Name the structure labelled B	
C	Name the structure labelled C	
D	Name the structure labelled D	
E	Name the structure labelled E	

Question 15

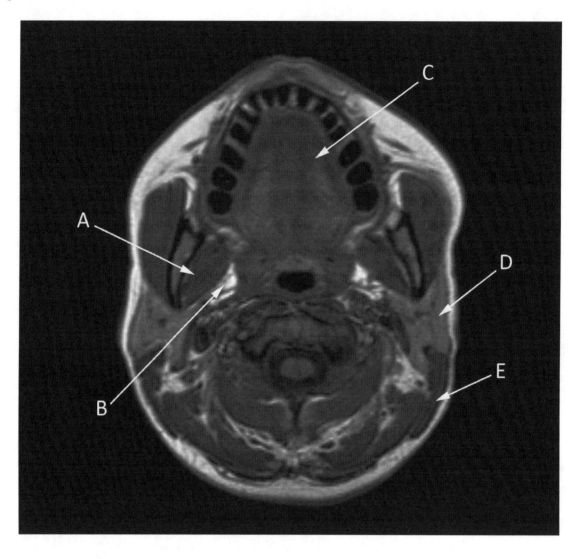

	QUESTION 15	WRITE YOUR ANSWER HERE
A	Name the structure labelled A	
B	Name the structure labelled B	
C	Name the structure labelled C	
D	Name the structure labelled D	
E	Name the structure labelled E	

Question 16

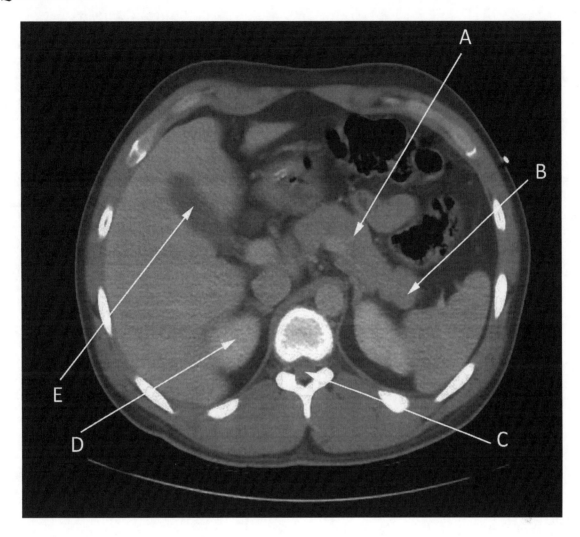

	QUESTION 16	WRITE YOUR ANSWER HERE
A	Name the structure labelled A	
B	Name the structure labelled B	
C	Name the structure labelled C	
D	Name the structure labelled D	
E	Name the structure labelled E	

Question 17

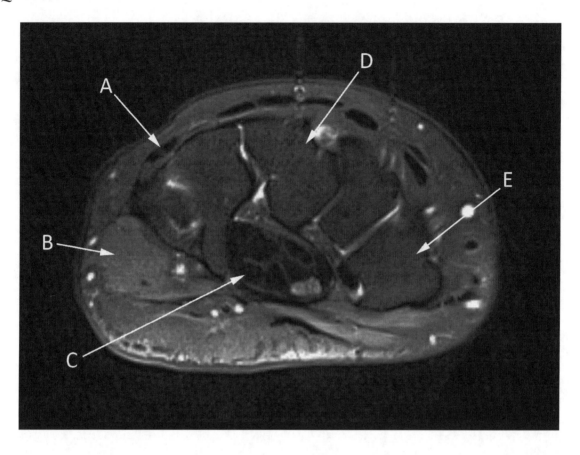

	QUESTION 17	WRITE YOUR ANSWER HERE
A	Name the structure labelled A	
B	Name the structure labelled B	
C	Name the structure labelled C	
D	Name the structure labelled D	
E	Name the structure labelled E	

Question 18

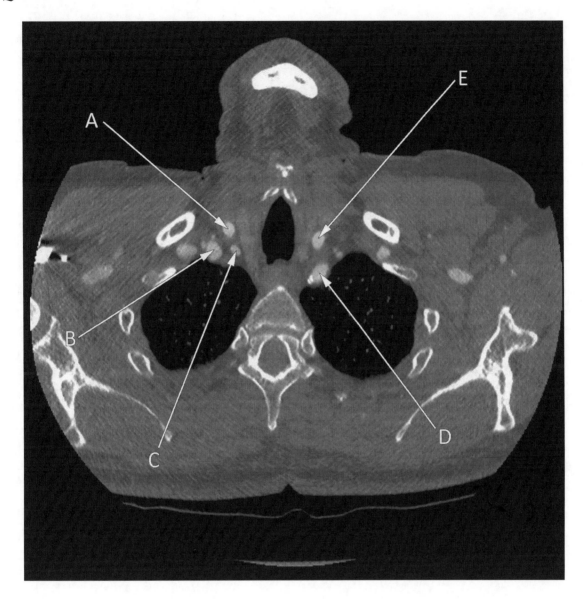

	QUESTION 18	WRITE YOUR ANSWER HERE
A	Name the vessel labelled A	
B	Name the vessel labelled B	
C	Name the vessel labelled C	
D	Name the vessel labelled D	
E	Name the vessel labelled E	

Question 19

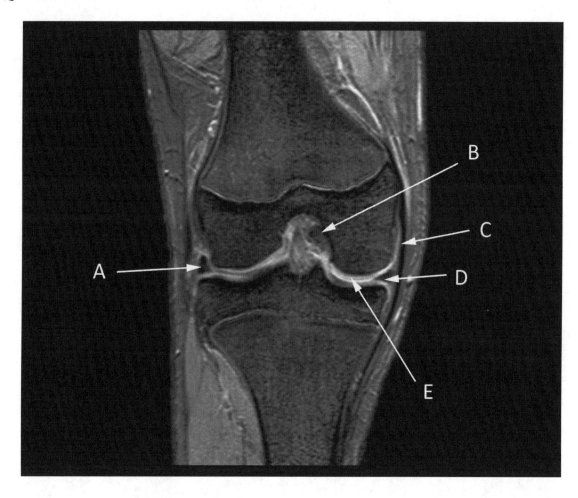

	QUESTION 19	WRITE YOUR ANSWER HERE
A	Name the structure labelled A	
B	Name the structure labelled B	
C	Name the structure labelled C	
D	Name the structure labelled D	
E	Name the structure labelled E	

Question 20

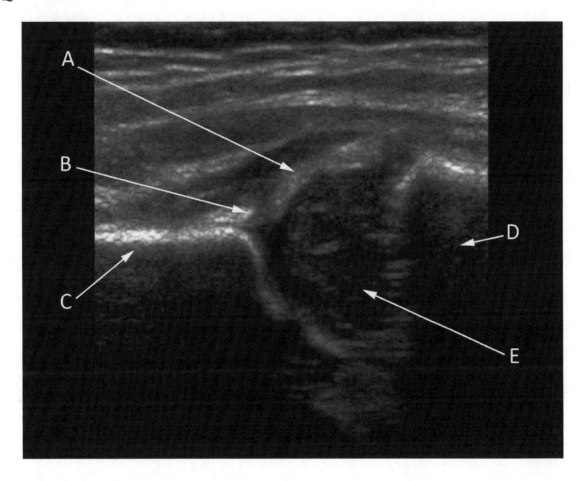

	QUESTION 20	WRITE YOUR ANSWER HERE
A	Name the structure labelled A	
B	Name the structure labelled B	
C	Name the structure labelled C	
D	Name the structure labelled D	
E	Name the structure labelled E	

Paper 18

Answers

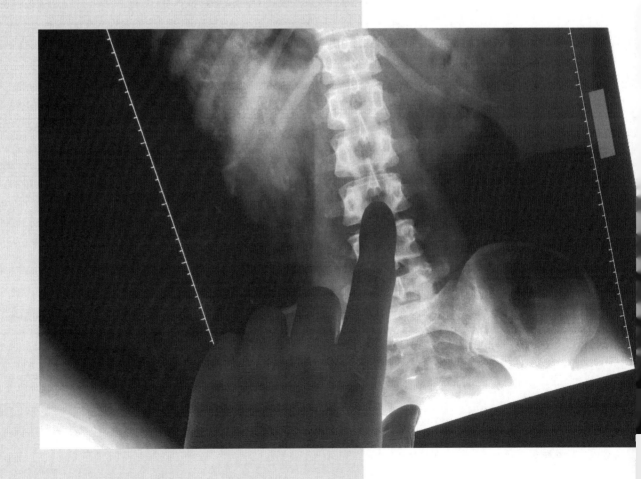

Question 1

A. Left atrium
B. Inferior vena cava
C. Right coronary artery
D. Right ventricle
E. Main pulmonary artery

Question 2

A. Torcular Herophili
B. Transverse sinus
C. Straight sinus
D. Superior sagittal sinus
E. Internal carotid artery

Question 3

A. Spleen
B. Stomach
C. Left kidney
D. Left iliacus muscle
E. Left psoas muscle

Question 4

A. Right spermatic cord
B. Neck of right femur
C. Right ischium
D. Left iliopsoas muscle
E. Left pectineus muscle

Question 5

A. Right main pulmonary artery
B. Right upper lobe pulmonary artery
C. Interlobar artery
D. Right superior pulmonary vein
E. Descending aorta

Question 6

A. Interphalangeal joint of the right thumb
B. Growth centre for right first metacarpal
C. Right scaphoid bone
D. Right lunate bone
E. Right ulnar epiphysis

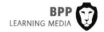

Question 7

A. Right pectineus muscle
B. Right obturator externus muscle
C. Right quadratus femoris muscle
D. Left common femoral artery
E. Right obturator internus muscle

Question 8

A. Right optic nerve
B. Right ethmoidal air cells
C. Left middle nasal turbinate
D. Left lamina papyracea
E. Left ostium of antrum

Question 9

A. Right acromio-clavicular joint
B. Right axillary vein
C. Right cephalic vein
D. Right subclavian vein
E. Right arm venogram

Question 10

A. Right upper lobe bronchus
B. Interlobar artery
C. Descending aorta
D. Left acromion
E. Left first rib

Question 11

A. Vertebral body (L4)
B. Right kidney – upper pole
C. Left crus of diaphragm
D. Left ureter
E. Left psoas muscle

Question 12

A. Left main bronchus
B. Left lower lobe pulmonary artery
C. Right upper lobe bronchus
D. Right lower lobe bronchus
E. Situs inversus

Question 13

A. Right masseter muscle
B. Right temporalis muscle
C. Right buccal fat space
D. Left lateral pterygoid muscle
E. Left medial pterygoid muscle

Question 14

A. Planum sphenoidal
B. Anterior clinoid
C. Pituitary fossa
D. Posterior clinoid
E. Clivus

Question 15

A. Right medial pterygoid muscle
B. Fat in right parapharyngeal space
C. Intrinsic muscles of tongue
D. Left parotid gland
E. Left sternocleidomastoid muscle

Question 16

A. Body of pancreas
B. Tail of pancreas
C. Spinal canal
D. Right kidney
E. Gallbladder

Question 17

A. Tendon of extensor carpi ulnaris muscle
B. Abductor digiti minimi muscle
C. Tendon of flexor digitorum superficialis muscle
D. Capitate
E. Trapezium

Question 18

A. Right common carotid artery
B. Right subclavian artery
C. Right vertebral artery
D. Left subclavian artery
E. Left common carotid artery

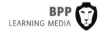

Question 19

A. Lateral meniscus
B. Posterior cruciate ligament
C. Medial collateral ligament
D. Medial meniscus
E. Articular cartilage

Question 20

A. Labrum
B. Cartilaginous acetabular roof
C. Ilium
D. Femoral neck
E. Femoral head

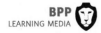

Paper 19

Question Bank

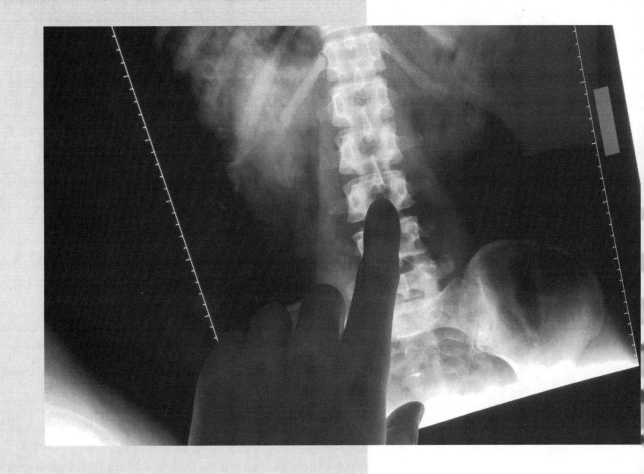

Question 1

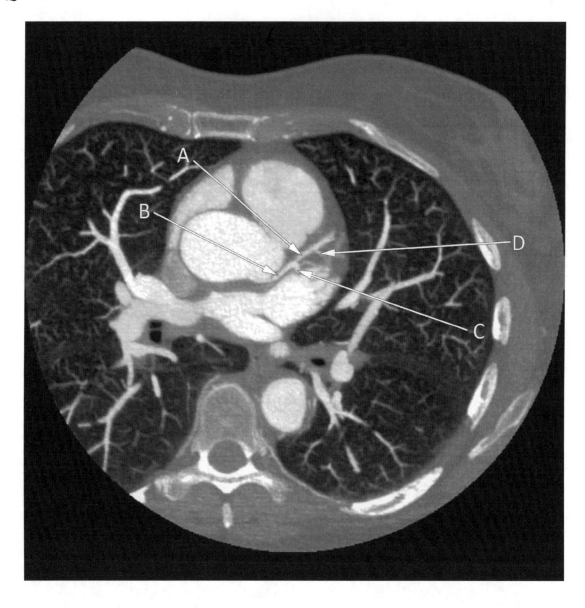

	QUESTION 1	WRITE YOUR ANSWER HERE
A	Name the vessel labelled A	
B	Name the vessel labelled B	
C	Name the vessel labelled C	
D	Name the vessel labelled D	
E	Where would a Ramus Intermedius vessel arise from?	

Question 2

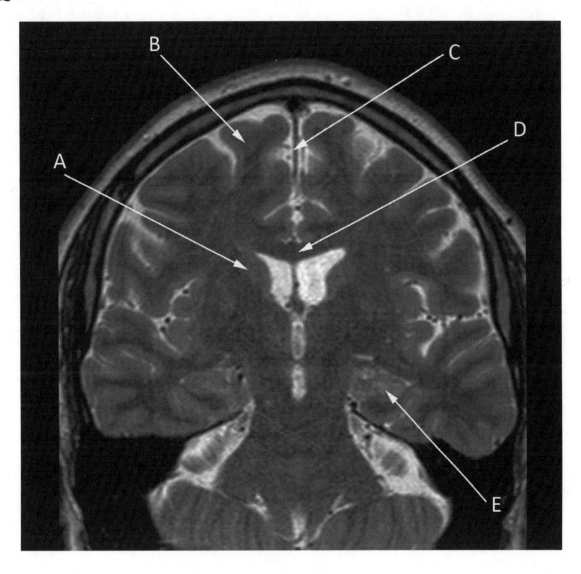

	QUESTION 2	WRITE YOUR ANSWER HERE
A	Name the structure labelled A	
B	Name the structure labelled B	
C	Name the structure labelled C	
D	Name the structure labelled D	
E	Name the structure labelled E	

Question 3

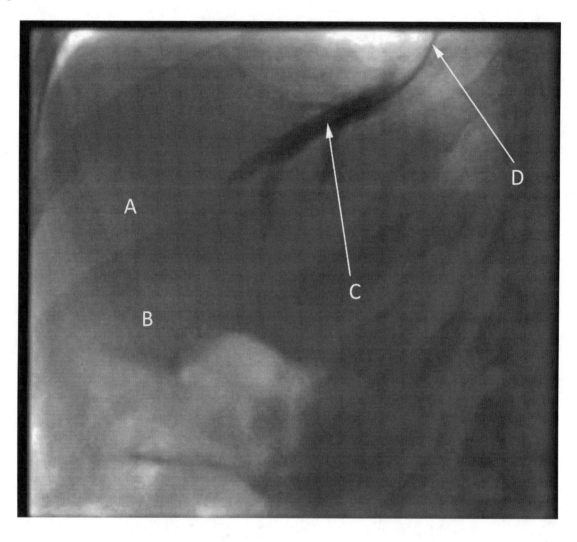

	QUESTION 3	WRITE YOUR ANSWER HERE
A	Name the structure labelled A	
B	Name the structure labelled B	
C	Name the structure labelled C	
D	Name the structure the catheter is in at this point (D)	
E	Name the investigation shown	

Question 4

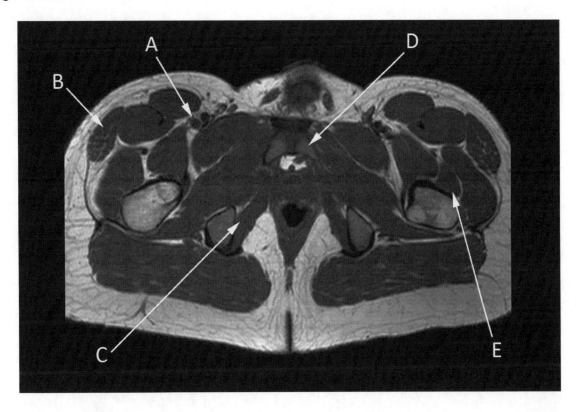

	QUESTION 4	WRITE YOUR ANSWER HERE
A	Name the structure labelled A	
B	Name the structure labelled B	
C	Name the structure labelled C	
D	Name the structure labelled D	
E	Name the structure labelled E	

Question 5

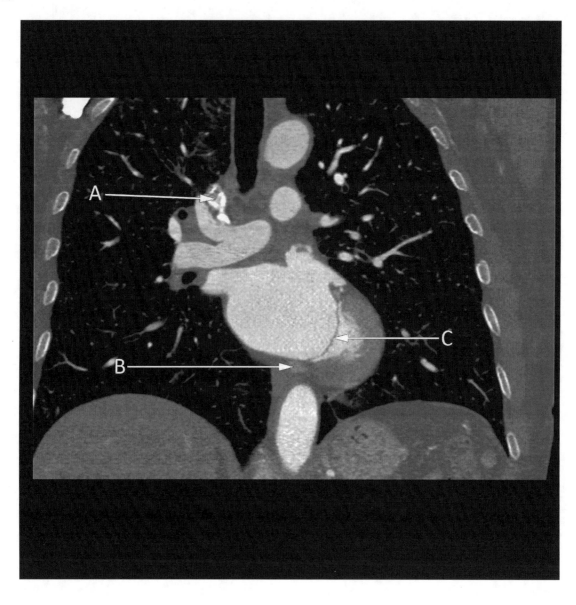

	QUESTION 5	WRITE YOUR ANSWER HERE
A	Name the vessel labelled A	
B	Name the vessel labelled B	
C	Name the structure labelled C	
D	Into which vessel does A drain?	
E	What does B drain into?	

Question 6

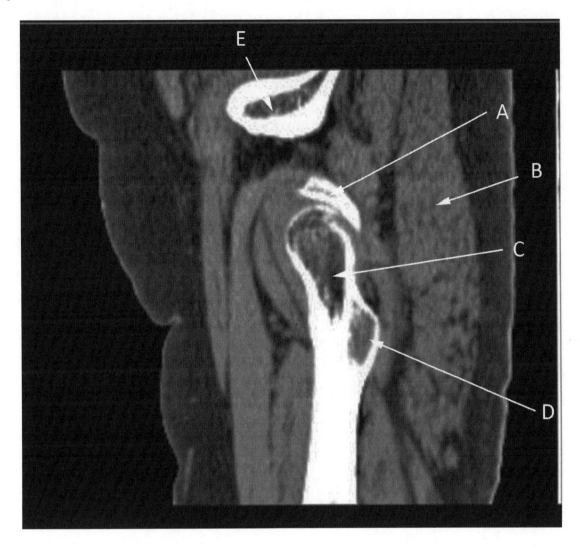

	QUESTION 6	WRITE YOUR ANSWER HERE
A	Name the structure labelled A	
B	Name the structure labelled B	
C	Name the structure labelled C	
D	Name the structure labelled D	
E	Name the structure labelled E	

Question 7

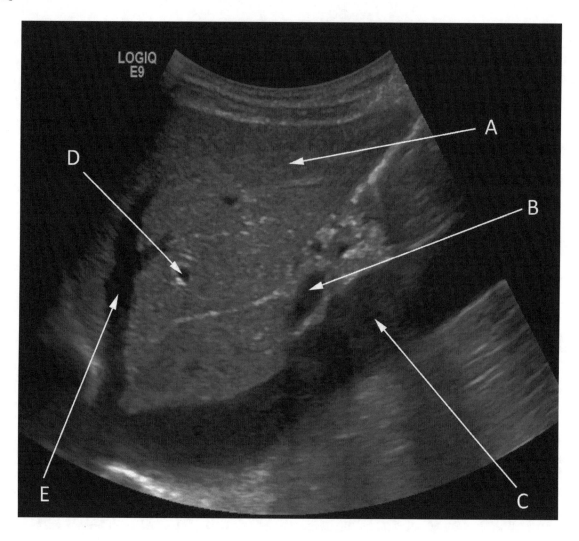

	QUESTION 7	WRITE YOUR ANSWER HERE
A	Name the structure labelled A	
B	Name the structure labelled B	
C	Name the structure labelled C	
D	Name the structure labelled D	
E	Name the structure labelled E	

Question 8

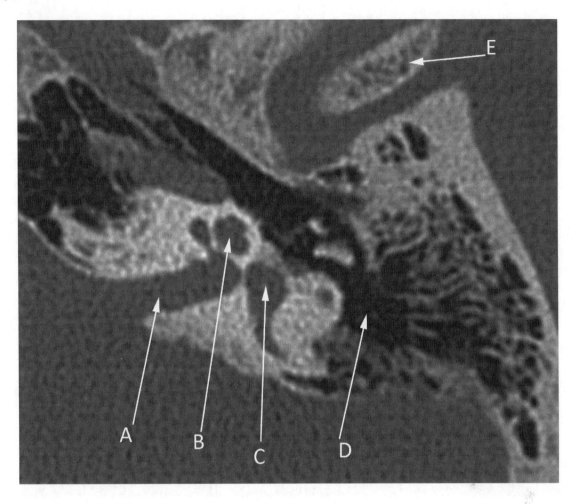

	QUESTION 8	WRITE YOUR ANSWER HERE
A	Name the structure labelled A	
B	Name the structure labelled B	
C	Name the structure labelled C	
D	Name the structure labelled D	
E	Name the structure labelled E	

Question 9

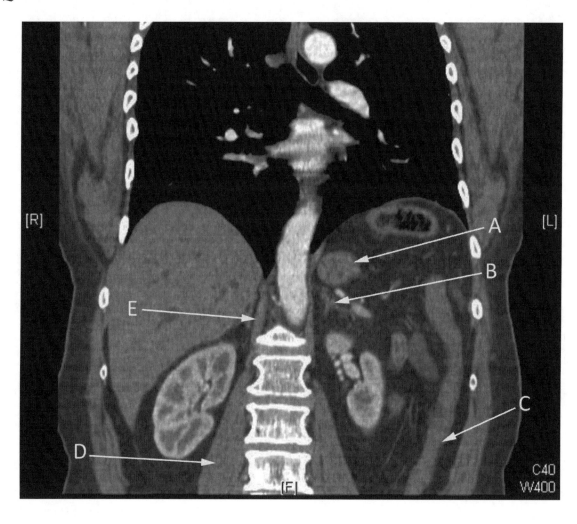

	QUESTION 9	WRITE YOUR ANSWER HERE
A	Name the structure labelled A	
B	Name the structure labelled B	
C	Name the structure labelled C	
D	Name the structure labelled D	
E	Name the structure labelled E	

Question 10

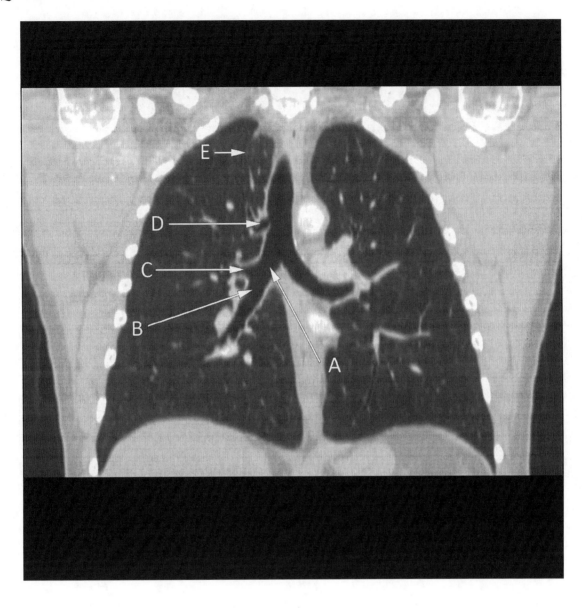

	QUESTION 10	WRITE YOUR ANSWER HERE
A	Name the structure labelled A	
B	Name the structure labelled B	
C	Name the structure labelled C	
D	Name the anatomical variant labelled D	
E	Name the anatomical variant labelled E	

Question 11

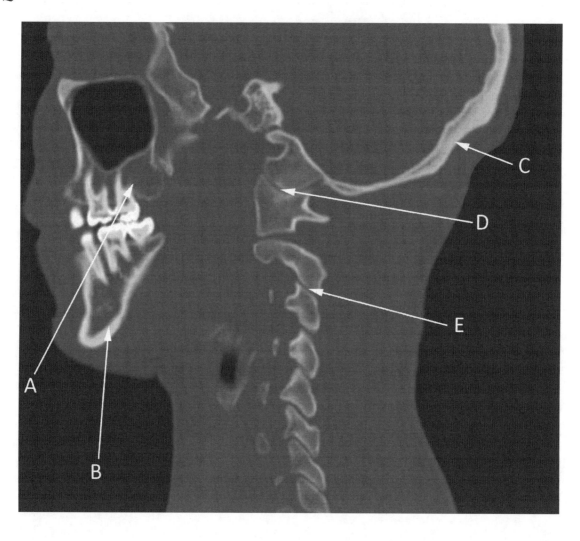

	QUESTION 11	WRITE YOUR ANSWER HERE
A	Name the structure labelled A	
B	Name the structure labelled B	
C	Name the structure labelled C	
D	Name the structure labelled D	
E	Name the structure labelled E	

Question 12

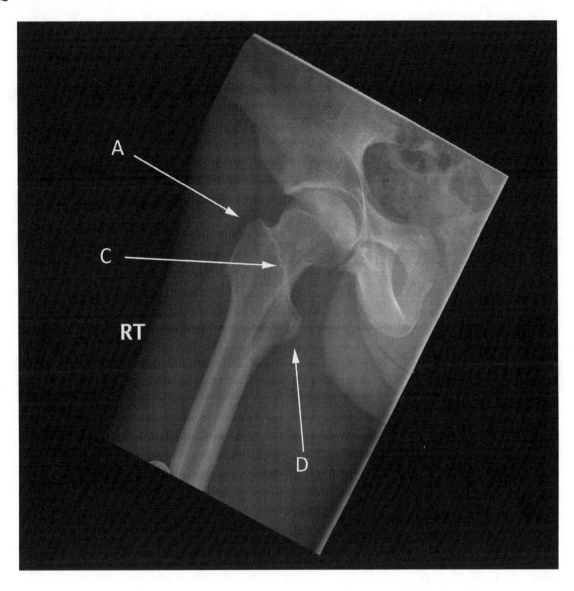

	QUESTION 12	WRITE YOUR ANSWER HERE
A	Name the structure labelled A	
B	What attaches to A?	
C	Name the structure labelled C	
D	Name the structure labelled D	
E	What attaches to D?	

Question 13

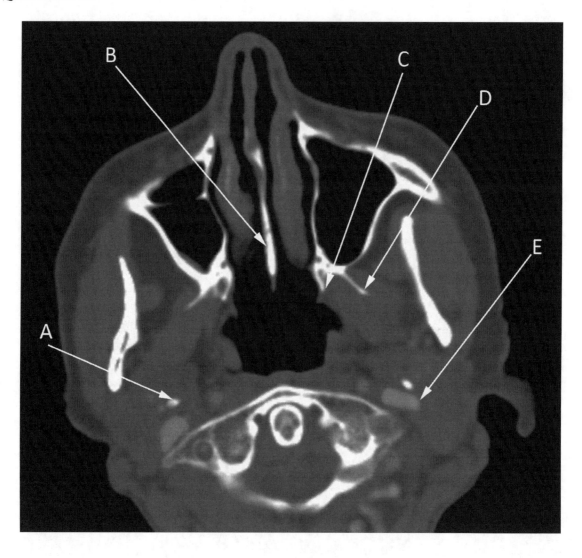

	QUESTION 13	WRITE YOUR ANSWER HERE
A	Name the structure labelled A	
B	Name the structure labelled B	
C	Name the structure labelled C	
D	Name the structure labelled D	
E	Name the structure labelled E	

Question 14

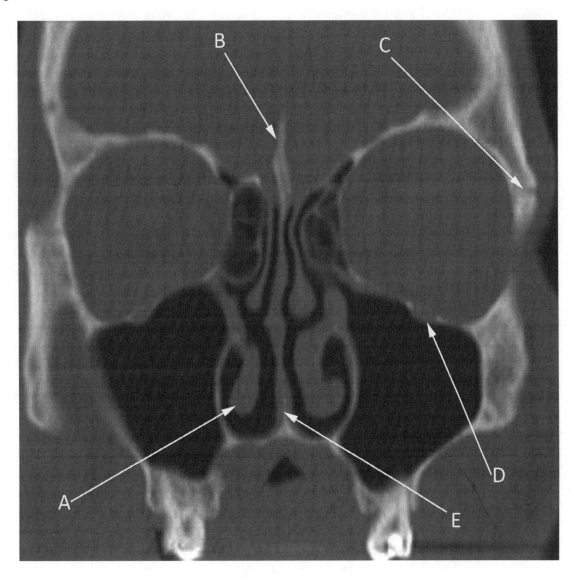

	QUESTION 14	WRITE YOUR ANSWER HERE
A	Name the structure labelled A	
B	Name the structure labelled B	
C	Name the structure labelled C	
D	Name the structure labelled D	
E	Name the structure labelled E	

Question 15

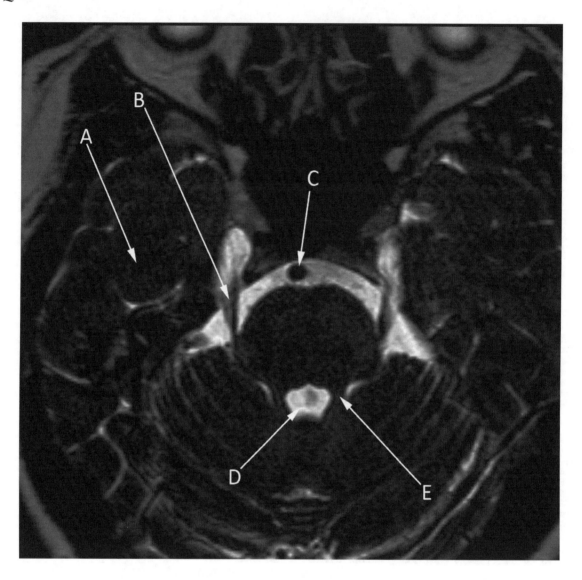

	QUESTION 15	WRITE YOUR ANSWER HERE
A	Name the structure labelled A	
B	Name the structure labelled B	
C	Name the structure labelled C	
D	Name the structure labelled D	
E	Name the structure labelled E	

Question 16

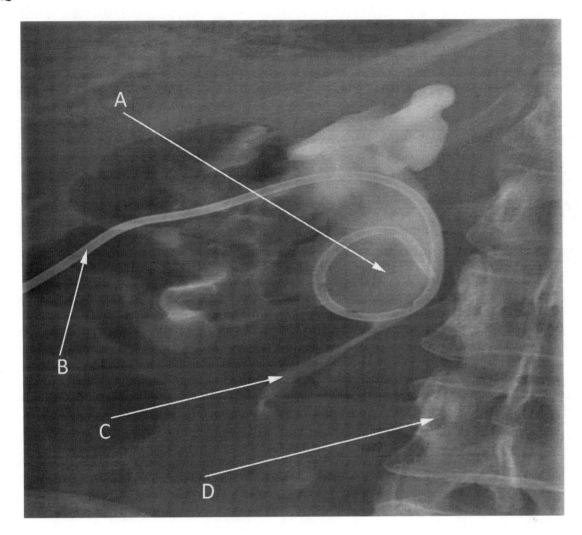

	QUESTION 16	WRITE YOUR ANSWER HERE
A	Name the structure labelled A	
B	Name the structure labelled B	
C	Name the structure labelled C	
D	Name the structure labelled D	
E	Name the investigation shown	

Question 17

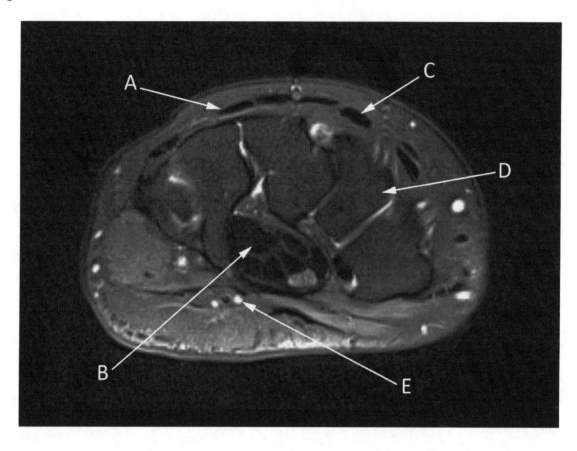

	QUESTION 17	WRITE YOUR ANSWER HERE
A	Name the structure labelled A	
B	Name the structure labelled B	
C	Name the structure labelled C	
D	Name the structure labelled D	
E	Name the structure labelled E	

Question 18

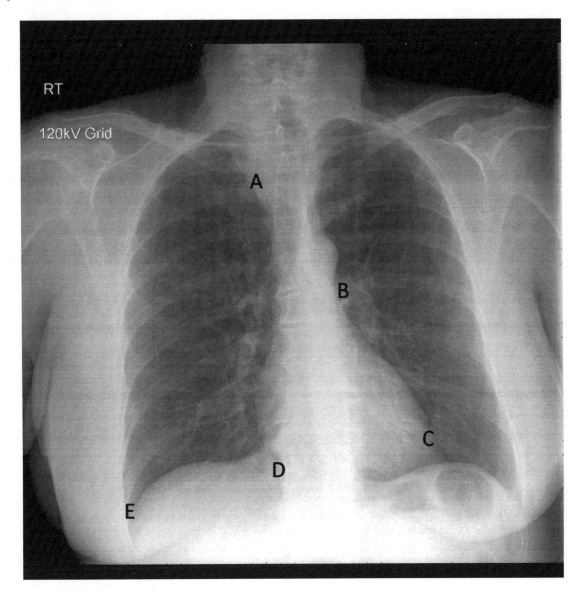

	QUESTION 18	WRITE YOUR ANSWER HERE
A	Name the vascular structure underlying A	
B	Name the structure labelled B	
C	Which heart chamber underlies label C?	
D	Name the vessel underlying D	
E	What region is E?	

Question 19

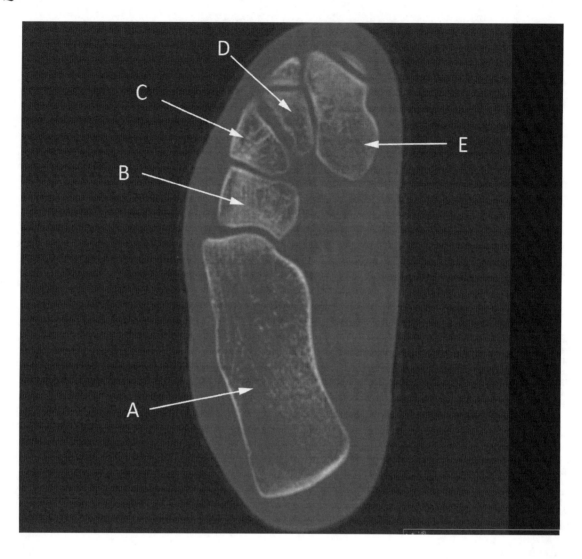

	QUESTION 19	WRITE YOUR ANSWER HERE
A	Name the structure labelled A	
B	Name the structure labelled B	
C	Name the structure labelled C	
D	Name the structure labelled D	
E	Name the structure labelled E	

Question 20

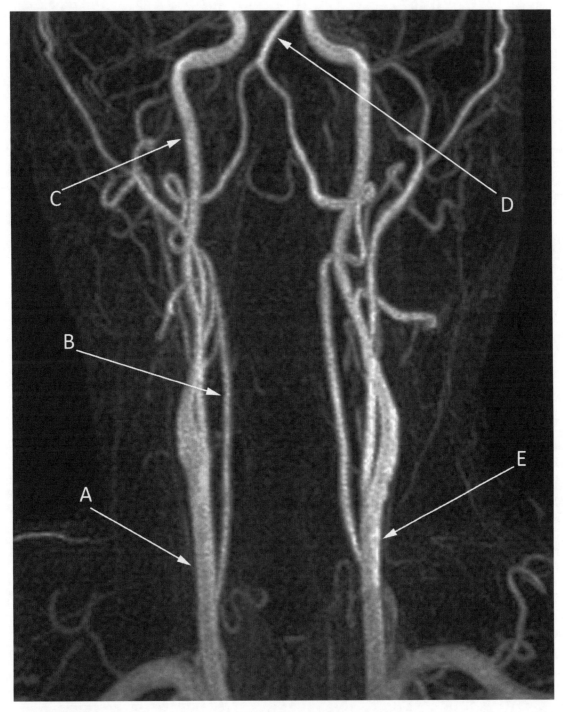

	QUESTION 20	WRITE YOUR ANSWER HERE
A	Name the structure labelled A	
B	Name the structure labelled B	
C	Name the structure labelled C	
D	Name the structure labelled D	
E	Name the structure labelled E	

BPP
LEARNING MEDIA

Paper 19

Answers

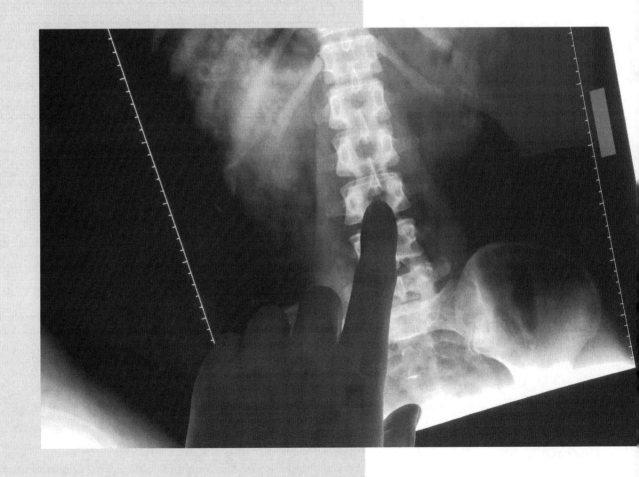

Question 1

A. Left anterior descending artery (LAD)
B. Left coronary artery / left main stem
C. Circumflex artery
D. Diagonal branch of LAD
E. Left main stem / left coronary artery

Question 2

A. Right caudate nucleus
B. Right superior frontal gyrus
C. Falx cerebri
D. Corpus callosum
E. Left hippocampus

Question 3

A. Right lobe of liver
B. Rib
C. Middle hepatic vein
D. IVC
E. Hepatic venogram

Question 4

A. Right common femoral artery
B. Right tensor fasciae latae
C. Right obturator internus
D. Left pubic bone
E. Left vastus intermedius

Question 5

A. Azygous vein
B. Coronary sinus
C. Mitral valve
D. Superior vena cava
E. Right atrium

Question 6

A. Acetabulum
B. Gluteus maximus muscle
C. Femoral neck
D. Greater trochanter
E. Ilium

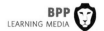

Question 7

A. Left lobe of liver
B. Gallbladder
C. IVC
D. Branch of portal vein
E. Left hepatic vein

Question 8

A. Internal auditory canal
B. Cochlea
C. Vestibule
D. Mastoid antrum
E. Mandibular condyle

Question 9

A. Stomach
B. Left adrenal
C. Descending colon
D. Right psoas muscle
E. Right diaphragmatic crus

Question 10

A. Right main bronchus
B. Bronchus intermedius
C. Right upper lobe bronchus
D. Accessory / tracheal / porcine bronchus
E. Azygous fissure

Question 11

A. Maxilla (alveolar process of)
B. Mandible
C. Occipital bone
D. Atlanto-occipital joint
E. C2/C3 facet joint

Question 12

A. Right greater trochanter
B. Right vastus lateralis, right piriformis muscle
C. Right intertrochanteric line
D. Right lesser trochanter
E. Right iliopsoas muscle

Question 13

A. Right styloid process
B. Vomer
C. Left medial pterygoid plate
D. Left lateral pterygoid plate
E. Left internal jugular vein

Question 14

A. Right inferior nasal turbinate
B. Crista galli
C. Left fronto-zygomatic suture
D. Left infra-orbital canal
E. Vomer

Question 15

A. Right temporal lobe
B. Right trigeminal nerve
C. Basilar artery
D. Fourth ventricle
E. Left superior cerebellar peduncle

Question 16

A. Renal pelvis
B. Catheter
C. Ureter
D. Pedicle
E. Nephrostogram / nephrostomy

Question 17

A. Tendon of extensor digitorum muscle
B. Tendon of flexor digitorum superficialis
C. Tendon of extensor carpi radialis brevis
D. Trapezoid bone
E. Ulnar artery

Question 18

A. Right brachiocephalic vein
B. Left main pulmonary artery
C. Left ventricle
D. Inferior vena cava
E. Right costophrenic angle

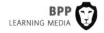

Question 19

A. Calcaneus
B. Cuboid
C. Lateral cuneiform
D. Intermediate cuneiform
E. Navicular

Question 20

A. Common carotid artery (right)
B. Vertebral artery (right)
C. Internal carotid artery (right)
D. Basilar artery
E. Common carotid (left)

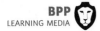

Paper 20

Question Bank

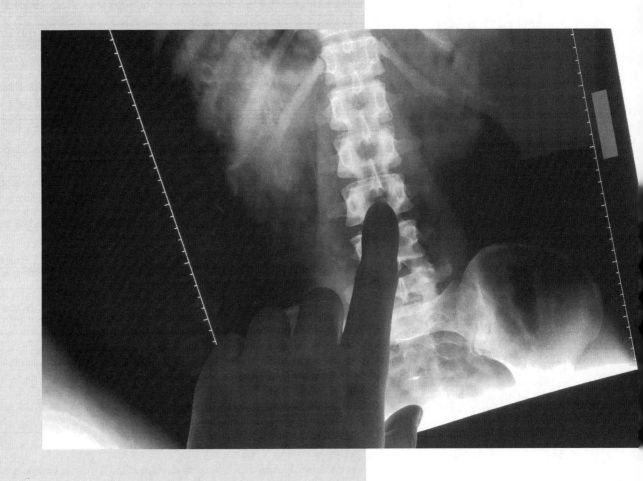

Question 1

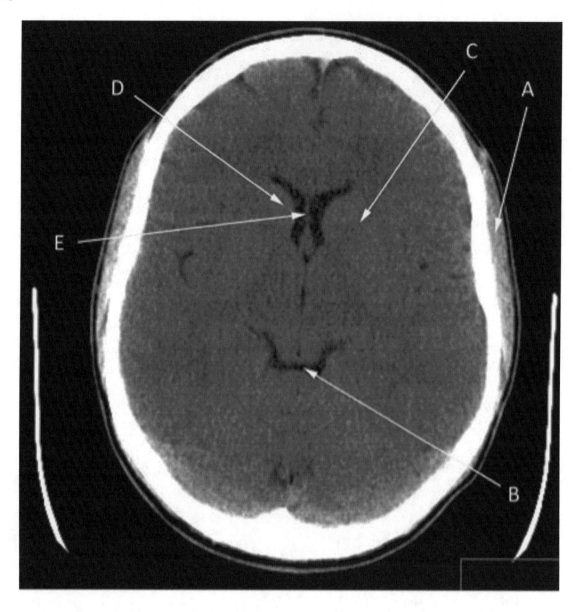

	QUESTION 1	WRITE YOUR ANSWER HERE
A	Name the structure labelled A	
B	Name the structure labelled B	
C	Name the structure labelled C	
D	Name the structure labelled D	
E	Name the structure labelled E	

Question 2

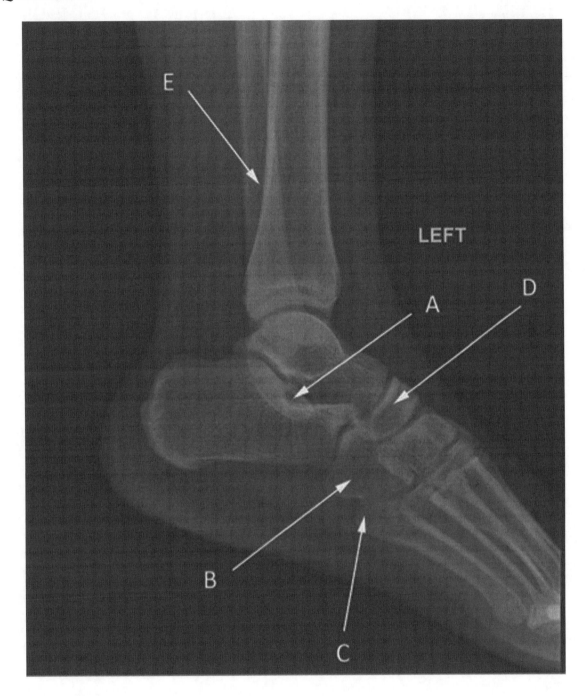

	QUESTION 2	WRITE YOUR ANSWER HERE
A	Name the structure labelled A	
B	Name the structure labelled B	
C	Name the structure labelled C	
D	Name the structure labelled D	
E	Name the structure labelled E	

Question 3

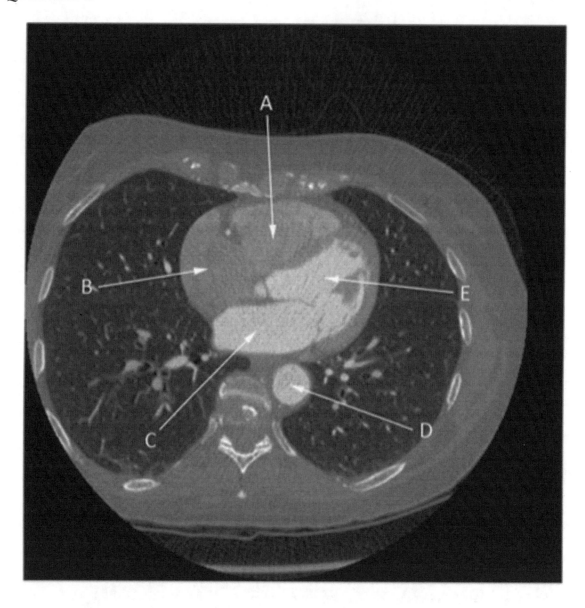

	QUESTION 3	WRITE YOUR ANSWER HERE
A	Name the structure labelled A	
B	Name the structure labelled B	
C	Name the structure labelled C	
D	Name the structure labelled D	
E	Name the structure labelled E	

Question 4

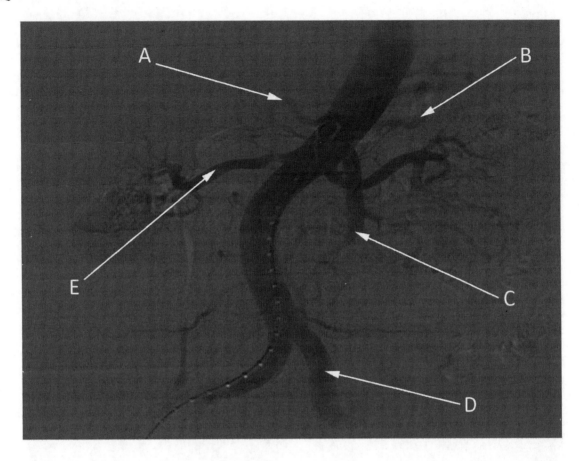

	QUESTION 4	WRITE YOUR ANSWER HERE
A	Name the structure labelled A	
B	Name the structure labelled B	
C	Name the structure labelled C	
D	Name the structure labelled D	
E	Name the structure labelled E	

Question 5

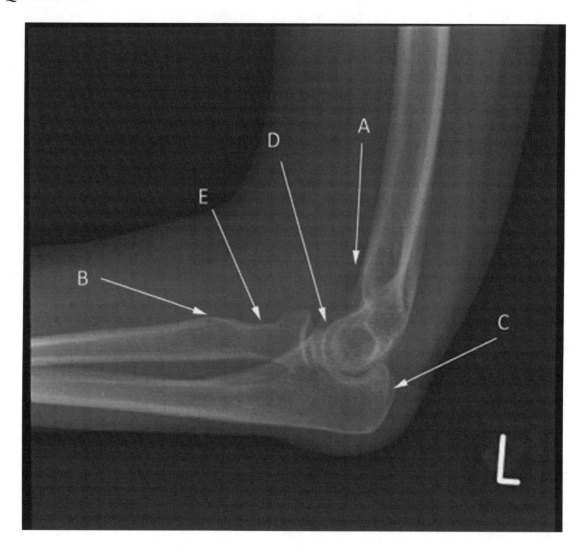

	QUESTION 5	WRITE YOUR ANSWER HERE
A	Name the structure labelled A	
B	Name the structure labelled B	
C	Name the structure labelled C	
D	Name the structure labelled D	
E	Name the structure labelled E	

Question 6

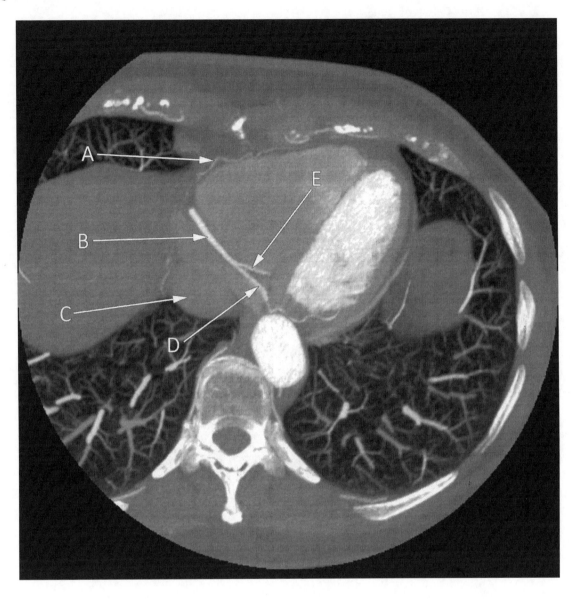

	QUESTION 6	WRITE YOUR ANSWER HERE
A	Name the vessel labelled A	
B	Name the vessel labelled B	
C	Name the structure labelled C	
D	Name the vessel labelled D	
E	Name the vessel labelled E	

Question 7

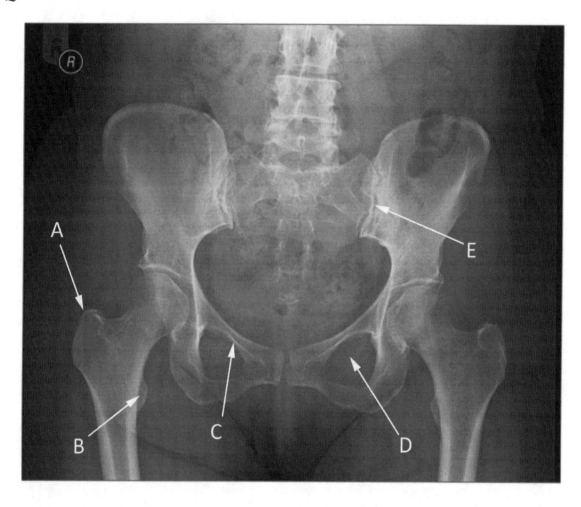

	QUESTION 7	WRITE YOUR ANSWER HERE
A	Name the structure labelled A	
B	Name the muscle that attaches to B	
C	Name the structure labelled C	
D	Name the structure labelled D	
E	Name the structure labelled E	

Question 8

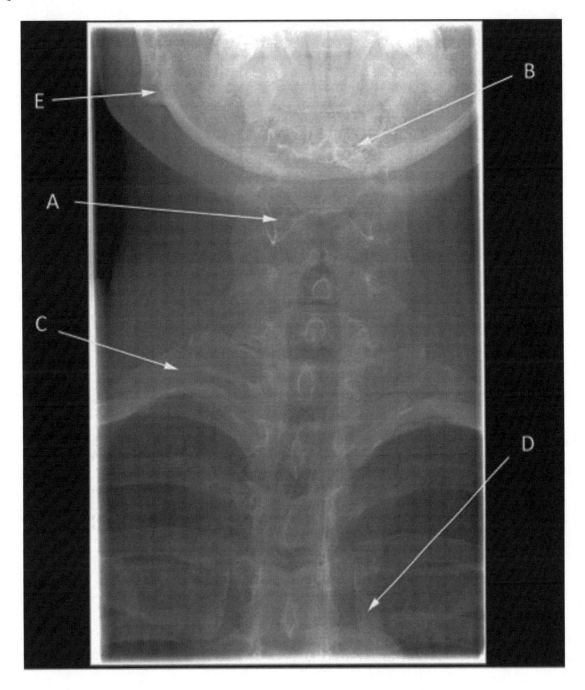

	QUESTION 8	WRITE YOUR ANSWER HERE
A	Name the structure labelled A	
B	Name the structure labelled B	
C	Name the structure labelled C	
D	Name the structure labelled D	
E	Name the structure labelled E	

Question 9

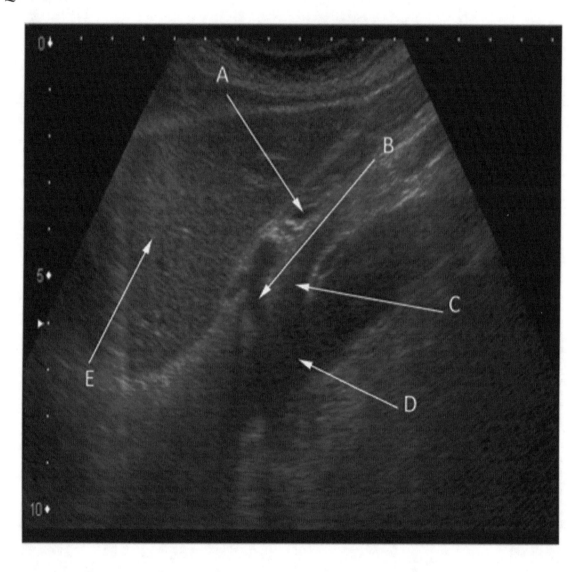

	QUESTION 9	WRITE YOUR ANSWER HERE
A	Name the structure labelled A	
B	Name the structure labelled B	
C	Name the structure labelled C	
D	Name the structure labelled D	
E	Name the structure labelled E	

Question 10

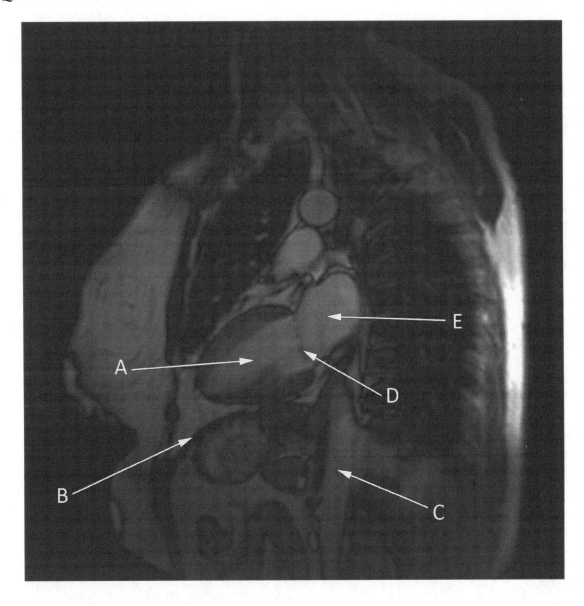

	QUESTION 10	WRITE YOUR ANSWER HERE
A	Name the structure labelled A	
B	Name the structure labelled B	
C	Name the structure labelled C	
D	Name the structure labelled D	
E	Name the structure labelled E	

Question 11

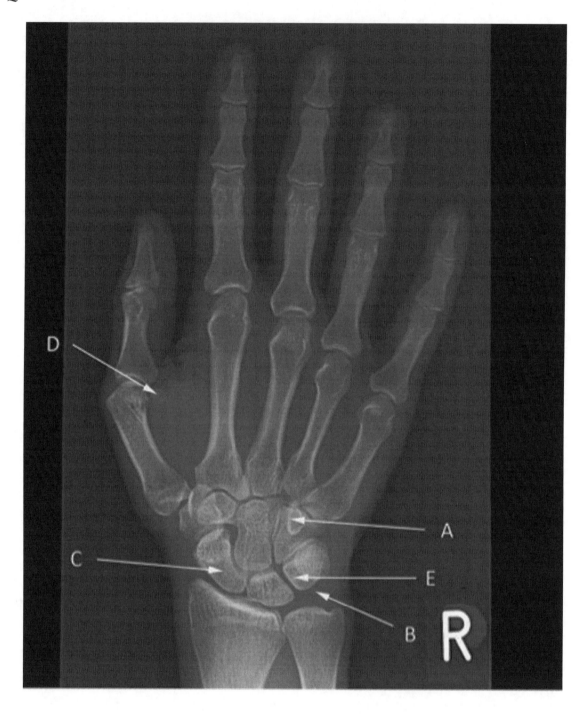

	QUESTION 11	WRITE YOUR ANSWER HERE
A	Name the structure labelled A	
B	Name the structure which occupies B	
C	Name the structure labelled C	
D	Name the structure labelled D	
E	Name the structure labelled E	

Question 12

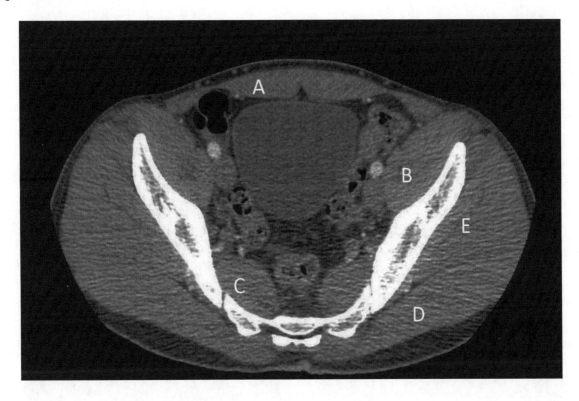

	QUESTION 12	WRITE YOUR ANSWER HERE
A	Name the structure labelled A	
B	Name the structure labelled B	
C	Name the structure labelled C	
D	Name the structure labelled D	
E	Name the structure labelled E	

Question 13

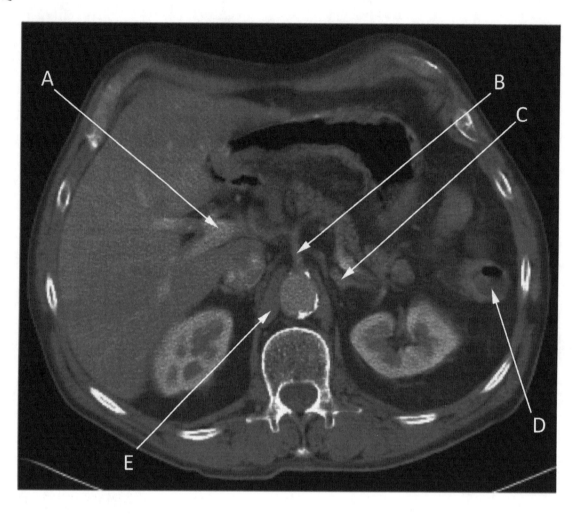

	QUESTION 13	WRITE YOUR ANSWER HERE
A	Name the structure labelled A	
B	Name the structure labelled B	
C	Name the structure labelled C	
D	Name the structure labelled D	
E	Name the structure labelled E	

Question 14

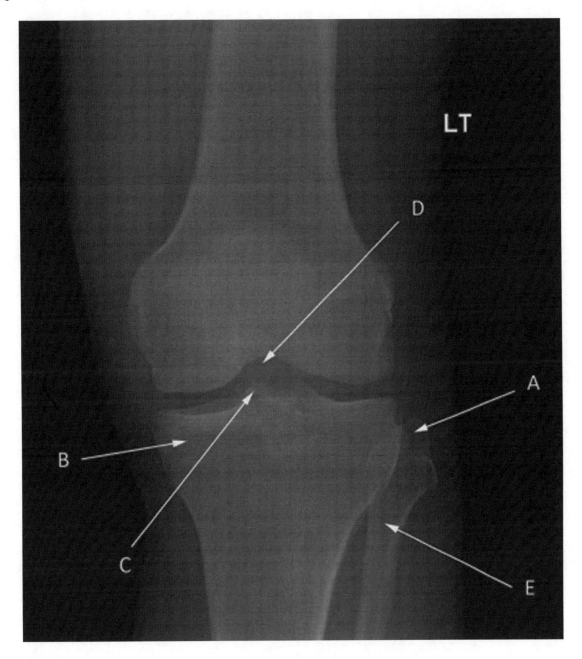

	QUESTION 14	WRITE YOUR ANSWER HERE
A	Name the structure labelled A	
B	Name the structure labelled B	
C	Name the structure labelled C	
D	Name the structure labelled D	
E	Name the structure labelled E	

BPP
LEARNING MEDIA

Question 15

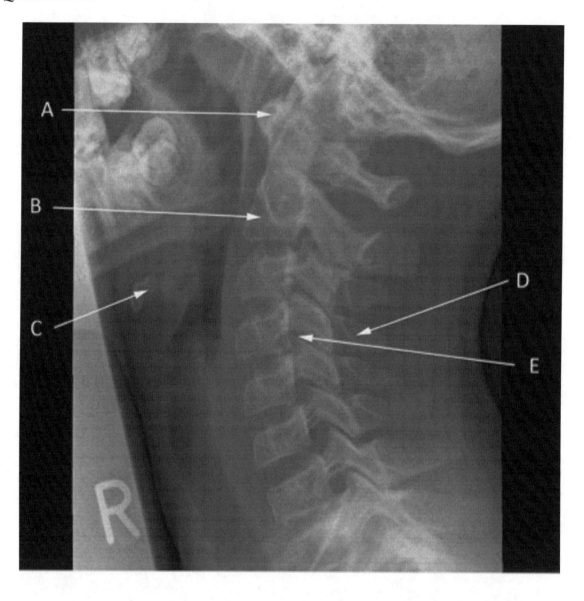

	QUESTION 15	WRITE YOUR ANSWER HERE
A	Name the structure labelled A	
B	Name the structure labelled B	
C	Name the structure labelled C	
D	Name the structure labelled D	
E	Name the structure labelled E	

Question 16

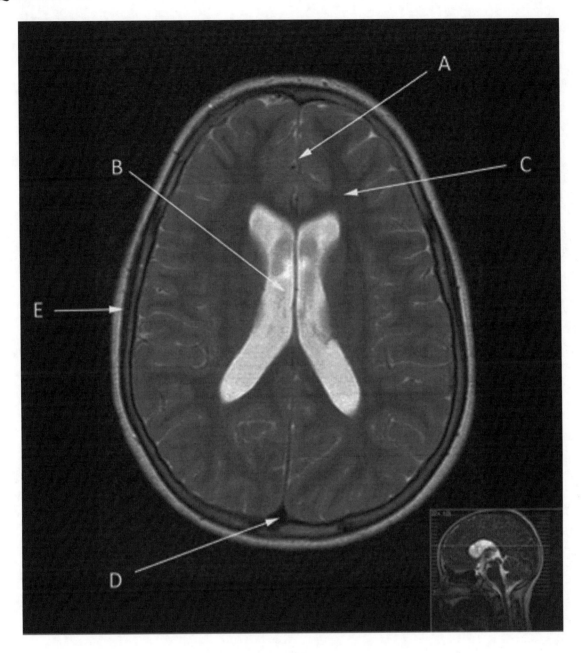

	QUESTION 16	WRITE YOUR ANSWER HERE
A	Name the structure labelled A	
B	Name the structure labelled B	
C	Name the structure labelled C	
D	Name the structure labelled D	
E	Name the structure labelled E	

Question 17

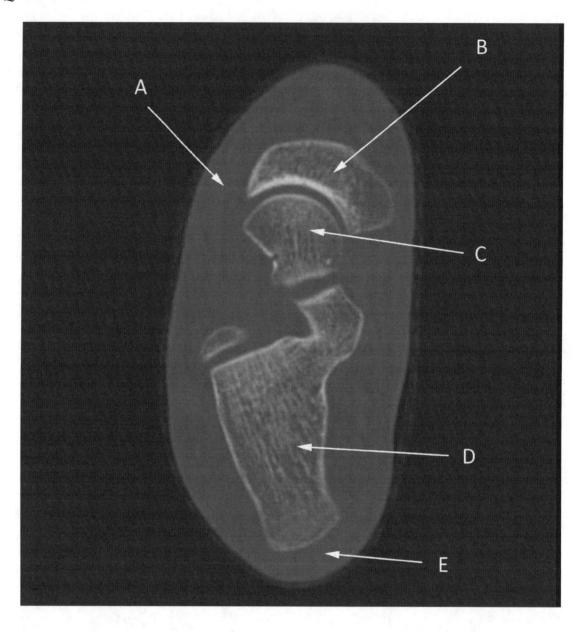

	QUESTION 17	WRITE YOUR ANSWER HERE
A	Name the structure labelled A	
B	Name the structure labelled B	
C	Name the structure labelled C	
D	Name the structure labelled D	
E	Name the structure labelled E	

Question 18

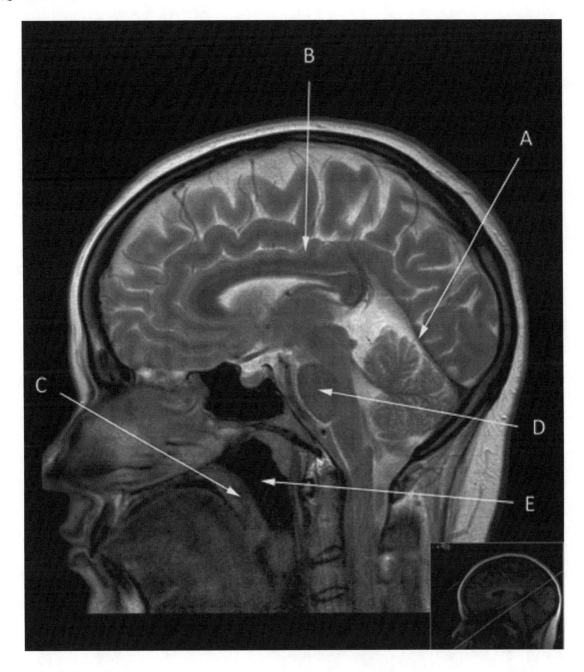

	QUESTION 18	WRITE YOUR ANSWER HERE
A	Name the structure labelled A	
B	Name the structure labelled B	
C	Name the structure labelled C	
D	Name the structure labelled D	
E	Name the structure labelled E	

Question 19

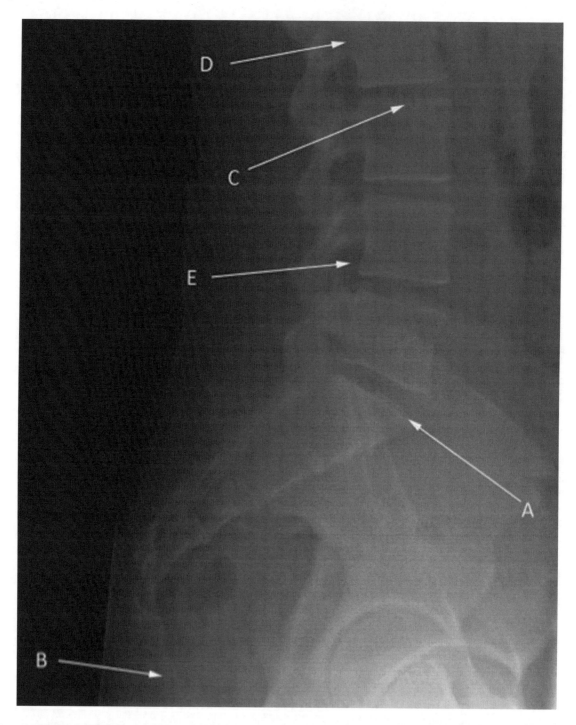

	QUESTION 19	WRITE YOUR ANSWER HERE
A	Name the structure labelled A	
B	Name the structure labelled B	
C	Name the structure labelled C	
D	Name the structure labelled D	
E	What exits at E?	

Question 20

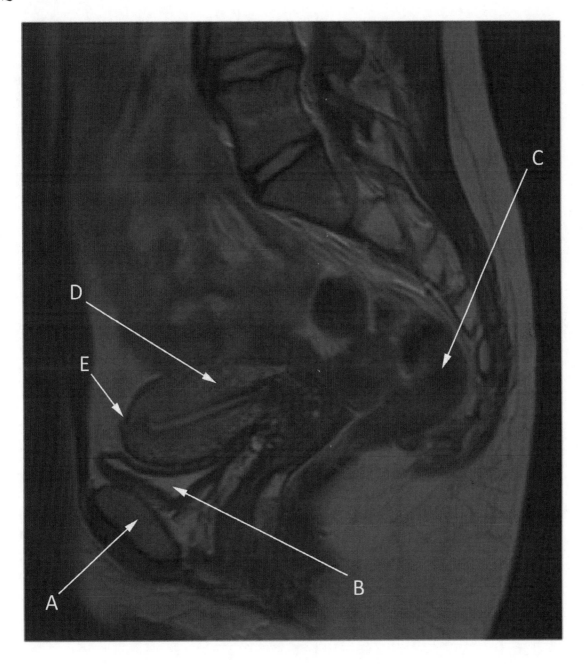

	QUESTION 20	WRITE YOUR ANSWER HERE
A	Name the structure labelled A	
B	Name the structure labelled B	
C	Name the structure labelled C	
D	Name the structure labelled D	
E	Name the structure labelled E	

Paper 20

Answers

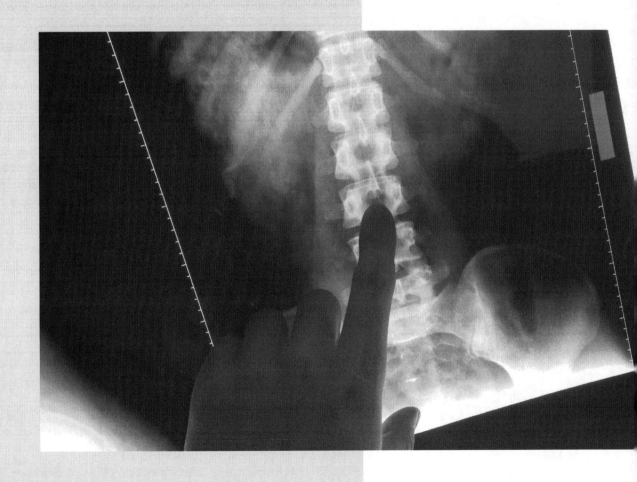

Question 1

A. Left temporalis muscle
B. Quadrigeminal cistern
C. Anterior limb of the left internal capsule
D. Right caudate nucleus
E. Septum pellucidum

Question 2

A. Sustentaculum tali of left calcaneus
B. Left cuboid
C. Tuberosity of base of left fifth metatarsal
D. Left navicular
E. Left fibula

Question 3

A. Right ventricle
B. Right atrium
C. Left atrium
D. Descending aorta
E. Left ventricle

Question 4

A. Common hepatic artery
B. Splenic artery
C. Superior mesenteric artery
D. Left common iliac artery
E. Right renal artery

Question 5

A. Left anterior fat pad
B. Left radial tuberosity
C. Left olecranon
D. Left capitellum
E. Left radial neck

Question 6

A. Acute marginal artery
B. Right coronary artery
C. Inferior vena cava
D. Posterolateral branch of the RCA
E. Posterior descending artery

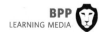

Question 7

A. Right greater trochanter
B. Right ilio-psoas muscle
C. Right superior pubic ramus
D. Left obturator foramen
E. Left sacro-iliac joint

Question 8

A. Valleculae
B. Piriform fossa
C. Right first rib
D. Medial end of left clavicle
E. Right mastoid process

Question 9

A. Splenic vein
B. Coeliac axis
C. Superior mesenteric artery
D. Aorta
E. Left lobe of liver

Question 10

A. Left ventricle
B. Left hemi diaphragm
C. Descending aorta
D. Mitral valve
E. Left atrium

Question 11

A. Right hook of hamate
B. Right triangular fibrocartilage
C. Right scaphoid
D. Sesamoid bone
E. Right triquetral

Question 12

A. Rectus abdominis muscle
B. Left iliacus muscle
C. Right psoas muscle
D. Left gluteus maximus muscle
E. Left gluteus medius muscle

Question 13

A. Portal vein
B. Coeliac axis
C. Left adrenal gland
D. Descending colon
E. Right crus of diaphragm

Question 14

A. Styloid process of left fibula
B. Medial condyle of left tibia
C. Tubercle of intercondylar eminence
D. Left intercondylar fossa
E. Neck of left fibula

Question 15

A. Anterior arch of atlas
B. Body of axis
C. Hyoid bone
D. Spinous process of C4
E. Facet joint of C4/C5

Question 16

A. Falx cerebri
B. Body of right lateral ventricle
C. Left corona radiata
D. Superior sagittal sinus
E. Outer table of calvarium

Question 17

A. Extensor digitorum brevis
B. Navicular
C. Head of talus
D. Calcaneum
E. Achilles' tendon

Question 18

A. Tentorium cerebelli
B. Cingulate gyrus
C. Soft palate
D. Pons
E. Nasopharynx

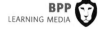

Question 19

A. Sacral promontory
B. Coccyx
C. Superior endplate of L3
D. Pedicle of L2
E. L4 nerve root

Question 20

A. Pubic bone
B. Urinary bladder
C. Distal sigmoid / recto-sigmoid junction
D. Myometrium
E. Fundus of uterus

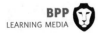

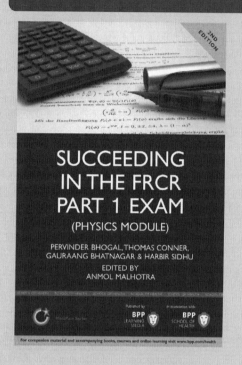
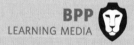

More titles in the Progressing your Medical Career Series

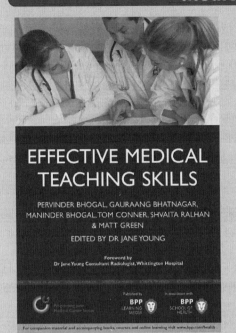

EFFECTIVE MEDICAL TEACHING SKILLS

PERVINDER BHOGAL, GAURAANG BHATNAGAR,
MANINDER BHOGAL, TOM CONNER, SHVAITA RALHAN
& MATT GREEN

EDITED BY DR JANE YOUNG

Foreword by
Dr Jane Young Consultant Radiologist, Whittington Hospital

£19.99
October 2011
Paperback
978-1-445379-55-5

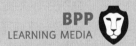

We can all remember a teacher that inspired us, encouraged us and helped us to excel. But what is it that makes a good teacher and are these skills that can be learned and improved?

As doctors and healthcare professionals we are all expected to teach, to a greater or lesser degree, and this carries a great deal of responsibility. We are helping to develop the next generation and it is essential to pass on the knowledge that we have gained during our experience to date.

This book aims to cover the fundamentals of medical education. It has been designed to be a guide for the budding teacher with practical advice, hints, tips and essential points of reflection designed to encourage the reader to think about what they are doing at each step.

By taking the time to read through this book and completing the exercises contained within it you should:

- Understand the needs of the learner

- Understand the skills required to be an effective teacher

- Understand the various different teaching scenarios, from lectures to problem based teaching, and how to use them effectively

- Understand the importance and sources of feedback

- Be aware of assessment techniques, appraisal and revalidation

This book aims to provide you with a foundation in medical education upon which you can build the skills and attributes to become a competent and skilled teacher.

More titles in the Progressing your Medical Career Series

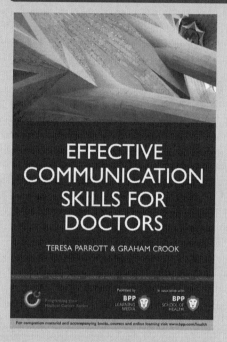

EFFECTIVE COMMUNICATION SKILLS FOR DOCTORS

TERESA PARROTT & GRAHAM CROOK

£19.99
September 2011
Paperback
978-1-445379-56-2

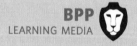

Would you like to know how to improve your communication skills? Are you looking for a clearly written book which explores all aspects of effective medical communication?

There is an urgent need to improve doctors' communication skills. Research has shown that poor communication can contribute to patient dissatisfaction, lack of compliance and increased medico-legal problems. Improved communication skills will impact positively on all of these areas.

The last fifteen years have seen unprecedented changes in medicine and the role of doctors. Effective communication skills are vital to these new roles. But communication is not just related to personality. Skills can be learned which can make your communication more effective, and help you to improve your relationships with patients, their families and fellow doctors.

This book shows how to learn those skills and outlines why we all need to communicate more effectively. Healthcare is increasingly a partnership. Change is happening at all levels, from government directives to patient expectations. Communication is a bridge between the wisdom of the past and the vision of the future.

Readers of this book can also gain free access to an online module which upon successful completion can download a certificate for their portfolio of learning/Revalidation/CPD records.

This easy-to-read guide will help medical students and doctors at all stages of their careers improve their communication within a hospital environment.

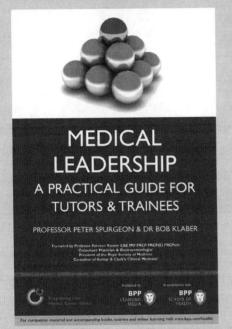
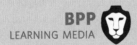

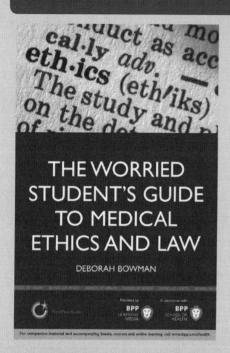
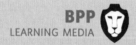

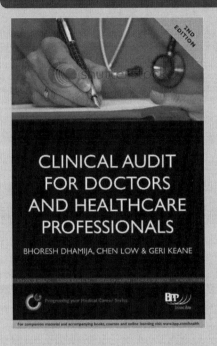
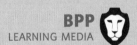

More Titles in the Progressing Your Medical Career Series

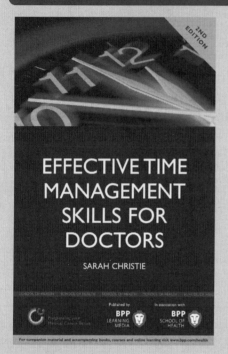

EFFECTIVE TIME MANAGEMENT SKILLS FOR DOCTORS

SARAH CHRISTIE

£19.99
October 2011
Paperback
978-1-906839-08-6

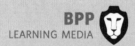
LEARNING MEDIA

Do you find it difficult to achieve a work-life balance? Would you like to know how you can become more effective with the time you have?

With the introduction of the European Working Time Directive, which will severely limit the hours in the working week, it is more important than ever that doctors improve their personal effectiveness and time management skills. This interactive book will enable you to focus on what activities are needlessly taking up your time and what steps you can take to manage your time better.

By taking the time to read through, complete the exercises and follow the advice contained within this book you will begin to:

- Understand where your time is being needlessly wasted

- Discover how to be more assertive and learn how to say 'No'

- Set yourself priorities and stick to them

- Learn how to complete tasks more efficiently

- Plan better so you can spend more time doing the things you enjoy

In recent years, with the introduction of the NHS Plan and Lord Darzi's commitment to improve the quality of healthcare provision, there is a need for doctors to become more effective within their working environment. This book will offer you the chance to regain some clarity on how you actually spend your time and give you the impetus to ensure you achieve the tasks and goals which are important to you.